Platelets

The Practical Approach Series

SERIES EDITORS

D. RICKWOOD
Department of Biology, University of Essex
Wivenhoe Park, Colchester, Essex CO4 3SQ, UK

B. D. HAMES
Department of Biochemistry and Molecular Biology
University of Leeds, Leeds LS2 9JT, UK

★ **indicates new and forthcoming titles**

Affinity Chromatography

Anaerobic Microbiology

Animal Cell Culture
(2nd edition)

Animal Virus Pathogenesis

Antibodies I and II

★ Antibody Engineering

★ Basic Cell Culture

Behavioural Neuroscience

Biochemical Toxicology

★ Bioenergetics

Biological Data Analysis

Biological Membranes

Biomechanics—Materials

Biomechanics—Structures and
Systems

Biosensors

★ Carbohydrate Analysis
(2nd edition)

Cell–Cell Interactions

The Cell Cycle

★ Cell Growth and Apoptosis

Cellular Calcium

Cellular Interactions in
Development

Cellular Neurobiology

Clinical Immunology

Crystallization of Nucleic
Acids and Proteins

★ Cytokines (2nd edition)

The Cytoskeleton

Diagnostic Molecular Pathology
I and II

Directed Mutagenesis

★ DNA Cloning 1: Core
Techniques (2nd edition)

★ DNA Cloning 2: Expression
Systems (2nd edition)

★ DNA Cloning 3: Complex
Genomes (2nd edition)

★ DNA Cloning 4: Mammalian
Systems (2nd edition)

Electron Microscopy in Biology

Electron Microscopy in
Molecular Biology

Electrophysiology

Enzyme Assays

Platelets
A Practical Approach

Edited by

STEVE P. WATSON

Department of Pharmacology, University of Oxford

and

KALWANT S. AUTHI

Thrombosis Research Institute, London

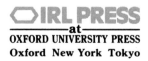

OXFORD UNIVERSITY PRESS
Oxford New York Tokyo

Oxford University Press, Walton Street, Oxford OX2 6DP

Oxford   New York
Athens   Auckland   Bangkok   Bombay
Calcutta   Cape Town   Dar es Salaam   Delhi
Florence   Hong Kong   Istanbul   Karachi
Kuala Lumpur   Madras   Madrid   Melbourne
Mexico City   Nairobi   Paris   Singapore
Taipei   Tokyo   Toronto

and associated companies in
Berlin   Ibadan

Oxford is a trade mark of Oxford University Press

Published in the United States
by Oxford University Press Inc., New York

Users of books in the Practical Approach Series are advised that prudent
laboratory safety procedures should be followed at all times. Oxford
University Press makes no representation, express or implied, in respect of
the accuracy of the material set forth in books in this series and cannot
accept any legal responsibility or liability for any errors or omissions
that may be made.

A catalogue record for this book is available from the British Library

Library of Congress Cataloging in Publication Data
(Data available)

ISBN 0 19 963538 2 (Hbk)
ISBN 0 19 963537 4 (Pbk)

Typeset by Footnote Graphics, Warminster, Wilts
Printed in Great Britain by Information Press, Ltd., Eynsham, Oxon

This book is dedicated to newly arrived sons of both Drs Kalwant Authi and Steve Watson. **Harmeet Singh Authi** *was born to Jaswinder Authi on March 22, 1995, and* **Callum Nicholas Watson** *to Anne Watson on March 23, 1995.*

Preface

In addition to the fundamental role in haemostasis, blood platelets represent a major model for the study of signal transduction pathways. Several important intracellular mechanisms were first observed in platelets including the ability of phorbol esters and diacylglycerols to activate protein kinase C, and the realization that integrins are capable of 'outside in' signalling. This volume represents a compilation of methods that will enable the laboratory worker to undertake many of the current experimental procedures used in the study of platelet function and signal transduction. The techniques described range from basic procedures such as platelet preparation and the monitoring of aggregation to newer techniques in cell biology, e.g. monitoring calcium in single cells and the use of PCR (despite the lack of a nucleus!). Each chapter has been prepared by an expert in the field and we are grateful for the thoroughness and enthusiasm with which they undertook this project.

Sadly during the preparation of this book Professor Michael Scrutton died. He was a major contributor to the platelet field and is perhaps best known for his work using semi-permeabilized platelets. He was particularly supportive to both of the editors and his premature death is a great loss to the field.

Oxford   S.P.W.
London   K.S.A.
November 1995

Contents

7. Identification, isolation, and characterization of platelet glycoproteins mediating platelet adhesion 131

John L. McGregor, Odile Gayet, Nathalie Mercier, Lilian McGregor, and Elza Chignier

8. Monoclonal antibodies to platelet cell surface antigens and their use 155

J. Michael Wilkinson

Contents

11. Study of proteins associated with the platelet
cytoskeleton   217

Joan E. B. Fox

12. Methods for measuring agonist-induced
phospholipid metabolism in intact human
platelets   235

Bruce J. Holub and Steve P. Watson

Contents

16. Platelet procoagulant activity and its measurement   319

Edouard M. Bevers, Paul Comfurius, Chris P. M. Reutelingsperger, and Robert F. A. Zwaal

17. The study of platelet function in other species   341

Alastair W. Poole

Contents

Contributors

KALWANT S. AUTHI
Thrombosis Research Institute, Emmanuel Kaye Building, Manresa Road, Chelsea, London SW3 6LR, UK.

EDOUARD M. BEVERS
Cardiovascular Research Institute Maastricht, University of Limburg, PO Box 616, 6200 MD Maastricht, The Netherlands.

JOAN S. BRUGGE
ARIAD Pharmaceuticals Inc., 26 Landsdowne Street, Cambridge, MA 02139–4234, USA.

ELKE BUTT
Medizinische Universitätsklinik, Labor Für Klinische Biochemie, Josef-Schneider Str. 2, 97080 Würzburg, Germany.

ELZA CHIGNIER
INSERM Unit 331, Thrombose-Hemostase, Université Claude Bernard, UFR Alexis Carrel, Rue Guillaume Paradin, 69372 Lyon Cedex 08, France.

EDWIN A. CLARK
ARIAD Pharmaceuticals Inc., 26 Landsdowne Street, Cambridge, MA 02139–4234, USA. Present address: Department of Biology, Massachusetts Institute of Technology, Cambridge, MA, USA.

KENNETH J. CLEMETSON
Theodor Kocher Institut, Universitat Bern, CH-3000 Bern 9, Postfach 99, Freiestrasse 1, Bern, Switzerland.

PAUL COMFURIUS
Cardiovascular Research Institute Maastricht, University of Limburg, PO Box 616, 6200 MD Maastricht, The Netherlands.

JORGE D. ERUSALIMSKY
Department of Medicine and The Cruciform Project, University College, University Street, London WC1E 6JQ, UK.

RICHARD W. FARNDALE
Department of Biochemistry, Tennis Court Road, Cambridge CB2 1QW, UK.

DENISE S. FERNANDEZ
Department of Biochemistry, Tennis Court Road, Cambridge CB2 1QW, UK.

Contributors

JOAN E. B. FOX
Department of Molecular Cardiology, Joseph-Jacob Center for Thrombosis and Vascular Biology, The Cleveland Clinic Foundation, 9500 Euclid Avenue, Cleveland, OH 44195, USA.

ODILE GAYET
INSERM Unit 331, Thrombose-Hemostase, Université Claude Bernard, UFR Alexis Carrel, Rue Guillaume Paradin, 69372 Lyon Cedex 08, France.

JON M. GERRARD
Department of Paediatrics, Health Sciences Centre, The University of Manitoba, 840 Sherbrook Street, Winnipeg, Manitoba R3A 1S1, Canada.

BRUCE J. HOLUB
Department of Nutritional Sciences, University of Guelph, Ontario N1G 2W1, Canada.

SARA J. ISRAELS
Department of Paediatrics, Health Sciences Centre, The University of Manitoba, 840 Sherbrook Street, Winnipeg, Manitoba R3A 1S1, Canada.

DEREK E. KNIGHT
MRC LMCV, University College, Gower Street, London WC1E 6BT, UK.

JOHN L. McGREGOR
INSERM Unit 331, Thrombose-Hemostase, Université Claude Bernard, UFR Alexis Carrel, Rue Guillaume Paradin, 69372 Lyon Cedex 08, France.

LILIAN McGREGOR
INSERM Unit 331, Thrombose-Hemostase, Université Claude Bernard, UFR Alexis Carrel, Rue Guillaume Paradin, 69372 Lyon Cedex 08, France.

ARCHIE McNICOL
Department of Oral Biology, Faculty of Dentistry, 780 Bannatyne Avenue, Winnipeg, Manitoba R3E 0W2, Canada.

JOHN F. MARTIN
Department of Medicine and the Cruciform Project, University College, University Street, London WC1E 6JQ, UK.

NATHALIE MERCIER
INSERM Unit 331, Thrombose-Hemostase, Université Claude Bernard, UFR Alexis Carrel, Rue Guillaume Paradin, 69372 Lyon Cedex 08, France.

ALAN D. MICHELSON
Center for Platelet Function Studies, University of Massachusetts Medical School, 55 Lake Avenue North, Worcester, MA 01655, USA.

ALASTAIR W. POOLE
Department of Pharmacology, School of Medical Sciences, University Walk, Bristol BS8 1TD, UK.

Contributors

CHRIS P. M. REUTELINGSPERGER
Cardiovascular Research Institute Maastricht, University of Limburg, PO Box 616, 6200 MD Maastricht, The Netherlands.

STEWART O. SAGE
Physiological Laboratory, Cambridge University, Downing Street, Cambridge CB2 3EG, UK.

MICHAEL C. SCRUTTON (deceased)
Division of Biomolecular Sciences, King's College, Campden Hill Road, London W8 7AH, UK.

SANFORD J. SHATTIL
Department of Vascular Biology, The Scripps Research Institute, 10666 North Torrey Pines Road, VB-5, La Jolla, CA 92037, USA.

KANWAR VIRDEE
Department of Biochemistry, Tennis Court Road, Cambridge CB2 1QW, UK.

ISOBEL A. WADMAN
Department of Biochemistry, Tennis Court Road, Cambridge CB2 1QW, UK.

ULRICH WALTER
Medizinische Universitätsklinik, Labor für Klinische Biochemie, Josef-Schneider Str. 2, 97080 Würzburg, Germany.

CHRISTINE L. WASUNNA
Department of Biochemistry, Tennis Court Road, Cambridge CB2 1QW, UK.

STEVE P. WATSON
Department of Pharmacology, University of Oxford, Mansfield Road, Oxford OX1 3QT, UK.

J. MICHAEL WILKINSON
The Wellcome Trust, 183 Euston Road, London NW1 2BE, UK.

ROBERT F. A. ZWAAL
Cardiovascular Research Institute Maastricht, University of Limburg, PO Box 616, 6200 MD Maastricht, The Netherlands.

Abbreviations

AA	arachidonic acid
ACD	acid–citric acid–dextrose
AM	acetoxymethyl ester
AP	aplastic human plasma
BSA	bovine serum albumin
βTG	β-thromboglobulin
cAMP	cyclic adenosine 3′-5′-phosphate
cAMP-PK	cAMP-dependent protein kinase
CCD	citrate–citric acid–dextrose
cPDE	cyclic nucleotide phosphodiesterase
CSF	colony-stimulating factor
DEPC	diethylpyrocarbonate
DG	diacylglycerol
DMSO	dimethyl sulfoxide
DOC	deoxycholate
DTT	dithiothreitol
EDTA	ethylenediaminetetraacetic acid
EM	electron microscopy
EPO	erythropoietin
FACS	fluorescence activated cell sorting
FAK	focal adhesion kinase
FAMEs	fatty acid methyl esters
FCS	fetal calf serum
Fg	fibrinogen
FITC	fluorescein isothiocyanate
FPLC	fast protein liquid chromatography
GAM	goat anti-mouse
GAP	GTPase activating protein
GLC	gas–liquid chromatography
GP	glycoprotein
GPRP	glycyl-L-prolyl-L-arginyl-L-proline
HR	high responder
IEF	isoelectric focusing
IL	interleukin
IP$_3$	inositol trisphosphate
LDH	lactate dehydrogenase
LIBS	ligand-induced binding sites
LR	low responder
mAb	monoclonal antibody
MBP	myelin basic protein

MK	megakaryocyte
MLC	myosin light chain
OPD	*o*-phenylene diamine
PA	phosphatidic acid
PBS	phosphate-buffered saline
PC	phosphatidylcholine
PCR	polymerase chain reaction
PE	phosphatidylethanolamine
PEG	polyethylene glycol
PF4	platelet factor 4
PG	prostaglandin
pI	isoelectric point
PI	phosphatidylinositol
PKC	protein kinase C
PKI	protein kinase inhibitor
PMA	phorbol myristate acetate
PMSF	phenyl methyl sulfonyl fluoride
PMT	photomultiplier tube
PPP	platelet-poor plasma
PRP	platelet-rich plasma
PS	phosphatidylserine
PTK	protein tyrosine kinase
PVA	poly (vinyl alcohol)
RGDS	Arg–Gly–Asp–Ser
RIA	radioimmunoasssay
RMCE	receptor-mediated Ca^{2+} entry
ROC	receptor-operated channel
RT	reverse transcriptase
SBFT	sodium-binding benzofuran isophthalate
SDS	sodium dodecyl sulfate
SDS–PAGE	SDS–polyacrylamide gel electrophoresis
SERCA	sarco-endoplasmic reticulum Ca^{2+}ATPase
SIN-1	morpholynosydnonimine hydrochloride
SMOC	second messenger-operated channel
SNP	sodium nitroprusside
TBV	total blood volume
TEA	triethanolamine
Tg	thapsigargin
TLC	thin-layer chromatography
TPA	tetradecanoylphorbol acetate
Tx	thromboxane
UA	uranyl acetate
vWF	von Willebrand's factor
WGA	wheat germ agglutinin

Platelet preparation and estimation of functional responses

ARCHIE McNICOL

1. Introduction

Human platelets are amongst the most widely studied cells in the body with a conservatively estimated 4000 articles published in 1993 alone. Clearly a vast number of investigators are presently isolating and successfully using platelets although the methods employed in many of these publications vary radically. The purpose of the present chapter is not to compare and contrast these multiple techniques but to provide reproducible protocols for the preparation of platelets and for assays of their functional responses. It should be noted that many of the more specialized techniques described in later chapters have particular requirements (e.g. specific buffers) not covered in this chapter.

2. Blood collection

Several general points should be borne in mind before blood donation:

(a) Many drugs are known to interfere with platelet function and therefore it is crucial to ensure that potential blood donors have not ingested such drugs during the previous 14 days (1). Several antiplatelet drugs such as aspirin (2), other non-steroidal anti-inflammatory drugs, and anti-histamines are available in over the counter preparations and donors often do not volunteer this information unless specifically asked.

(b) The blood should be drawn in a relaxed atmosphere. A busy laboratory is often not the ideal environment, especially for a first time, tense donor. Several investigators advocate that blood be drawn from fasting donors. Severe lipaemia may interfere with the apparent aggregatory response of platelets (3). However if plasma-free platelet suspensions are to be used fasting is not necessary.

(c) During the preparation procedure, the platelets should only be manipulated with, and stored in, polyethylene, polycarbonate, or siliconized glass. In the last case, the silicone should be applied to ensure complete and irreversible coverage of the glassware, which should then be thoroughly washed before use (4).

(d) It is preferable to maintain platelets either at room temperature or at 37°C during all manipulations.

(e) In common with all bodily fluids, blood products should be regarded as potentially hazardous. Gloves should be worn when drawing blood and during all manipulative procedures. Blood products should be regarded as biohazardous and handled according to individual institute's regulations.

2.1 Blood collection methods

Blood should be collected from a forearm vein. Venous occlusion, by a tourniquet, may be required although care should be taken to avoid stasis or anoxia (4). Following blood collection, venous pressure must be relieved before the needle is removed and the donor is encouraged to apply pressure to the site of venipuncture with a cotton swab for several minutes.

2.1.1 Syringes

(a) Blood may be drawn into syringes. The appropriate amount of anticoagulant (see below) should be added to the syringe before attachment of the Butterfly-type needle.

(b) Butterfly-type, Vacutainer brand blood collection sets (Becton Dickinson) with 21 gauge needles are suitable for this method.

(c) Contamination of the sample with thrombin generated during venipuncture may be reduced by discarding the first 2 ml of blood drawn (4).

(d) The blood should be drawn into the syringes in an even manner to avoid vortexing, and thoroughly and continuously mixed with the anticoagulant. To facilitate mixing 20 ml, or larger, syringes should be used.

(e) If larger quantities of blood are required the syringes must be changed and during this procedure it is important to compress the tubing to prevent loss.

2.1.2 Vacutainers

Blood may also be drawn into a Vacutainer collection system (Becton Dickinson). These evacuated vessels contain the appropriate volume of anticoagulant and are used in conjunction with Vacutainer brand blood collection sets and adapters. This affords the advantage of an enclosed system. However the blood is drawn by vacuum and this rapid turbidity may cause a certain degree of platelet activation. Furthermore the ratios of blood to anticoagulant are inflexible. Available anticoagulants include liquid EDTA, powdered EDTA, heparin, and sodium citrate.

2.1.3 Free flow

To avoid any form of turbidity, platelets may be obtained by simply allowing the blood to flow freely into an anticoagulant. Several points should be remembered when using this method:

(a) Venous occlusion is required and a larger gauge needle (18 or 19) recommended.

(b) The needle should be attached to tubing prior to venipuncture, and the other end of the tubing placed in a plastic tube below the level of the appropriate anticoagulant solution.

(c) Following venipuncture the blood should be allowed to flow into the anticoagulant. This procedure prevents vortexing in the collection tube and therefore reduces activation.

(d) Thorough mixing of the platelets with the anticoagulant is difficult during the bleeding procedure and must be carried out immediately afterwards.

2.2 Anticoagulants

A number of anticoagulants are available. The appropriate choice depends largely on what aspect of platelet function is to be ultimately examined. Heparin, for example, has been widely used as an anticoagulant. However some heparin preparations cause platelet aggregation (5,6).

Inhibition of coagulation by chelating divalent cations is the method of choice for most investigators. EDTA has been used but is not ideal as it both affects cell surface adhesive receptors and may deplete intracellular calcium stores. Any one of three citric acid based anticoagulants may be used:

- sodium citrate
- citrate–citric acid–dextrose (CCD)
- acid–citric acid–dextrose (ACD)

All three are made in distilled water and may be stored at 4°C for several weeks (*Table 1*).

Suitable ratios of blood to anticoagulant are:

- blood : sodium citrate (9 : 1, v/v)
- blood : CCD (9 : 1, v/v)
- blood : ACD (8.1 : 1.9, v/v)

Platelet-rich plasma (PRP) (see Section 3.1) prepared from blood using either sodium citrate or CCD as the anticoagulant may be used directly in functional studies. In contrast, the pH of ACD (approximately pH 4.5) lowers that of the PRP to a level which is incompatible with aggregation, and in this case the platelets must be isolated into a plasma-free, washed suspension (Section 3.2).

Table 1. Composition of anticoagulants[a]

	Trisodium citrate	Citric acid (monohydrate)	Glucose	Reference
Sodium citrate	3.8	–	–	7
CCD[b]	2.94	2.10	2.45	9
ACD	2.5	1.37	2.0	10

[a] All values expressed in g/100 ml.
[b] pH to 6.5 before use.

3. Preparation of platelet suspensions

3.1 Preparation of platelet-rich plasma

The preparation of PRP from whole blood is achieved by centrifugation. Reported centrifugation conditions vary widely, although 800 g for 5 min and 200 g for 20 min at room temperature give reproducibly good separations (8,10). Three distinct phases are seen:

(a) Packed red cells, accounting for the lower 50–80% of the total volume. This shows individual variability but in general is greater in males than females.

(b) A thin band of white blood cells, or 'buffy coat'.

(c) Straw-coloured PRP.

The PRP should be aspirated using a plastic pipette and transferred to a fresh plastic tube. Care should be taken not to disturb either the buffy coat or red cells to prevent contamination of the platelet preparation. Platelet counts in PRP are normally 350 000 to 500 000 platelets/μl.

3.2 Isolation of platelets from PRP

In many experiments, citrated plasma is not an ideal medium in which to study platelet function due to factors such as plasma protein content, calcium chelation, and platelet agglutination by the action of thrombin. Under such circumstances plasma-free platelet preparations are preferred.

The buffers chosen for plasma-free platelet studies depend upon the experimental objectives. *Table 2* lists those buffers mentioned in this chapter. In each case all of the components, except glucose and bovine serum albumin (BSA), can be combined in 100 ml of distilled water to form a 10 × concentrate stock which may be stored at 4°C for several weeks. Prior to use the buffers are warmed to 37°C, glucose and BSA added, the volume corrected with distilled water, and the pH adjusted with 1 M HCl or 1 M NaOH as required.

Table 2. Composition of buffers[a]

	Buffer I[b]	Buffer II[c]	Buffer III[d]
NaCl	7.83 (134)	8.18 (140)	5.26 (90)
NaHCO$_3$	1.01 (12.0)	0.84 (10.0)	–
KCl	0.22 (2.9)	0.19 (2.5)	0.38 (5.0)
Na$_2$HPO$_4$	0.09 (0.34)	0.13 (0.50)	–
MgCl$_2$	0.20 (1.0)	0.20 (1.0)	–
Hepes	2.38 (10.0)	–	–
Na$_3$ citrate	–	6.46 (22.0)	10.58 (36.0)
Na$_2$ EDTA	–	–	3.72 (10.0)
Glucose	0.90 (5.0)	0.1 (0.55)	0.9 (5.0)
BSA	0.3 g/100 ml	0.35 g/100 ml	–
pH	7.4	6.5	6.5
Reference	11	3	12

[a] Values given as g/litre (mM in brackets), except BSA.
[b] Buffer I is an excellent general purpose buffer which maintains the structural, and functional, integrity of washed platelets, and which supports most functional responses (e.g. aggregation, secretion).
[c] Buffer II is a useful wash buffer due to the citrate component. In particular buffer II is recommended for use during the second platelet wash in the presence of apyrase (Section 3.2.1*ii*b).
[d] Buffer III contains both citrate and EDTA and is useful as a wash buffer, particularly when dealing with a large number of platelets (i.e. platelet concentrates).

3.2.1 Centrifugation

i. Basic method

Platelets can be isolated from PRP by centrifugation. This involves pelleting of the platelets and subsequent resuspension in a suitable buffer. It is important to note that a degree of activation may take place during the centrifugation. If ACD was used in the initial PRP preparation procedure, no further anticoagulant will be required. However if sodium citrate or CCD were used, an additional agent should be added at this stage to minimize this activation. The choice of inhibitor may include:

(a) CCD (1 : 9, v/v).

(b) Prostacyclin (300 nM) (13) which acts by elevating platelet cAMP. This is a transient increase and the platelets should not be used for experimental purposes for 30 min after the use of prostacyclin. Indeed the use of prostacyclin may be inappropriate for certain biochemical studies.

Centrifuge the PRP at 2000 *g* for 12 min at room temperature to yield a platelet pellet. Aspirate and discard the supernatant then gently resuspend the platelets in the chosen buffer. The platelets should resuspend easily and be seen swirling when the tube is gently shaken. The presence of platelet clumps at this stage represents a large degree of platelet activation and, if present, the preparation should be discarded.

ii. Additional centrifugation

In general at this point platelets can be used in functional assays. However in some experimental conditions an additional washing step is required. These include situations where residual plasma proteins may interfere with drug action, where desensitization by platelet-derived ADP compromises its subsequent use as an exogenous agonist, the preparation of platelets into a high potassium buffer suitable for permeabilization studies (Chapter 3), and the removal of excess radiolabel. The second centrifugation can involve either repeating the basic method, or incubating the platelets in the presence of the ADP scavenger apyrase, which preserves the response of the platelets to ADP.

(a) Resuspend the platelet pellet in buffer I and add one of the following anticoagulants:

   • ACD (1 : 9, v/v)

   • CCD (1 : 9, v/v)

   • prostacyclin (300 nM)

   Centrifuge the platelets at 800 g for 15 min at room temperature. Remove and discard the supernatant and resuspend the platelet pellet as outlined above.

(b) Resuspend the platelet pellet in buffer II to which 2 mM $CaCl_2$ and 0.1 mg/ml apyrase (Sigma, A6132) are added. Apyrase converts released ADP to the inactive AMP. Incubate the platelets for 15 min at 37°C, then centrifuge at 800 g for 15 min at room temperature. Remove and discard the supernatant and resuspend the platelet pellet as outlined above.

3.2.2 Gel filtration

A plasma-free platelet suspension may also be prepared by passing PRP through a gel filtration column of either Sepharose 2B or Biogel A–150. This is a gentler method of isolating platelets from PRP. Gel filtered platelets are more quiescent and are generally in better condition than platelets prepared by centrifugation. However it should be stressed that it is impossible to concentrate the platelets using this technique.

Protocol 1.   Gel filtered platelets

Equipment and reagents

• Siliconized glass column
• 0.9% NaCl
• Acetone

• Buffer I (*Table 2*)
• Sepharose 2B (Sigma, Cat. No. 2B–300)

A. *Column preparation*

1. Prepare a siliconized glass column containing a nylon microfilament disc of 52 μm mesh (14).

2. Wash the Sepharose 2B in acetone (3–4 vol.) followed by 0.9% NaCl (5–6 vol.).

3. Pour the packing material into the column. It is important to avoid air bubbles in the poured column; in this instance the column should be re-packed.

4. Connect polyethylene tubing to the bottom of the column and regulate outflow by means either of a two-way stopcock or a bulldog clip.

5. The column should be used at room temperature.

B. *Isolation of platelets*

1. Apply buffer I (2–3 vol.) to column and allow to pass through. During this pre-equilibration period alter the flow rate to approximately 1 ml/min.

2. When the equilibrating buffer has entered the gel, apply the PRP directly on to, and allow to enter, the gel.

3. Add more buffer.

4. Collect the eluate which will be clear in the absence of platelets.

5. Platelets are eluted as an opaque fraction prior to plasma proteins.

C. *Maintenance of column*

1. Pass several volumes of buffer I through the column to remove all plasma proteins.

2. The column may be stored for several days at 4°C in buffer I in the absence of glucose or BSA.

3. Supplement the buffer with 0.2% sodium azide for long-term storage, however it is important to thoroughly pre-wash the column prior to subsequent use.

3.3 Isolation of platelets from hospital concentrates

Platelets can be prepared from hospital platelet concentrates. These preparations tend to be less responsive *in vitro* to exogenously added agonists than fresh platelets. However even outdated concentrates are good sources of platelet proteins. The anticoagulant used by most Blood Banks is citrate based although other components, such as preservatives, are present and the proportions vary.

Protocol 2. Isolation of platelets from concentrates[a]

Reagents

- 0.25 M EDTA
- Buffer III (*Table 2*)

Method

1. Decant the concentrate into 50 ml centrifuge tubes.
2. Add 20 µl of 0.25 M EDTA/ml of platelets, giving a final concentration of 5 mM EDTA, and mix thoroughly.
3. Centrifuge at 1500 *g* for 15 min at room temperature.
4. Discard the supernatant. Note that this is potentially biohazardous.
5. Resuspend the pellet in buffer III at a volume equivalent to that of the original concentrate.
6. Centrifuge at 1500 *g* for 15 min at room temperature.
7. Discard the supernatant and resuspend the pellet in buffer III at a volume equivalent to that of the original concentrate.
8. Remove contaminating erythrocytes by centrifugation; accelerate to 1500 *g*, maintain for 10 sec, then switch off. Decant the supernatant to a fresh tube. This stage may be repeated as often as necessary. However, excessive centrifugation will result in platelet loss.
9. Centrifuge at 1500 *g* for 15 min at room temperature.
10. Discard the supernatant and resuspend the pellet in an appropriate buffer.

[a] From ref. 12.

3.4 Counting of isolated platelets

Certain experimental conditions may require the enumeration of platelets in the final suspension. The methods mentioned below have been previously described in detail (15).

3.4.1 Platelet counting by phase microscopy

Phase microscopy is a labour-intensive technique which is only recommended when other methods are unavailable or unsuitable (e.g. abnormal platelet size).

A 1% ammonium oxalate solution should be prepared and filtered. Add 50 µl of the platelet suspension to 950 µl of 1% ammonium oxalate and mix thoroughly. This will cause the lysis of any remaining erythrocytes. Apply 20 µl of the suspension to each side of the haemocytometer and leave undisturbed for 15 min. Examine the haemocytometer under a phase micro-scope (×400 magnification). The platelets present in all 25 of the small squares in the centre of each chamber of the haemocytometer should be counted. The mean value gives a platelet count $\times 10^3/\mu l$.

3.4.2 Platelet counting by semi-automated counter

Platelet counting can be carried out using a semi-automated, Coulter-type counter. The instrument quantifies particles based on impedance or optical density and requires precalibration to exclude background noise and micro-particles, as well as larger erythrocytes and leucocytes. Dilution of the platelet suspension into the manufacturer's isotonic medium is required. If the concentration of the washed suspension is similar to PRP then a dilution of 1 in 5000 (2 µl in 10 ml) to 1 in 10 000 (1 µl in 10 ml) is required. Counting should be performed according to the manufacturer's instructions and the appropriate dilution factors applied to obtain the final platelet count.

3.4.3 Platelet counting by electronic particle analysis

Platelet counting can be carried out using electronic particle analysers. Such counters are available in routine haematology laboratories rather than platelet research laboratories. Cells are detected on the basis of impedance or optical density. Any particle within a defined size range (normally 2–20 fl) is identified as a platelet. Such counters utilize 50–100 µl of a washed platelet suspension and manufacturer's instructions should be followed. In addition the presence and abundance of contaminating leucocytes and erythrocytes can be evaluated. This instrument will also determine platelet counts from both whole blood and PRP, therefore recovery efficiencies of platelet isola-tion techniques can be determined.

4. Functional responses: aggregation and shape change

Platelet aggregation follows, and is dependent upon, many biochemical and biophysical events and is therefore a relatively late index of platelet activa-tion. However aggregation is regarded as an important and sensitive assay of the functional viability of isolated platelets. Furthermore, in clinical settings aggregation can be used in the initial screen for several platelet dysfunctions (16). Several techniques have been developed to monitor platelet aggrega-tion including the measurement of light transmission (Section 4.1) and impedance (Section 4.2). Both techniques are based on the formation of an aggregate, the size of which is proportional to the extent of aggregation.

Two additional methods which have been used are single cell disappear-ance (Section 4.3) and the measurement of fibrinogen binding (Section 4.4). These technically more involved techniques are independent of the size of the platelet aggregate formed, and therefore can be used to assess the early stages of aggregation. In contrast, the multiple phases of the aggregation response (Section 4.1) cannot be distinguished under these conditions.

4.1 Monitoring platelet aggregation by light transmission

Aggregation can be monitored by measuring light transmission through a stirred platelet suspension (17). Following the addition of an agonist, platelet activation proceeds in a multi-step process. Several agonists initially cause the platelets to change shape which decreases light transmission (*Figure 1*). As aggregation occurs, the platelets form small clumps leading to an increase in light transmission. The aggregation profile can sometimes be divided into two phases (*Figure 1*):

(a) Primary aggregation, which is a reversible process.

(b) Secondary aggregation, which is irreversible and for weak agonists (e.g. ADP, 5-HT) is dependent on granule release and thromboxane production.

Several companies (e.g. Chrono-log, Helena Laboratories, Payton Scientific) supply aggregometers with various degrees of sophistication. Each has the capability to compare light transmission through a stirred platelet suspension

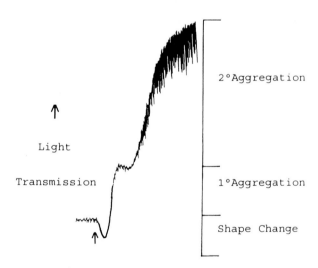

Figure 1. Components of platelet aggregation as monitored by light transmission. A platelet sample is stirred in an aggregometer and light transmission is measured. Following the addition of an agonist (↑) the light transmission transiently decreases, consistent with platelet shape change. The subsequent increase in light transmission reflects platelet aggregation. Initial aggregation (1° aggregation) is due to the effects of the initiating agonist. A small plateau may be observed before 2° aggregation occurs. The 2° aggregation is associated with granule release and thromboxane production.

to that through a control blank and display the results either on a chart recorder or computer. Conventionally, aggregometers are calibrated so that there is about 10% transmission though the unactivated platelet suspension and about 90% transmission through the blank. Some aggregometers have the capacity to calibrate automatically whereas others require manual adjustment. Multiple channel aggregometers allow processing of several experimental conditions simultaneously. Certain aggregometers (Chrono-log lumi-aggregometer) can concomitantly measure luminescence as required for ATP release (Section 5.2.2).

Aggregation cuvettes and stir bars are also commercially available. The cuvettes and siliconized stir bars are disposable. Reusable Teflon covered stir bars are also available, however care must be taken to thoroughly wash them to prevent contamination. Consecutive washing with 1 M HCl, water and methanol, followed by a thorough rinse with water is advised.

Aggregation may be measured in either PRP, from blood drawn in CCD anticoagulant, or in washed platelets resuspended in buffer I. Platelet density can range from 2.5×10^6 platelets per microlitre to as low as 200 000 platelets per microlitre. If PRP is being studied, this dilution should be done with the donors own platelet-poor plasma (PPP). PPP is obtained by centrifugation of PRP at 3000 g for 10 min.

The method for monitoring aggregation in a single channel aggregometer with an auto-set feature is detailed in *Protocol 3*. The basic concept for other aggregometers is similar and individual manuals should be consulted for calibration methods.

Protocol 3. Monitoring platelet aggregation by light transmission

Equipment and reagents

- Aggregometer, chart recorder
- 100 mM CaCl$_2$
- Cuvettes, stir bars
- Platelet suspension, blank

Method

1. Allow the aggregometer cuvette chamber to reach 37 °C. Set the stirrer to 800 r.p.m.[a]

2. Aliquot 400 µl[b] of the platelet suspension into cuvettes and incubate at 37 °C.

3. Aliquot 400 µl of the appropriate blank into a cuvette and place in the appropriate chamber (often designated 'PPP').

4. Add a clean stir bar to the platelet suspension and place in the appropriate chamber (often designated 'PRP').

5. If required, add 4 µl of 100 mM CaCl$_2$ to washed platelets to give a

---

11

Protocol 3. *Continued*

    final concentration of 1 mM CaCl$_2$.[c,d] Do not add CaCl$_2$ if PRP is being used.

6. Turn on the chart recorder at 1 cm/min.

7. Press the auto-set button. The chart recorder pen will deflect to indicate 90% transmission. Release the auto-set button and the pen will return to baseline.

8. Monitor for 1–5 min to ensure that the baseline is stable.

9. Add the agonist; with most agonists maximum aggregation occurs within 2–3 min.

10. Several indices of aggregation may be measured, although they all should correlate:[e]

    • maximal rate
    • maximal extent
    • extent at a given time after agonist addition

[a] A range of stirring speeds (700–1200 r.p.m.) can be used.
[b] Other volumes may be used. Smaller volumes may require a small spacer which will elevate the sample into the light path.
[c] If shape change is being monitored specifically, 4 μl of 100 mM EGTA should be added rather than CaCl$_2$ at this stage. Chelation of calcium prevents the progression of the platelet response from shape change to aggregation.
[d] If the effects of weak agonists, such as ADP, on washed platelets are to be examined, 4 μl of 10 mg/ml fibrinogen (Sigma, F8630) should be added.
[e] Some aggregometers have the capacity to calculate these parameters directly.

4.2 Impedance

An alternative method of measuring platelet aggregation is by monitoring electrical impedance (18). This technique allows aggregation to be determined in whole blood, however it can also be used in PRP or plasma-free platelet suspensions.

Impedance measurements depend on changes in electrical resistance between two electrodes in a platelet suspension. Platelets form a monolayer coat on electrodes placed in the suspension. Following activation, platelets aggregate onto this initial monolayer impairing the electrical conduction. This aggregation can be monitored as an increase in impedance and observed on either a chart recorder or computer screen. Chrono-log Corporation manufacture specific Whole Blood Aggregometers, some of which have the capacity to also measure luminescence as required for ATP release (Section 5.2.2).

Whole blood should be drawn into sodium citrate or CCD and, if required, PRP or plasma-free platelet suspensions prepared (Section 2). *Protocol 3* should be followed using a 1 ml sample omitting steps 3 and 7, and measuring impedance. Step 5, the addition of CaCl$_2$, should also be omitted if either whole blood or PRP are being used.

Aggregation monitored by impedance has been reported to correlate well with that measured by light transmission (18).

4.3 Monitoring platelet aggregation by single cell disappearance

A full discussion of single cell disappearance is presented elsewhere (19), however, briefly it requires the counting of platelets (Section 3.4) both before and after the addition of an agonist. This can be done in PRP or washed platelets and the reaction time should be short (200 msec). Mixing may be achieved either:

(a) In an aggregometer cuvette (Section 4.1).

(b) By a quenched flow technique. The platelets and the agonist are mixed from separate syringes by injection through a T-piece into a common Teflon reaction tubing. The tubing is of a predetermined length corresponding to the reaction time (reaction time = tube length/flow rate).

In both cases aggregation is terminated by fixation (four volumes of 1% glutaraldehyde) and single platelets counted (Section 3.4). Comparison of the platelet counts pre- and post-agonist addition gives an accurate evaluation of platelet aggregation.

4.4 Monitoring platelet aggregation by fibrinogen binding

An important component of the platelet aggregation response is the binding of fibrinogen to the αIIb/β$_3$ integrin on activated platelets. The interaction serves to consolidate the aggregate. Fibrinogen binding domains are hidden on resting platelets and therefore the exposure of such sites is used as an index of platelet aggregation. The expression of the fibrinogen binding domain, following stimulation by an agonist, can be detected by either:

(a) ^{125}I–labelled fibrinogen (20).

(b) FACS analysis (Chapter 6) using a detection antibody raised against activated αIIb/β$_3$ (21)*.

5. Functional responses: secretion

Platelets contain four distinct intracellular storage granules (22):

(a) Alpha granules contain adhesive molecules (including fibrinogen, fibro-nectin, thrombospondin), growth factors (β-transforming growth factor, platelet-derived growth factor), coagulation factors (V, VII), and other proteins (platelet factor 4, platelet basic protein, β-thromboglobulin, connective tissue activating protein III, neutrophil activating peptide 2).

(b) Dense granules contain 5-HT, ATP, ADP, calcium, and pyrophosphate.

(c) Lysosomes contain acid proteases, acid glycosidases, acid phosphatases, and aryl sulfatases.

(d) Peroxisomes contain catalase.

With the possible exception of peroxisomes, platelet activation by a number of agonists is associated with release of granular contents. Methods to stimulate the specific release from the individual granule species have been devised (23–25), although overlap does occur. Release can be measured in many ways, and the protocols presented here provide selected methods to monitor release of constituents representative of alpha granules, dense granules, and lysosomal granules. Release can be measured from platelets in PRP or washed preparations. Studies can be done in conjunction with aggregation (*Protocol 3*) or simply by incubation in a shaking water-bath at 37 °C. The latter case is less time-consuming and gives similar results.

5.1 Alpha granule release: β-thromboglobulin

Measurement of β-thromboglobulin is achieved using a commercially available radioimmunoassay (RIA) kit (Amersham Corporation). The kit is self-contained, can determine 19 samples in duplicate, and has a sensitivity range of 10–225 ng/ml. It should be noted however that the kit is designed for plasma levels of β-thromboglobulin and, in experimental situations, where stimulated washed platelets are used, dilutions of the releaseate may be required. The kit uses [^{125}I]β-thromboglobulin and the appropriate facilities and precautions are required.

Protocol 4. Assay of β-thromboglobulin release from platelet α granules

Equipment and reagents

- Ice-cold ACD
- Microcentrifuge
- Sonicator (or Triton)
- β-Thromboglobulin RIA kit
- Washed platelets

Method

1. Release can be measured in 400 μl platelet samples in a water-bath or aggregometer.

2. Following incubation with agonist, terminate the release by addition of ice-cold ACD (400 μl) and transferring the entire sample to a microcentrifuge tube. The samples may be stored at 4 °C for 1 h although

---

more immediate centrifugation (step 4) and aspiration (step 5) are preferential.

3. Add 400 µl of ACD to 400 µl of unstimulated platelets and lyse platelets. This sample will be used to determine the total β-thromboglobulin present. Lysis can be achieved by:

   - microprobe (3×20 sec) sonicator
   - a bath sonicator
   - addition of 8 µl of Triton (final concentration of 1%)

4. Centrifuge the samples at 10 000 g for 10 min.

5. Carefully aspirate and retain the supernatant. This may be stored for several days at 4°C prior to assay. For longer periods storage should be at –20°C.

6. All samples should be diluted in 0.9% saline prior to assay. The dilution factor depends on the experimental conditions, however 1/10 and 1/100 are recommended initially.

7. The assay should be carried out following the manufacturers instructions.

8. The results are expressed as ng β-thromboglobulin/ml. These values should then be multiplied by the appropriate dilution factors.

9. If desired, per cent secretion can be determined by:

$$\frac{\text{value in sample} - \text{value in control}}{\text{total value} - \text{value in control}} \times 100.$$

Although this technique is simple and reproducible there are several drawbacks:

(a) The form of β-thromboglobulin detected by this assay may not be a single species (26).

(b) It is not a continuous measurement and so a specific time point must be chosen.

(c) The assay size is limited to 19 samples performed in duplicate, including an unstimulated control and a total β-thromboglobulin level. Although antibody dilution may be possible, several kits may be required for a series of experiments.

(d) Kits are expensive.

5.2 Dense granule release

5.2.1 [^{3}H] or [^{14}C]5-HT

A radiotracing technique for the measurement of 5-HT release from dense granules is presented in *Protocol 5* (27). This technique is a non-continuous measurement and requires termination of release at specific time points. Appropriate caution should be exercised when handling radioactive material.

Protocol 5. Assay of 5-HT release from platelet dense granules using [^{3}H] or [^{14}C]5-HT

Equipment and reagents

- PRP
- Scintillation fluid
- [^{3}H] or [^{14}C]5-HT binoxalate
- Microcentrifuge
- 88% formic acid or 99.5% acetic acid

- Buffer I (*Table 2*)
- 0.1% glutaraldehyde in White's Saline (Chapter 14)[a]
- ACD

Method

1. Add 0.5 µCi of either [^{3}H] or [^{14}C]5-HT binoxalate per 1 ml of PRP and incubate at 37°C (30–60 min).[b]

2. Add ACD (1 ml of ACD per 9 ml of PRP) and centrifuge at 1500 *g* for 12 min at room temperature.

3. Discard the supernatant as radioactive waste.

4. Resuspend the platelet pellet in buffer I.

5. Carry out the experiment on 400 µl samples.

6. At the appropriate time, terminate the release by adding 400 µl of glutaraldehyde solution, transfer to microcentrifuge tubes, and place on ice.

7. Centrifuge all samples at 10 000 *g* for 10 min.

8. Remove 400 µl aliquots of supernatant to scintillation vials for counting.

9. Carefully aspirate and discard the remaining supernatant as radioactive waste.

10. Invert tubes on a paper towel and allow to drain. The paper towel should be discarded as radioactive waste.

11. Add 100 µl of 88% formic acid or 99.5% acetic acid to tube and incubate at 37°C for 1 h to digest pellet.

12. Transfer the digested pellet to a scintillation vial for counting.

13. Calculate the apparent per cent release (APR)[c] per sample by:

$$\frac{[\text{counts in supernatant (step 8)} \times 2]}{[\text{counts in pellet (step 12)}] + [\text{counts in supernatant} \times 2]} \times 100$$

14. Calculate the corrected per cent release:[d]

$$\frac{[\text{APR of sample}] - [\text{APR of control}]^e}{100 - [\text{APR of control}]} \times 100.$$

[a] An alternative fixative is 6% glutaraldehyde in sodium phosphate buffer. Mix 12 ml of 50% glutaraldehyde with 88 ml of phosphate buffer (100 ml of 0.2 M NaH_2PO_4, 400 ml of Na_2HPO_4, 500 ml of H_2O; pH 7.3).
[b] Approximately 90% of the 5-HT is accumulated by the platelets.
[c] This value includes 5-HT that was not taken up or which has been spontaneously released; it should be less than 5%.
[d] Stimulation by 1 U/ml thrombin for 1 min releases 90–95% 5-HT.
[e] The APR of the control sample should be less than 10%. It is advised that several control samples be taken during the course of an experiment.

It is also possible to measure 5-HT release in PRP. *Protocol 5* should be followed omitting steps 2–4. Qualitatively similar results will be obtained using both techniques, however the APR of the PRP control sample (background) will be appreciably higher than in washed platelets.

5.2.2 ATP release by luciferin–luciferase

A non-radiolabelling, continuous monitoring method of measuring dense granule ATP release is presented in *Protocol 6* (28,29). The basis of this reaction is the emission of light following the interaction of the firefly extract substrate luciferin with the enzyme luciferase in the presence of ATP. The emitted light can be detected and quantified. This technique is not limited to individual time points as the luminescence is determined continuously. Several companies (e.g. Chronolog) manufacture aggregometers with the capacity to simultaneously measure luminescence, however non-aggregometer luminescence detection apparatus is equally effective.

The luciferin and luciferase reagents can be:

(a) Obtained pre-mixed from companies such as Sigma (L0633), Chronolog (product number 395), and DuPont. Supplier's instructions should be followed to reconstitute the reagent. Immediate aliquoting of this material and storage at –20 °C is recommended. Single aliquots should be thawed as required. Re-freezing and thawing is not recommended. For most studies 10 µl of the mixture is sufficient.

(b) The individual components can be obtained separately and prepared:

   i. Dissolve 1 mg of luciferase (Boehringer Mannheim, 411–532) in 1 ml 0.5 M Tris acetate (9.06 g/100 ml water, pH 7.5) at 4 °C. Allow to stand for 10 min then aliquot into glass vials for storage at –20 °C. Prior to use, dilute 1 : 100 in 0.5 M Tris acetate and use 20 µl per sample.

   ii. Prepare a stock 3.6 mM luciferin solution by dissolving 10 mg D-(–)-luciferin (Boehringer Mannheim, 411–400) in 10 ml of 0.5 M Tris acetate. This is light-sensitive, and therefore aliquot into dark glass

17

bottles and store at –20 °C. Thaw when required and use 20 µl per sample. Discard any excess; do not re-freeze.

Protocol 6. Assay of ATP release by luciferin–luciferase[a,b]

Equipment and reagents
- Lumiaggregometer
- Cuvettes, stir bars
- 1 mM CaCl$_2$
- Luciferin–luciferase solution(s)
- 1 mM ATP
- PRP or washed platelets

Method

1. See *Protocol 1*, steps 1–7.

2. Add the luciferin–luciferase solution(s) and close the lid to a ensure light-free environment.

3. Monitor for 30 sec. The baseline should be steady.

4. Open the lid, quickly add the agonist, and close the lid.

5. When the maximal deflection (i.e. ATP release) has been reached, open the lid and rapidly add 0.4 µl of 1 mM ATP standard to give a final concentration of 1 µM ATP. Close the lid.

6. Measure the distance from the baseline to the first plateau—this is the agonist-induced ATP release.[c]

7. Measure the distance elicited by the standard ATP.

8. Calculate peak ATP release[d] in µM by:

$$\frac{\text{agonist-induced distance (step 11)}}{\text{standard ATP distance (step 12).}}$$

[a] This protocol is designed for use with a luminescence aggregometer although any luminscence detection equipment can be employed.
[b] PRP or washed platelets can be used as required. The mean ATP release in PRP, with a corrected platelet count of 200 000/µl, in response to 1 U/ml thrombin in a normal population is in the range of 1.89–5.45 µM (29).
[c] Low luminescence levels may be corrected by either increasing the sensitivity of the detection system or increasing the amount of luciferin–luciferase used.
[d] Due to hydrolysis of released ATP the value obtained is peak release rather than total release.

5.3 Lysosomal granule release

Several lysosomal granule constituents can be monitored. A method for quantifying β-glucuronidase by a fluorescent assay of the enzyme activity is presented in *Protocol 7* (30) using 4-methylumbelluferyl β-D-glucuronide as the phosphatase substrate.

Protocol 7. Assay of β-glucuronidase release from platelet lysosomes

Equipment and reagents

- Solution A: 0.292 g of NaCl in 10 ml of distilled water
- Solution B: dissolve 5.253 g of citric acid (monohydrate) and 13.4 g of $Na_2HPO_4.7H_2O$ in 25 ml of distilled water and pH to 4.5—this must be prepared fresh each day
- Solution C: dissolve 1.88 g of glycine in 90 ml of distilled water, add 2.08 ml of 10 M NaOH, pH to 10.3, and adjust to 100 ml
- Ice-cold CCD
- Microcentrifuge
- Sonicator
- Fluorometer

- Washed platelets in buffer I
- Standard 4-methylumbelliferone (Sigma, M1381): dissolve 1.76 mg/1 ml of solution A to achieve a 10 mM stock solution of 4-methylumbelliferone—add 5 μl of 10 mM 4-methylumbelliferone to 495 μl of solution A to achieve a 17.6 μg/ml or 0.1 nmoles/μl working solution (solution D)
- 4-methylumbelliferyl β-D-glucuronide (Sigma, M9130) substrate: dissolve 4.3 mg/1 ml of solution A to achieve a 10 mM 4-methylumbelliferyl β-D-glucuronide solution (note that 1 ml of 10 mM 4-methylumbelliferyl β-D-glucuronide solution is sufficient for approx. 15 samples)

Method

1. See *Protocol 4*, steps 1–5 using CCD rather than ACD to terminate release. This includes unstimulated controls and lysed samples to determine total β-glucuronidase levels.

2. Prepare standard curve (see *Table 3*).

3. To assay, combine the following in order at 37°C:
   - 50 μl of solution B
   - 100 μl of sample supernatant or standard
   - 50 μl of 10 mM 4-methylumbelliferyl β-D-glucuronide

4. Incubate at 37°C for 2 h.

5. Terminate the reaction by adding 2 ml of solution C.

6. Determine the fluorescence at 360 nm excitation and 446 nm emission.

7. Subtract the blank from all values.

8. Draw a standard curve and read unknown values.

6. Measurement of thromboxane release

A central component of agonist-induced platelet activation is the release of arachidonic acid from membrane phospholipids and its subsequent conversion to the pro-aggregatory product thromboxane A_2 (22). Several methods have been developed to measure the release of the stable metabolite of

Table 3. Preparation of standard curve for β-glucuronidase assay

Tube	Enzyme	Water	Concentration[a]
1	100 μl of solution D	100 μl	50
2	100 μl of tube 1	100 μl	25
3	100 μl of tube 2	100 μl	12.5
4	100 μl of tube 3	100 μl	6.25
5	100 μl of tube 4	100 μl	3.125
6	100 μl of tube 5	100 μl	1.562
7	100 μl of tube 6	100 μl	0.781
8	–	100 μl	0

[a] Final concentration expressed as pmoles/μl.

thromboxane A_2, thromboxane B_2, from stimulated platelets. Two such methods are described here:

- an *in vitro* radiolabelling technique
- a quantitative ELISA assay

6.1 Measurement of radiolabelled thromboxane

Protocol 8 outlines a procedure for the preparation of arachidonate pre-labelled platelets, and the extraction and separation by thin-layer chromatography (TLC) of the released product (10). Several points should be noted:

(a) Either [^{14}C]arachidonic acid (specific activity: 56 mCi/mol) or [^{3}H]arachidonic acid (specific activity: 200 Ci/mol) can be used.

(b) An in depth analysis of TLC techniques is beyond the scope of this chapter (see ref. 31).

(c) All work with solvents and iodine should be carried out in a fume-hood.

Protocol 8. Assay of released thromboxane B_2 from platelets pre-labelled with radioactive arachidonic acid

Equipment and reagents

- [^{14}C]Arachidonic acid or [^{3}H]arachidonic acid
- PRP
- Nitrogen
- Liquid nitrogen
- Ethyl acetate
- 1 M HCl
- Heating block
- Chloroform, methanol, acetic acid
- TLC tank
- Iodine
- Silica gel Si250 TLC plates
- Scintillation fluid

A. Labelling

1. Add [^{14}C]arachidonic acid (1 μCi/ml) or [^{3}H]arachidonic acid (2 μCi/ml) to a plastic tube and evaporate to dryness under nitrogen.

---

2. Centrifuge PRP at 1500 *g* for 12 min at room temperature to yield a platelet pellet. Aspirate and retain the supernatant at 37 °C.

3. Rapidly resuspend the pellet in 1/4 vol. of supernatant. Add 1/10 vol. of ACD.

4. Add the platelet suspension to the radiolabel and incubate at 37 °C for 1 h.

5. Add an equal volume of supernatant and 1/10 vol. of ACD.

6. Centrifuge at 1500 *g* for 12 min at room temperature to yield a platelet pellet. Aspirate and discard the supernatant as radioactive waste.

7. Resuspend the pellet in buffer I.

8. Carry out the experiment on 400 µl samples and terminate release by transferring the entire sample to a plastic tube and immersing in liquid nitrogen.

B. *Extraction*

1. Thaw the sample and add 1.8 ml of ethyl acetate and mix thoroughly. Vigorous mixing for 10 min is recommended to ensure proper extraction.

2. Centrifuge at 1000 *g* for 5 min to separate phases.

3. Remove and retain the upper phase.

4. Repeat steps 1–3 combining the two upper phases.

5. Add 30 µl of 1 M HCl to the lower phase.

6. Add 1.8 ml of ethyl acetate, vortex, and mix thoroughly.

7. Centrifuge at 1000 *g* for 5 min to separate the phases.

8. Remove the upper phase and combine with step 4.

9. Discard the lower phase as radioactive waste.

10. Dry the combined upper phases under nitrogen in a heated block which does not exceed 50 °C.

C. *Separation[a]*

1. Resuspend the samples in 100 µl of ethyl acetate.

2. Separation is carried out on Silica gel Si250 TLC plates which have been heat activated at 100 °C for 1 h.

3. The mobile phase is 90 ml of chloroform, 8 ml of methanol, 1 ml of acetic acid, and 0.8 ml of distilled water (29). The tank does not require pre-equilibration with the solvent. Depending on the ambient conditions, a 20 cm plate may take 1 h.

Protocol 8. *Continued*

4. The unsaturated metabolites are visualized by exposure to iodine vapour. The R_f values for thromboxane B_2 and arachidonic acid in this system are 0.30 and 0.78 respectively.[b]

5. Remove the appropriate bands from the plate by scraping and quantify by liquid scintillation counting.

---

[a] Further details on TLC techniques are found in Chapter 12.

[b] Several other arachidonic acid metabolites are separated using this system, including HHT and 12-HETE. Arachidonate-containing phospholipids remain at the origin and triglycerides run at the solvent front (10,31).

6.2 Measurement of thromboxane release by ELISA

A method for the measurement of thromboxane B_2 by ELISA is described in *Protocol 9* using commercially available mouse antisera (Cayman Chemicals). This gives reproducible quantitative values for thromboxane production but involves lengthy methodologies and standardization. Therefore only investigators who intend to use this technique on a routine basis are advised to adopt it; others are directed towards commercially available assays (e.g. Cayman Chemicals) or radiolabelling methods (*Protocol 8*).

Protocol 9. ELISA of thromboxane B_2 released from platelets

Equipment and reagents

- Glycine
- Thromboxane B_2 (Cayman Chemicals)
- Bovine serum albumin
- 2.8 mM indomethacin
- Acetonitrile
- Tween 20 (Sigma, P1397)
- Dialysis tubing
- Antithromboxane B_2 IgG (Cayman, 419032)
- Ice-cold ACD
- Microcentrifuge

- Microtitre plates
- Microtitre plate reader
- Na_2CO_3, $NaHCO_3$, NaN_3, NaCl, $KH_2PO_4.H_2O$, KCl, $MgCl_2$, $ZnCl_2$
- 1-Ethyl-3-(3-diethylaminopropyl) carbodiimide–HCl (Sigma, E7750)
- Goat anti-mouse IgG alkaline phosphatase conjugate (Sigma, A–1418)
- Alkaline phosphate substrate tablet (Sigma, 104–105)

A. Preparation of materials

1. Prepare coating buffer: dissolve 1.59 g of Na_2CO_3, 2.93 g of $NaHCO_3$, and 0.2 g of NaN_3 in 1 litre of distilled water (the pH should be 9.6).

2. Prepare coating conjugate: dissolve 9 mg of thromboxane B_2 in 0.5 ml of acetonitrile : water (95 : 5, v/v) then add 8.5 ml of distilled water. Adjust the pH to 5.5 then add 18 mg of 1-ethyl-3-(3-diethyl-aminopropyl) carbodiimide–HCl. Incubate at room temperature for 1 h then add 18 mg of bovine serum albumin and stir gently until dissolved. Incubate at room temperature for 2 h then overnight at 4°C.

Transfer to a dialysis bag and dialyse against distilled water for 24 h with several changes of water. Remove to aliquots of 2 mg/ml which are diluted 1 in 20 000 in coating buffer prior to use (32).

3. Prepare phosphate-buffered saline (PBS): dissoive 32.0 g of NaCl, 0.8 g of $KH_2PO_4.H_2O$, 0.8 g of KCl, and 0.8 g of NaN_3 in 4 litres of distilled water and pH to 7.4.

4. Prepare PBS–Tween washing buffer: add 1 ml of Tween 20 to 2 litres of PBS.

5. Prepare BSA–PBS: dissolve 1 g of bovine serum albumin in 100 ml of PBS.

6. Prepare substrate buffer: dissolve 7.51 g of glycine, 0.20 g of $MgCl_2$, and 0.14 g of $ZnCl_2$ in 1 litre of distilled water. Adjust the pH to 10.4 with NaOH.

7. Dilute antithromboxane B_2 IgG to 1/2000 in coating buffer. This is a mouse monoclonal antibody; if antibodies from other species are used, the secondary antibody used in part C, step 10 must be altered accordingly. 10 ml will be required for each 96-well microtitre plate.

B. Sample preparation

1. See *Protocol 4*, steps 1–5. Terminate release by adding 400 µl of ice-cold ACD containing 100 µl of 2.8 mM indomethacin.

2. All samples should be diluted in 0.9% saline prior to assay. The dilution factor depends on the experimental conditions however 1/10 and 1/100 are recommended initially.

C. Assay

1. Add 200 µl of diluted coating conjugate to each well of a microtitre plate. Ensure no bubbles are trapped. Incubate at 4 °C overnight.

2. Add 6 µl of 1 µg/ml thromboxane B_2 to 1 ml of BSA–PBS to give a 6 ng/ml (or 600 pg/100 µl) stock. Prepare the standard curve (*Table 4*).

3. Empty the wells by rapidly flipping the plate over and gently tapping it against a paper towel.

4. Add 200 µl of freshly prepared bovine serum albumin (10 mg/ml in coating buffer) to each well and incubate at room temperature for 1 h. Empty the wells (see step 10).

5. Wash the plate with PBS–Tween by filling all wells with PBS–Tween, shaking for 30 sec, and emptying. This should be carried out three times.

6. Leave the wells in column 1 of the plate empty to serve as controls. Add 100 µl of the standard curve to the wells in columns 2, 3, and 4 of the corresponding row (i.e. standard 1 goes to row 1, standard 2 goes to row 2, etc.).

Protocol 9. *Continued*

7. Add 100 µl of unknown samples (from part A, steps 1–7) to the remaining 64 wells. Duplicates of samples are recommended (32 unknown samples per plate).

8. Add 100 µl of antithromboxane B_2 IgG to all wells except those in row 1. Gently shake the plate at room temperature for 1 h, then overnight at 4°C. It is important that there is no spillage from one well to another, therefore the plate should not be rocked.

9. Wash the plate with PBS–Tween (see step 5).

10. Dilute the goat anti-mouse IgG alkaline phosphatase conjugate (Sigma, A–1418) 1/1000 in PBS–Tween. 20 ml will be required per plate. If an antithromboxane antibody raised in rabbits was used then a goat anti-rabbit IgG alkaline phosphatase conjugate (Sigma, A–7778) should be used at this point.

11. Add 200 µl of the appropriate alkaline phosphatase conjugate to each well and shake gently for 2 h at room temperature.

12. Wash the plate with PBS–Tween (see step 5).

13. Dissolve one 5 mg alkaline phosphate substrate tablet in 5 ml substrate buffer. 20 ml will be required per plate. Add 200 µl to each well. Incubate at 37°C until colour develops (this time will vary from 10 min to several hours). The plate should not be exposed to light during this period.

14. Absorbance at 405 nm should be determined using a microtitre plate reader using row 1 for background calibration.

15. Draw a standard curve and read unknown values. All values are pg thromboxane B_2/100 µl. The appropriate dilution factors should then be applied.

Table 4. Preparation of standard curve for measurement of thromboxane by ELISA

Tube	Thromboxane B_2	BSA–PBS	Concentration[a]
1	900 µl of stock	–	600
2	300 µl of tube 1	600 µl	200
3	300 µl of tube 2	600 µl	66.67
4	300 µl of tube 3	600 µl	22.22
5	300 µl of tube 4	600 µl	7.41
6	300 µl of tube 5	600 µl	2.47
7	300 µl of tube 6	600 µl	0.82
8	300 µl of tube 7	600 µl	0.27

[a] Final concentration expressed as pg/100 µl.

References

1. Weiss, H. J. (1972). *Prog. Hemostasis Thromb.*, **1**, 199.
2. Leist, E. R. and Banwell, J. G. (1974). *N. Engl. J. Med.*, **291**, 710.
3. Zucker, M. B. (1989). In *Methods in enzymology* (ed. J. Hawiger), Vol. 169, pp. 117–33. Academic Press, San Diego, CA, USA.
4. Mustard, J. F., Kinlough-Rathbone, R., and Packham, M. A. (1989). In *Methods in enzymology* (ed. J. Hawiger), Vol. 169, pp. 3–11. Academic Press, San Diego, CA, USA.
5. Eika, C. (1972). *Scand. J. Haematol.*, **9**, 248.
6. Eika, C. (1972). *Scand. J. Haematol.*, **9**, 480.
7. MacIntyre, D. E. and Pollock, W. K. (1983). *Biochem. J.*, **212**, 433.
8. Gerrard, J. M., Beattie, L. L., McCrae, J. M., and Singhroy, S. (1987). *Biochem. Cell Biol.*, **65**, 642.
9. Aster, R. H. and Jandl, J. H. (1964). *J. Clin. Invest.*, **43**, 843.
10. McNicol, A., Saxena, S. P., Becker, A. B., Brandes, L. J., and Gerrard, J. M. (1991). *Platelets*, **2**, 215.
11. Murayama, T., Kajiyama, Y., and Nomura, Y. (1990). *J. Biol. Chem.*, **265**, 4290.
12. Gerrard, J. M., Lint, D. W., Sims, P. J., Wiedmer, T., Fugate, R. D., McMillan, E., *et al.* (1991). *Blood*, **77**, 101.
13. Moncada, S., Radomski, M., and Vargas, J. R. (1982). *Br. J. Pharmacol.*, **75**, 165P.
14. Timmons, S. and Hawiger, J. (1989). In *Methods in enzymology* (ed. J. Hawiger), Vol. 169, pp. 11–21. Academic Press, San Diego, CA, USA.
15. Bessman, D. (1989). In *Methods in enzymology* (ed. J. Hawiger), Vol. 169, pp. 164–72. Academic Press, San Diego, CA, USA.
16. Rendu, F. and Dupuy, E. (1991). In *Blood cell biochemistry* (ed. J. R. Harris), Vol. 2, pp. 77–112. Plenum Publishing Corp.
17. Born, G. V. R. (1962). *Nature*, **194**, 927.
18. Cardinal, D. C. and Flower, R. J. (1980). *J. Pharmacol. Meth.*, **3**, 135.
19. Frojmovic, M. M., Milton, J. G., and Gear, A. L. (1989). In *Methods in enzymology* (ed. J. Hawiger), Vol. 169, pp. 134–49. Academic Press, San Diego, CA, USA.
20. van Willigen, G. and Akkerman, J. N. (1992). *Blood*, **79**, 82.
21. Frojmovic, M., Wong, T., and van de Ven, T. (1991). *Biophys. J.*, **59**, 815.
22. McNicol, A. and Gerrard, J. M. (1995). In *Advances in molecular and cell biology* (ed. E. G. Lapetina). JAI Press, Greenwich, CT, USA.
23. Lages, B. (1986). In *Platelet responses and metabolism I* (ed. H. Holmsen), pp. 115–44. CRC Press, Boca Raton, FL, USA.
24. Kaplan, K. L. (1986). In *Platelet responses and metabolism I* (ed. H. Holmsen), pp. 145–75. CRC Press, Boca Raton, FL, USA.
25. Nishibori, M., Cham, B., McNicol, A., Shalev, A., Jain, N., and Gerrard, J. M. (1993). *J. Clin. Invest.*, **91**, 1775.
26. Holt, J. C. and Niewiarowski, S. (1989). In *Methods in enzymology* (ed. J. Hawiger), Vol. 169, pp. 224–33. Academic Press, San Diego, CA, USA.
27. Gerrard, J. M., Beattie, L. L., Park, J., Israels, S. J., McNicol, A., Lint, D. W., *et al.* (1989). *Blood*, **74**, 2405.
28. Machin, S. J. and Preston, E. (1988). *J. Clin. Pathol.*, **41**, 1322.
29. Israels, S. J., McNicol, A., Robertson, C., and Gerrard, J. M. (1990). *Br. J. Haematol.*, **75**, 118.

30. Hoehn, S. K. and Kanfer, J. N. (1978). *Can. J. Biochem.*, **56,** 352.
31. Salmon, J. A. and Flower, R. J. (1982). In *Methods in enzymology* (ed. W. E. M.Lands and W. L. Smith), Vol. 86, pp. 477–93. Academic Press, San Diego, CA, USA.
32. Maclouf, J. (1982). In *Methods in enzymology* (ed. W. E. M. Lands and W. L. Smith), Vol. 86, pp. 273–86. Academic Press, San Diego, CA, USA.

Cellular model systems to study megakaryocyte differentiation

JORGE D. ERUSALIMSKY and JOHN F. MARTIN

1. Introduction

In recent years the study of megakaryocyte (MK) differentiation has generated considerable interest. This is due to the fact that it is now widely recognized that changes in platelet reactivity are determined in the MK during thrombopoiesis and that MKs change in pathological conditions (1). For a long time substantial progress in the study of MK differentiation has been hampered by both the unavailability of specific megakaryocyte colony-stimulating factors (MK–CSF) and by the difficulties in obtaining pure populations of both mature MKs and their progenitors in ample supply. The latter problem has been partially circumvented by the application of techniques which do not require a large number of cells, such as flow cytometry, dynamic video imaging, *in situ* hybridization, and the polymerase chain reaction. In addition, the use of megakaryoblastic cell lines, although not the real thing, provide enough homogeneous material for biochemical analysis. Most of the techniques described here may not necessarily apply directly to the study of signal transduction during MK differentiation. However they have an integral role in any approach to identifying and characterizing molecular mechanisms related to the biology of this lineage.

2. Megakaryocytopoiesis—an overview

MKs originate in the bone marrow from pluripotent stem cells through a complex differentiation process involving stem cell commitment, mitotic amplification of committed progenitors, nuclear polyploidization, and cytoplasmic maturation leading to the production of platelets. This process is physiologically controlled by a serum factor which stimulates the bone marrow to produce mature MKs in response to platelet consumption (2). The existence of a humoral regulator of megakaryocytopoiesis has been postulated for a long time, but its identity has been established only recently (3–6). This factor, known as c-Mpl ligand or thrombopoietin, stimulates haematopoietic progenitors to proliferate and differentiate into mature MKs, and when injected into animals, increases platelet production dramatically. In addition to c-Mpl ligand, a variety of pleiotropic haematopoietic growth factors, including interleukin (IL)-3, IL-6, IL-11, granulocyte/macrophage colony-stimulating factor (GM–CSF), leukaemia inhibitory factor, oncostatin M, stem cell factor, and erythropoietin (EPO), synergistically promote the growth and maturation of human MKs (reviewed in refs 2,7). *In vitro*, phorbol esters, in combination with cytokines which stimulate proliferation, also stimulate MK maturation (8,9). Furthermore, phorbol esters cause terminal megakaryocytic differentiation of erythroid and mekaryoblastic leukaemic cell lines (see *Table 1*).

A distinctive feature of MK differentiation is the process of nuclear polyploidization. After cessation of proliferation and before cytoplasmic fragmentation takes place, MKs undergo a variable number of endomitotic cycles. As in normal mitosis, during MK endomitosis the nuclear membrane breaks down, mitotic spindles are formed, and condensed chromosomes can be identified in metaphase. After this stage, however, there seems to be a diversion from the normal mitotic pathway which results in the restitution of the nuclear membrane and the inhibition of nuclear and cellular division. Thus, the cell becomes polyploid by allowing many rounds of DNA replication without completion of the intervening mitosis.

The ploidy of bone marrow MKs usually ranges from 4n to 64n, with 16n being the modal ploidy under normal physiological conditions in all the mammals studied. In humans this ploidy distribution may change under pathological conditions, as shown in patients with cancer, platelet disorders, and cardiovascular disease (reviewed in ref. 1).

3. Purification of megakaryocytes from human bone marrow

Mature MKs are by nature unstable cells. Several factors contribute to this instability including a relatively large size (mean diameter of ~ 35 μm), an intrinsic mechanical fragility which is a consequence of the normal mechanism of cytoplasmic fragmentation, and a tendency to aggregate caused by their platelet-like reactivity. These features, combined with the fact that MKs comprise less than 0.1% of all nucleated bone marrow cells, make their purification a daunting task. However, several practical precautions help to increase the yields and quality of MK preparations:

(a) The use of prostaglandin E_1 (PGE_1) throughout the preparative procedure inhibits MK reactivity.

(b) Cutting down the number of washing steps minimizes fragmentation.

(c) The use of solutions containing high concentrations of bovine serum albumin (BSA) during centrifugation facilitates the resuspension of pellets and thus, reduces mechanical trauma and aggregation.

Various methods for the purification of MKs from bone marrow samples have been developed. These can be divided into two categories:

(a) Enrichment techniques.

- Percoll density gradient centrifugation. This method is described in Section 3.2.
- Counterflow centrifugal elutriation (10). In this method, cells are separated according to size in a specially designed centrifuge rotor. The purity of recovered MKs varies between 5–20%. One disadvantage of this technique is that it is biased towards large MKs.

(b) Purification to homogeneity.

- Fluorescence activated cell sorting (11). This method generates pure preparations of viable MKs. However, it requires expensive equipment and specialized technical assistance.
- Magnetic immunoselection. This method is described in Section 3.3.

3.1 Preparation of human bone marrow suspensions

Bone marrow may be obtained from patients with no evidence or history of haematological disease or infections after informed written consent has been obtained in accordance with hospital ethics regulations. Samples are usually obtained under local anaesthesia by aspiration from the iliac crest. In the UK this procedure is performed by medical personnel. Alternatively, marrow can be collected in the same way by sternal aspiration before cardiac surgery. Aspirates are diluted and filtered within 30 min of collection (*Protocol 1*).

Protocol 1. Preparation of single cell suspensions from bone marrow aspirates

Equipment and reagents

- 2.8 mM PGE_1 (Sigma, P5515): dissolve in ethanol (1 mg/ml) and store at 4°C
- Modified ACD-A anticoagulant solution: 38 mM citric acid, 75 mM trisodium citrate, 139 mM D-glucose, and 12.5 mM EDTA. Sterilize by autoclaving at 126°C for 30 min and store at 4°C in 1 ml aliquots. Just prior to use add 5 μl of 2.8 mM PGE_1 for each millilitre of anticoagulant.
- 150 μm mesh monofilament nylon filter (Baltex PA-150/51, G. Bopp & Co. Ltd, UK)

- MK buffer: Ca^{2+}/Mg^{2+}-free Dulbecco's phosphate-buffered saline (PBS) containing 3% BSA (fraction V; Sigma, A6793), 5.5 mM D-glucose, and 10.2 mM trisodium citrate, adjusted to pH 7.3 and an osmolarity of 295 mosm/litre. Filter through 0.45 μm pore filter using positive pressure. Store at 4°C and use within one month. Add PGE_1 (2.8 μM) just prior to use.
- Sterile sternal/iliac crest biopsy needle (Horwell Ltd, UK), plastic syringe, 50 ml polypropylene centrifuge tubes (Falcon, 2070)

Method

Perform all steps at room temperature.

1. Aspirate 4 ml of marrow using a sternal/iliac crest biopsy needle into a plastic syringe containing 1 ml modified ACD-A anticoagulant solution.

Protocol 1. *Continued*

2. Dilute the bone marrow aspirate with 5 ml MK buffer. Pipette up and down gently several times until an homogeneous suspension is obtained.

3. Filter the marrow suspension through a 150 μm mesh monofilament nylon filter collecting the sample into a 50 ml centrifuge tube.

Femoral heads obtained during orthopaedic surgery may also be used as sources of bone marrow (protocols may be found in ref. 12).

3.2 Percoll discontinuous density gradient fractionation

MKs are less dense than other bone marrow nucleated cells by virtue of their having unique intracytoplasmic membrane structures, namely the demarcation membrane and the surface connected canalicular system. This physical difference can be exploited to obtain MK enriched cell suspensions from bone marrow using Percoll density gradient centrifugation (*Protocol 2*). The following protocol is developed from that reported by Tomer *et al.* (11).

Protocol 2. MK enrichment by Percoll discontinuous density gradient centrifugation

Equipment and reagents

- Bone marrow cell suspension (from *Protocol 1*)
- Percoll (ρ = 1.13 g/ml; Sigma, P-1664)
- 1.5 M NaCl
- MK buffer (see *Protocol 1*)
- MK buffer/0.3% BSA: MK buffer containing 0.3% BSA (fraction V; Sigma, A6793)
- Polypropylene conical centrifuge tubes, 15 ml capacity (Falcon, 2096)
- Bench-top refrigerated centrifuge

Method

1. Prepare 10 ml Percoll (ρ = 1.06 g/ml)[a] by mixing 4.17 ml Percoll (ρ = 1.13 g/ml) with 4.83 ml double distilled water and 1 ml 1.5 M NaCl.

2. Divide the Percoll (ρ = 1.06 g/ml) into two centrifuge tubes, then layer carefully the cell suspension over the Percoll (5 ml into each tube), and finally overlay each tube with 3 ml MK buffer/0.3% BSA.

3. Centrifuge at 400 g for 20 min at room temperature.

4. Aspirate and discard the upper layer. Collect the cells from the interface between the Percoll and the intermediate layer and all of the remaining intermediate layer.

5. Mix the collected cells with 2 vol. of ice-cold MK buffer and centrifuge at 300 g for 10 min at 4°C.

6. Aspirate the supernatants and resuspend the cell pellets in MK buffer to a final volume of ~ 0.3 ml. Keep the cells on ice until further use.

7. Sample an aliquot of 5 μl into 95 μl MK buffer, mix with 100 μl 0.4% Trypan blue solution, and count the cells in a haemocytometer. After counting, if necessary, adjust the cell concentration to $\sim 1.0 \times 10^7$ cells/ml.

[a] Proportions are calculated according to the formula $V_0 = V(\rho - 0.1 \times \rho_{10} - 0.9)/ \rho_0 - 1$, where V_0 is the volume of stock Percoll, V is the volume of final working solution, ρ is the desired density of the working solution, ρ_0 is the density of the stock Percoll, and ρ_{10} is the density of 1.5 M NaCl (1.058 g/ml).

It should be emphasized that the success of this method is often predetermined by the quality of the marrow sample itself. This is largely dependent on donor related factors (in general younger patients have more red marrow) and also to some extent on the degree of experience of the doctor performing the aspiration. As a practical guide a thick marrow sample will produce the best yields. A thin, runny sample is a sign of excessive peripheral blood contamination. Good quality bone marrow aspirates have $\sim 1 \times 10^8$ nucleated cells with a MK frequency of $\sim 0.05\%$. In these cases the procedure outlined in *Protocol 2* yields $\sim 5 \times 10^4$ MKs with a purity of $\sim 1.5\%$.

3.3 Magnetic immunoselection

In this method MKs are first labelled with an antiplatelet mouse monoclonal antibody (mAb), then they are rosetted with magnetizable polystyrene beads (Dynabeads M-450) which are conjugated to a secondary sheep anti-mouse immunoglobulin, and finally they are isolated with a magnet. *Protocol 3* was originally designed in our laboratory as a single-step method for the rapid isolation of MKs from unfractionated bone marrow suspensions (13). We use the mAb Plt-1 which reacts with the glycoprotein complex GPIIb–IIIa (CD41), a surface antigen, whose expression is restricted to platelets and their precursors.

Protocol 3. Immunomagnetic isolation of MKs

Equipment and reagents

- Bone marrow aspirate (see *Protocol 1*)
- MK buffer/0.3% BSA (see *Protocol 2*)
- Dynabeads M-450 coated with sheep anti-mouse IgG (Dynal, 110.01): wash as described by the manufacturers and dilute 15 times in MK buffer/0.3% BSA (2.7×10^7 beads/ml)
- Magnetic particle concentrator (MPC) (Dynal Ltd, UK)
- Plt-1 mAb (Coulter Immunology, UK): dissolve as described by the manufacturers (0.25 mg/ml) and store at –20°C in 0.25 ml aliquots
- Polypropylene 14 ml round-bottom tubes, 50 ml conical tubes
- 150 μm mesh monofilament nylon filter (Baltex PA-150/51, G. Bopp & Co. Ltd, UK)

Method

1. Dilute the bone marrow aspirate to a final volume of 45 ml with ice-cold MK buffer/0.3% BSA in a 50 ml polypropylene tube; mix gently.

31

Protocol 3. *Continued*

2. Filter the marrow suspension through a 150 µm mesh monofilament nylon filter collecting the sample into a clean 50 ml tube which is kept on ice.

3. Add 0.25 ml Plt-1 mAb and incubate at 4°C for 30 min with gentle continuous mixing, ensuring that the cells are kept in suspension.

4. Add 50 µl Dynabeads, incubate for another 30 min as in step 3, and then aliquot the cell suspension into five round-bottom tubes (~ 9 ml/tube).

5. Place the tubes in the MPC for 2 min and then aspirate the supernatant whilst the tubes are still in contact with the magnet.

6. Remove the tubes from the MPC, resuspend the remaining cells with 5 ml ice-cold MK buffer/0.3% BSA per tube, pool the cells, and then redistribute them into four tubes.

7. Collect the rosetted cells with the MPC as in step 5.

8. Repeat steps 6 and 7 three more times, ensuring that each time the number of tubes is reduced by one (i.e. the last wash is done in one tube).

9. Resuspend the cells in 0.5 ml MK buffer/0.3% BSA and count them.

From one bone marrow aspirate this method usually yields $2.5–5 \times 10^4$ cells with a purity of 85–95%. This amount of cells is suitable for analysis by immunocytochemistry, *in situ* hybridization, and the polymerase chain reaction. Magnetic immunoselection can also be used in combination with pre-enrichment by Percoll density gradient centrifugation (*Protocol 2*) whenever purity reaching 100% is required, at the expense of some cell loss (see for example ref. 14). One disadvantage of this method is that the presence of the large beads bound to the cells is incompatible with flow cytometric analysis. Bead removal from MKs may be attempted by enzymatic release with chymopapain (15).

4. Identification of megakaryocytes by two colour flow cytometry

Flow cytometry is an essential tool for MK analysis in clinical studies (16) and for the investigation of the effects that haematopoietic growth factors have on their development (15,17). *Protocols 4* and *5* are part of a two colour fluorescence technique used routinely in our laboratory for the analysis of MK ploidy distribution in human bone marrow. The technique can be also adapted for the analysis of MK development in liquid cultures.

4.1 Fluorescent staining

The essence of this method is to label the MK with a selective fluorescent label. We use direct labelling with fluorescein isothiocyanate (FITC)-conjugated mAb Y2/51 which recognizes the glycoprotein (GP) IIIa (CD61). GPIIa forms part of the heterodimeric fibrinogen receptor complex GPIIb–IIIa, an integrin expressed exclusively on the surface of platelets, MKs, and their precursors. As the second fluorescent label we use propidium iodide (PI) which binds to DNA (and also RNA) and thus stains all the nucleated cells. PI staining is performed in the presence of RNase A and the detergent saponin. Saponin is chosen because it permeabilizes efficiently the plasma and nuclear membrane while maintaining sufficient integrity to enable cellular discrimination on the basis of morphology (18). In addition, the protocol includes a mild fixation with paraformaldehyde to prevent washing off the antibody during incubation with RNase A.

Protocol 4. Two colour fluorescent staining of MKs

Equipment and reagents

- MK enriched cell suspension in MK buffer at 1×10^7 cells/ml (Section 3.2)
- FITC-conjugated Y2/51 anti-human GPIIIa antibody (Dako, UK)
- FITC-conjugated mouse IgG1 control antibody (Dako, UK)
- Phosphate-buffered saline (PBS)
- 1% paraformaldehyde (BDH, 29447): dissolve 0.5 g in 50 ml PBS at 60°C and adjust pH to 7.4 with 1 M NaOH—store at 4°C for up to two weeks
- Refrigerated bench-top centrifuge and 15 ml polypropylene conical tubes

- 1000 U/ml RNase A (Sigma, R5125): dissolve protein in 10 mM Tris–HCl, 1 mM EDTA pH 7.5, heat at 95°C for 15 min to inactivate any contaminating DNase, and store at –20°C in 50 μl aliquots
- 5 mg/ml PI (Molecular Probes): dissolve in PBS and store at 4°C protected from light (note this substance is a mutagen: handle according to local safety regulations)
- DNA staining solution: PBS containing 2 mM $MgCl_2$, 0.2% BSA, 0.05% saponin, 0.05 mg/ml PI, and 10 U/ml RNase A (PI and RNase A are added just prior to use from 100-fold concentrated stock solutions)

Method

Filter all solutions through 0.22 μm filters and keep at 4°C. Carry out all incubations and washing steps at 4°C. Perform incubations in the dark.

1. Aliquot cells and FITC-conjugated antibodies (Ab) as follows:

Tube	Cells	Control Ab	Y2/51 Ab
1	47.5 μl	–	–
2	47.5 μl	2.5 μl	–
3	190.0 μl	–	10 μl

2. Mix well and incubate for 45 min with occasional swirls.

3. Add 5 ml PBS and centrifuge at 200 *g* for 5 min.

4. Aspirate the supernatants and resuspend the pellets in 0.5 ml PBS. Add 0.5 ml 1% paraformaldehyde and leave on ice for 1 h.

Protocol 4. *Continued*

5. Add 5 ml PBS and centrifuge at 200 *g* for 5 min.

6. Aspirate the supernatants and resuspend the pellets in 1 ml DNA staining solution.

7. Incubate overnight and analyse the next morning.

The use of a fluorescence microscope equipped with illumination and filter combinations for fluorescein and PI may be helpful to assess the success of the staining prior to analysis by flow cytometry. MKs are easily identified by the diffuse green fluorescence of the cell surface and the strong red fluorescence of the multilobed nuclei.

4.2 Cytofluorimetric analysis

A Becton Dickinson FACScan flow cytometer connected to a Consort 32 computer system is used in the following protocol. Data are recorded and analysed using the LYSYS II software program. The detailed running of the instrument is beyond the scope of this chapter. The instructions given in *Protocol 5* are intended for workers with some experience in flow cytometry (see also Chapter 6). Equivalent instruments with a wide diameter nozzle are equally appropriate.

Protocol 5. Data acquisition using the FACScan flow cytometer

Equipment
- FACScan flow cytometer (Becton Dickinson)

Method

1. Set-up the instrument for acquisition. Adjust photomultiplier settings and gains to record forward scatter (FSC), side scatter (SSC), fluorescein fluorescence (FL1), and PI fluorescence (FL2) of each cell. Set the fluidics flow rate to 'low'. The table below shows the initial settings that we routinely use with our instrument.

	FSC	SSC	FL1	FL2
Detectors	E-1	270V	400V	250V
Amplifier gains	5.0	2.5	log	log

2. Run tube No. 1 in set-up mode. Using a dot plot of FL1 versus FL2, correct electronically for spillage of the red fluorescence signal into the green fluorescence detector. Adjust the analyser threshold on the FL2 channel to exclude subcellular debris and to include all cells with a DNA content of 2n or greater.

3. Run tube No. 2 in set-up mode. Using a dot plot of FL1 versus FL2, set a live gate which excludes all the non-specific green fluorescence.

4. Run tube No. 3 in set-up mode and perform the following adjustments:

    (a) Check that the sample flow rate falls within 1000–2000 cells/sec. If necessary adjust the cell concentration by diluting the sample with PBS.

    (b) Using a dot plot of FL1 versus FL2, correct electronically the spillage of green fluorescence into the red fluorescence detector. This is done by aligning, parallel to the FL1 axis, all the cells with different levels of green fluorescence within the 4n ploidy subset.

    (c) If necessary adjust the boundaries of the live gate so that polyploid cells with a dim green fluorescence are not excluded.

5. Switch the FACScan to acquisition mode. Run the rest of tube No. 3 and acquire at least 10 000 events within the live gate in list mode (this usually corresponds to running 500 000 cells through the cytometer).

In the protocol outlined above the position of the live gate for data acquisition is set to include all the MKs, including those with a lower level of cell surface associated green fluorescence. Unavoidably, this gate also includes 2n and 4n non-megakaryocytic cells with a relatively high degree of non-specific fluorescence and/or autofluorescence. However the majority of these non-megakaryocytic cells can be gated out at a later stage during data analysis. Following data acquisition, a two parameter display of FSC (a parameter related to cell size) versus FL1 is used to identify the MK population (*Figure 1*). In this display MKs appear as a distinct subset comprising the largest most fluorescent cells. To establish the DNA ploidy distribution, an analysis gate is set around this cell population, and all the cells within this gate are depicted in a DNA histogram (the *y* axis indicates cell number; the *x* axis indicates PI fluorescence intensity in log scale). Histograms are divided into compartments that approximate the different ploidy classes in terms of DNA content using the 2n and 4n peaks of the ungated cells as internal references. Boundaries of DNA compartments are determined manually by setting markers at the nadirs between peaks. The frequency of cells in each DNA compartment is calculated by dividing the number of cells in the compartment by the total number of cells in the histogram.

In some bone marrow samples a two parameter display of FSC versus FL1 does not result in a clear cut separation between the MK population and the rest of the marrow cells. In these cases positioning of the analysis gate is somewhat arbitrary. As a result, the ploidy distribution may be slightly altered due to the inclusion of 2n and 4n non-megakaryocytic cells or to the

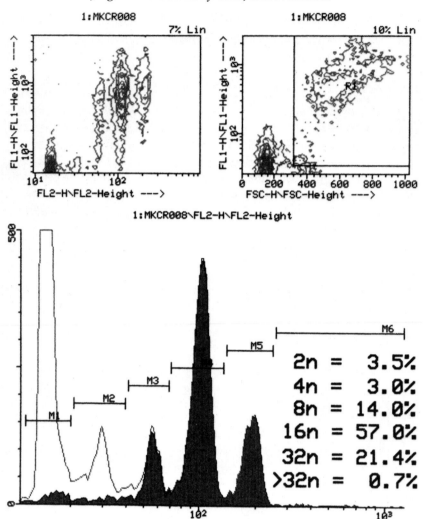

Figure 1. Flow cytometric analysis of MKs from normal human bone marrow. Contour plots of FL1 versus FL2 (upper *left* panel) and of FSC versus FL1 (upper *right* panel). Note on the *right* the position of the analysis gate (R1) which surrounds the population of large GPIIIa⁺ cells. The bottom panel displays a DNA histogram of 5600 gated cells. The ungated cells are represented by the non-shaded tracing.

exclusion of some 8n cells. The presence of activated platelets adhering to monocytes may constitute a potential cause of this problem. Under the fluorescence microscope these monocyte/platelet conjugates display a distinctive dotted pattern of green fluorescence. This problem is usually more manifest in bone marrow aspirates which are heavily contaminated with peripheral blood.

5. Cellular model systems to study megakaryocyte differentiation

MK differentiation has been studied using both human and rodent cells. Although many aspects of megakaryocytopoiesis are common to both types of cells, it should be emphasized that some of the observations made in one system do not necessarily apply to the other. One example is the detection of acetylcholinesterase activity which appears as an early megakaryocytic marker in the mouse but not in man.

Two different types of culture systems have been used to study MK differentiation. One involves the growth of MK colonies in a soft gel matrix and the other is a straightforward liquid culture technique in which MKs are grown in suspension. A large body of work using these two *in vitro* techniques has established that MKs require for their development two classes of trophic factors or activities (2,19). One, a MK colony-stimulating activity affects mainly the proliferation of progenitors. The other, a terminal differentiation (thrombopoietin-like) activity acts on more mature cells, including promegakaryoblasts and MKs, stimulating an increase in cellular size, DNA content, and the synthesis of platelet-specific constituents. Conditioned media from various transformed cell lines and human plasma have been used as sources of MK colony-stimulating activity. Similarly, sources of maturation activities have included conditioned media from macrophages, bone marrow stromal cells, and lung cells, as well as plasma from patients with aplastic marrows.

Recently, c-Mpl ligand, a specific humoral regulator of megakaryocytopoiesis, has been obtained in recombinant form (3,4). This molecule has all the properties attributed to the putative MK–CSF and those of thrombopoietin as well, accounting for both the proliferation and maturation activities present in thrombocytopenic plasma (3–6). Several other defined haematopoietic growth factors also affect MK differentiation (reviewed in ref. 7). Among these, IL-3 is the most efficient colony-stimulating factor, while IL-6 is a potent maturation factor. It should be noted, however, that the division between proliferation and maturation factors, in practice is not clear cut and these factors, often acting in synergistic combinations, have overlapping roles influencing megakaryocytopoiesis at various differentiation stages.

5.1 Growth of megakaryocyte colonies on semi-solid media

Several clonogenic assays have been developed for the growth of MK colonies from myeloid progenitors. These assays differ mainly in the semi-solid matrix used (agar, methyl cellulose, or fibrin), the source of growth factors (serum, plasma, conditioned media, and/or recombinant growth factors), and the method used to identify the colonies. These assays have been instrumental to identify the haematopoietic growth factors which affect MK differentiation at the progenitor level. MK colony assays are not suitable however, for the detailed analysis of terminal megakaryocytic differentiation.

5.2 Megakaryocyte differentiation in liquid cultures

More recently, conditions have been defined for the growth of MKs in liquid media. This technique, when combined with flow cytometry, allows the study of early and late stages of megakaryocytopoiesis. The protocol outlined below has been adapted from the method originally described by Vainchenker and his colleagues (20).

Protocol 6. Growth of MKs in liquid culture

Equipment and reagents

- Umbilical cord blood: 30–50 ml are collected at the time of delivery (usually by Caesarean section) using 50 U/ml preservative-free heparin (Sigma, 210–6) as anticoagulant—keep at room temperature and process within 1 h
- Hepes-buffered α-medium: α-medium (Gibco, 22561) containing 0.1% BSA (tissue culture grade; Sigma, A8412) and 25 mM Hepes buffer (Gibco, 15630)—store at 4°C and use within two weeks
- Basic culture medium: Iscove's modified Dulbecco's medium (Gibco, 21980) containing 1% BSA (Sigma, A8412), 100 U/ml penicillin, 100 μg/ml streptomycin, and 4 mM glutamine—store at 4°C and use within two weeks

- Ficoll–paque (ρ = 1.077 g/ml; Pharmacia Biosystems Ltd)
- Aplastic human plasma (AP): obtain blood from patients with severe thrombocytopenia (usually individuals who have had a bone marrow transplantation within the previous two weeks). Use preservative-free heparin (40 U/ml) as anticoagulant. Remove the cells by two consecutive centrifugations at 3000 g for 15 min at 4°C. If necessary, to ensure sterility filter the supernatant through a 0.22 μm low protein binding filter. Store at –20°C in 1 ml aliquots.
- 50 ml conical centrifuge tubes (Falcon), 150 mm plastic tissue culture Petri dishes (Nunc), 25 cm² tissue culture flasks (Costar)

Method

Perform all steps under sterile conditions.

1. Add an equal volume of Hepes-buffered α-medium (warmed to room temperature) to the umbilical cord blood and mix well.

2. Gently layer the diluted blood over an equal volume of Ficoll–paque and centrifuge at 400 g for 30 min at room temperature.

3. Collect the low density cells from the interface and wash them three times in Hepes-buffered α-medium, centrifuging at 300 g for 12 min at 4°C.

4. Resuspend the cells (2 x 10⁶/ml) in basic culture medium supplemented with 10% AP and plate on plastic Petri dishes at a depth of ~ 1 cm. Incubate for 2 h at 37°C in a tissue culture incubator under 5% CO_2.

5. Transfer the non-adherent cells to a centrifuge tube and rinse the Petri dish with 1/10 vol. of culture medium to recover loosely attached cells. Adjust the cell concentration to 1 x 10⁶ cells/ml.

6. Dispense 10 ml aliquots of the cell suspension into 25 cm^2 tissue culture flasks and incubate at 37 °C in a tissue culture incubator under 5% CO_2.

7. After 12 days of culture harvest the non-adherent cells and follow *Protocols 4* and *5* to assess MK development by flow cytometry.

1. After the 12 day incubation period, the frequency of MKs (GPIIIa$^+$ cells) in the non-adherent fraction of bone marrow cultures ranges between 10–30%. Of these, the majority are in the 2n and 4n ploidy class, with 8n and 16n cells representing only 7–20%. Occasionally, cells with a ploidy higher than 16n can be found in some cultures. An important factor in the successful culture of MKs is the source of human plasma. Although normal plasma supports MK growth, plasma from patients with aplastic marrows, which is rich in MK colony-stimulating activity, is much more effective (17). Further addition of IL-3 (10–100 U/ml) consistently increases the yield of MKs. However, in this case the increase in ploidy may be somewhat reduced.

2. Recently, recombinant c-Mpl ligand has been shown to stimulate megakaryocytopoiesis in liquid media containing fetal calf serum (FCS) (3). MKs can also be grown in serum-free media (5,21). This allows the study of differentiation under defined growth conditions and in particular, it eliminates the interference caused by inhibitory molecules such as TGF-β1 (21,22). Still one of the limitations of the liquid culture system is that some cytokines may be produced endogenously (23) and this makes it difficult to study the specific effects of individual growth factors.

3. The above mentioned problem can be partially alleviated by growing cultures of CD34$^+$ cells (15). This population of cells, which in umbilical cord blood constitutes ~ 5% of the mononuclear cell fraction, is greatly enriched in MK progenitors. In our laboratory we usually separate CD34$^+$ cells using a magnetic immunoselection technique developed by Miltenyl Biotech, Germany. The method consists of first coating the cells with an anti-CD34 mouse mAb (QBEND/10), then attaching super-paramagnetic microbeads conjugated with a secondary anti-mouse immunoglobulin, and finally purifying the CD34$^+$ cells on a column using a magnetic cell separator (MiniMACS, Miltenyl Biotech). Detailed instructions are provided by the manufacturer. In our hands, 35 ml of cord blood yield ~ 2×10^6 CD34$^+$ cells with a purity of greater than 90%. Other investigators use immunomagnetic separation with Dynabeads (Dynal, Norway) followed by chymopapain treatment (15).

6. Leukaemic cell lines expressing megakaryocytic features

One of the disadvantages of using MK cultures to study signal transduction is that they do not provide a source of homogeneous cellular material. This

Table 1. Human cell lines which express MK markers

Cell line	Phenotype	References	
		Characterization	Phorbol ester effect
UT-7	Multipotent factor-dependent	24,25	24
M-07E	Multipotent factor-dependent	26,27	Not reported
K562	Erythroleukaemic	28,29	30
HEL	Erythro/megakaryocytic	31–33	33,34
DAMI	Erythro/megakaryocytic	35	35
CMK	Erythro/megakaryocytic	36	36,37
MEG-01	Megakaryocytic	38	39

problem can be partially circumvented by the use of continuous cell lines that have phenotypic properties of MK precursors (*Table 1*). These cells are arrested at different stages of lineage development and express MK/platelet markers including α granule proteins and the surface glycoprotein IIb/IIIa. Moreover, for the majority of these cell lines it has been shown that treatment with phorbol esters induces further megakaryocytic development, resulting in nuclear polyploidization and in an increase in the expression of platelet/MK constituents.

Although UT-7 has been initially regarded as a megakaryoblastic cell line (24), in fact it represents an earlier pluripotent progenitor stage. Indeed, besides undergoing megakaryocytic maturation, these cells are also capable of eosinophilic and basophilic differentiation when cultured with GM–CSF or IL-3, and of erythroid differentiation when cultured with EPO (25). This pluripotent capacity is likely to be encountered also in M-07E, a cytokine-dependent cell line which displays similar phenotypic characteristics to those found in UT-7 (26,27). M-07E cells proliferate in response to c-Mpl ligand (5), but it is not yet known whether this cytokine can also induce megakaryocytic differentiation in these pluripotent cell lines.

Besides platelet-specific proteins, the more lineage restricted cell lines K562, HEL, DAMI, and CMK express also erythroid markers such as glycophorin A or globin. In addition, in K562 and HEL cells the erythroid phenotype can be further enhanced by treatment with chemical inducers such as haemin (31,32,40). This bipotential quality presumably reflects a close relationship between erythroid and megakaryocytic differentiation.

DAMI and CMK cells are capable of limited further megakaryocytic maturation when treated with haematopoietic growth factors. DAMI cells respond to EPO, IL-3, and IL-6 (41), whereas CMK cells respond to IL-3, GM–CSF, EPO, IL-6, and c-Mpl ligand (5,37,42). However, none of the differentiation effects observed in these cells are comparable to those seen after phorbol ester treatment. In particular, haematopoietic growth factors have so far not been shown to induce endomitosis in either these, or any other megakaryoblastic cell line.

Specific details of culture conditions used in our laboratory for the growth and induction of terminal megakaryocytic differentiation of HEL cells are given in *Protocol 7*. Details of the conditions for other cell lines are given in the references found in *Table 1*. The references also provide extensive documentation on the marker proteins present in the respective cell lines.

Protocol 7. Culture of HEL cells and induction of terminal differentiation

Equipment and reagents

- R/D medium: A 1:1 mixture of RPMI 1640 (Gibco, 31870) and Dulbecco's modified Eagle's medium (Gibco, 41966) supplemented with 0.1% BSA (tissue culture grade; Sigma, A8412), 1% Nutridoma HU (Boehringer Mannheim), 2 mM glutamine, 50 U/ml penicillin, 50 µg/ml streptomycin, and 0.125 µg/ml amphotericin B—store at 4°C and use within two weeks

- 2 mM phorbol 12-myristate 13-acetate (PMA) (Sigma, P8139): dissolve in ethanol and store dark at –20°C
- Tissue culture flasks, 25 cm² and 75 cm²

Method

1. Dilute exponentially growing cells to a density of 1×10^5/ml in R/D medium.[a]

2. Incubate flasks at 37°C under 5% CO_2/95% air in a humidified incubator.

3. To maintain the cells in exponential growth, subculture every three to four days, repeating steps 1 and 2.

4. To induce differentiation, adjust the concentration of exponentially growing cells to 2×10^5/ml. Incubate in R/D medium plus 10 nM PMA for three days as described in step 2.

5. Harvest the cells by centrifugation and assess differentiation.

[a] Cells previously grown in medium containing FCS are weaned from the serum gradually by subculturing every three to four days into fresh medium containing increasing proportions of R/D medium.

Megakaryocytic differentiation can be assessed by flow cytometry after staining the cells with FITC-conjugated Y2/51 anti-GPIIIa mAb (see *Protocol 4*). In our hands HEL cells undergo a threefold increase in the expression of GPIIIa when induced with PMA as described here.

7. Signal transduction studies

7.1 Involvement of protein kinase C in megakaryocyte differentiation

A major biochemical effect of phorbol esters is the activation of protein kinase C (PKC). PKC comprises a family of phospholipid-dependent serine/

threonine kinases which are activated by intracellular diacylglycerol. Phorbol esters bypass the transmembrane signal transduction pathways which generate diacylglycerol and activate PKC directly. PKC activation triggers a cascade of phosphorylation events leading to the activation of MAP kinases which in turn lead to changes in the expression and/or activity of nuclear transcription factors controlling genes involved in growth and differentiation.

In addition to their effect on megakaryoblastic cell lines (*Table 1*), phorbol esters have been shown to mimic the action of thrombopoietin-like activities in human bone marrow cultures (9). Although it is tempting to speculate that thrombopoietin-like activities, including c-Mpl ligand, might induce MK differentiation via the activation of PKC, at least two other equally relevant possibilities should be taken into consideration. First, at present there is no evidence that PKC is the sole target of phorbol esters. Therefore, it is possible that some effects of these compounds are mediated through unidentified pathways independently of PKC activation. Secondly, phorbol esters have been shown to induce cytokine expression in megakaryoblastic cells (43,44). Some of these cytokines may affect MK differentiation in an autocrine or paracrine fashion (23) raising the possibility that the effect of phorbol esters might be indirect.

7.2 Other signal transduction pathways

Cell lines expressing megakaryocytic features have been used to study a variety of signal transduction mechanisms, including those involving G proteins and receptor tyrosine kinases (45–48). However, characterization of the pathways relevant to MK differentiation awaits identification of the signal transduction events elicited by stimulation the *c-mpl*-encoded receptor. c-Mpl is a member of the haematopoietic growth factor receptor superfamily (49–51). The cytoplasmic domain has no protein kinase or phosphatase motifs, but contains sequences implicated in signal transduction (50,51). It is not known yet whether c-Mpl constitutes a single chain receptor or if it is the signal transducing β-subunit of an heterodimeric entity. *c-mpl* transcripts have been detected by PCR in CD34[+] haematopoietic cells, megakaryocytes, and platelets (52). In addition, *c-mpl* mRNA is expressed in various cell lines including UT-7, M-07E, TF-1, KU812, HEL, and DAMI, but not in K562 or MEG-01 (52). Among the positive cell lines, so far, only M-07E and KU812 cells are known to express a functional receptor.

An interesting development in this field is the finding of a novel intracytoplasmic tyrosine kinase (matk) which is predominantly expressed in cells of the megakaryocytic lineage and is up-regulated in these cells during phorbol ester-induced differentiation (53). Work on megakaryoblastic cell lines has also provided evidence for the involvement of the GATA family of transcription factors in the process of MK differentiation (54,55). The pathways leading from the haematopoietic growth factor receptors that regulate megakaryocytopoiesis to these transcription factors remain to be elucidated.

As c-Mpl ligand becomes more widely available it it will advance a great deal our understanding of these mechanisms.

Note added in proof: Various laboratories have recently reported that c-Mpl ligand stimulates tyrosine phosphorylation of proteins implicated in cytokine signal transduction, including the Janus kinase JAK2, and several members of the signal transducers and activators of transcription (STAT) family (56–60).

References

1. Erusalimsky, J. D. and Martin, J. F. (1993). *Eur. J. Clin. Invest.*, **23**, 1.
2. Hoffman, R. (1989). *Blood*, **74**, 1196.
3. de Sauvage, F. J., Hass, P. E., Spencer, S. D., Malloy, B. E., Gurney, A. L., Spencer, S. A., *et al.* (1994). *Nature*, **369**, 533.
4. Lok, S., Kaushansky, K., Holly, R. D., Kuijper, J. L., Lofton-Day, C. E., Oort, P. J., *et al.* (1994). *Nature*, **369**, 565.
5. Kaushansky, K., Lok, S., Holly, R. D., Broudy, V. C., Lin, N., Bailey, M. C., *et al.* (1994). *Nature*, **369**, 568.
6. Wendling, F., Maraskovsky, E., Debili, N., Florindo, C., Teepe, M., Titeux, M., *et al.* (1994). *Nature*, **369**, 571.
7. Gordon, M. S. and Hoffman, R. (1992). *Blood*, **80**, 302.
8. Long, M. W., Smolen, J. E., Szczepanski, P., and Boxer, L. A. (1984). *J. Clin. Invest.*, **74**, 1686.
9. Long, M. W., Hutchinson, R. J., Gragowski, L. L, Heffner, C. H., and Emerson, S. G. (1988). *J. Clin. Invest.*, **82**, 1779.
10. Gewirtz, A. M. (1987). In *Modern methods in pharmacology*, Vol. 4, pp. 1–17. Alan R. Liss Inc.
11. Tomer, A., Harker, L. A., and Burstein, S. (1987). *Blood*, **70**, 1735.
12. Coutinho, L. H., Gilleece, M. H., De Wynter, E. A., Will, A., and Testa, N. G. (1993). In *Haemopoiesis: a practical approach* (ed. N. G. Testa and G. Molineux), pp. 75–106. Oxford University Press, New York.
13. Gladwin, A. M., Carrier, M. J., Beesley, J. E., Lelchuk, R., Hancock, V., and Martin, J. F. (1990). *Br. J. Haematol.*, **76**, 333.
14. Tanaka, H., Ishida, Y., Kaneko, T., and Matsumoto, N. (1989). *Br. J. Haematol.*, **73**, 18.
15. Debili, N., Massé, J. M., Katz, A., Guichard, J., Breton-Gorius, J., and Vainchenker, W. (1993). *Blood*, **82**, 84.
16. Tomer, A., Friese, P., Conklin, R., Bales, W., Archer, L., Harker, L. A., *et al.* (1989). *Blood*, **74**, 594.
17. Debili, N., Hegyi, E., Navarro, S., Katz, A., Mouthon, M.-A., Breton-Gorius, J., *et al.* (1991). *Blood*, **77**, 2326.
18. Jacob, M. C., Favre, M., and Bensa, J.-C. (1991). *Cytometry*, **12**, 550.
19. Long, M. W. (1993). *Stem Cells*, **11**, 33.
20. Debili, N., Kieffer, N., Nakazawa, M., Guichard, J., Titeux, M., Cramer, E., *et al.* (1990). *Blood*, **76**, 368.
21. Berthier, R., Valiron, O., Schweitzer, A., and Marguerie, G. (1993). *Stem Cells*, **11**, 120.

Jorge D. Erusalimsky and John F. Martin

22. Mitjavila, M. T., Vinci, G., Villeval, J. L., Kieffer, N., Henri, A., Testa, U., *et al.* (1988). *J. Cell Physiol.*, **134,** 93.

23. Navarro, S., Debili, N., Le Couedic, J.-P., Klein, B., Breton-Gorius, J., Doly, J., *et al.* (1991). *Blood*, **77,** 461.

24. Komatsu, N., Nakauchi, H., Miwa, A., Ishihara, T., Eguchi, M., Moroi, M., *et al.* (1991). *Cancer Res.*, **51,** 341.

25. Hermine, O., Mayeux, P., Titeux, M., Mitjavila, M.-T., Casadevall, N., Guichard, J., *et al.* (1992). *Blood*, **80,** 3060.

26. Avanzi, G. C., Lista, P., Giovinazzo, B., Miniero, R., Saglio, G., Benetton, G., *et al.* (1988). *Br. J. Haematol.*, **69,** 359.

27. Avanzi, G. C., Brizzi, M. F., Giannotti, J., Ciarletta, A., Yang, Y. C., Pegoraro, L., *et al.* (1990). *J. Cell Physiol.*, **145,** 458.

28. Lozzio, C. and Lozzio, B. B. (1975). *Blood*, **45,** 321.

29. Gewirtz, A. M., Burger, D., Rado, T. A., Benz, E. J.Jr., and Hoffman, R. (1982). *Blood*, **60,** 785.

30. Tetteroo, P. A. T., Massaro, F., Mulder, A., Schreuder-van Gelder, R., and von dem Borne, A. E. G. (1984). *Leuk. Res.*, **8,** 197.

31. Martin, P. and Papayannopoulou, T. (1982). *Science*, **216,** 1233.

32. Papayannopoulou, T., Nakamoto, B., Kurachi, S., and Nelson, R. (1987). *Blood*, **70,** 1764.

33. Tabilio, A., Rosa, J.-P., Testa, U., Kieffer, N., Nurden, A. T., Del Canizo, M. C., *et al.* (1984). *EMBO J.*, **3,** 453.

34. Long, M. W., Heffner, C. H., Williams, J. L., Peters, C., and Prochownik, E. V. (1990). *J. Clin. Invest.*, **85,** 1072.

35. Greenberg, S. M., Rosenthal, D. S., Greeley, T. A., Tantravahi, R., and Handin, R. I. (1988). *Blood*, **72,** 1968.

36. Sato, T., Fuse, A., Eguchi, M., Hayashi, Y., Ryo, R., Adachi, M., *et al.* (1989). *Br. J. Haematol.*, **72,** 184.

37. Komatsu, N., Suda, T., Moroi, M., Tokuyama, N., Sakata, Y., Okada, M., *et al.* (1989). *Blood*, **74,** 42.

38. Ogura, M., Morishima, Y., Ohno, R., Sato, Y., Hirabayashi, N., Nagura, H., *et al.* (1985). *Blood*, **66,** 1384.

39. Ogura, M., Morishima, Y., Okumura, M., Hotta, T., Takamoto, S., Ohno, R., *et al.* (1988). *Blood*, **72,** 49.

40. Rutheford, T. R., Clegg, J. B., and Weatherall, D. J. (1979). *Nature*, **280,** 164.

41. Greenberg, S. M. and Chandrasekhar, C. (1991). *Exp. Hematol.*, **19,** 53.

42. Fuse, A., Kakuda, H., Shima, Y., Van Damme, J., Billiau, A., and Sato, T. (1991). *Br. J. Haematol.*, **77,** 32.

43. Avraham, H., Vannier, E., Chi, S. Y., Dinarello, C. A., and Groopman, J. E. (1992). *Int. J. Cell Cloning*, **10,** 70.

44. Navarro, S., Mitjavila, M. T., Katz, A., Doly, J., and Vainchenker,W. (1991). *Exp. Hematol.*, **19,** 11.

45. Kanakura, Y., Druker, B., Cannistra, S. A., Furukawa, Y, Torimoto, Y., and Griffin, J. D. (1990). *Blood*, **76,** 706.

46. Kanakura, Y., Druker, B., DiCarlo, J. B., Cannistra, S. A., and Griffin, J. D. (1991). *J. Biol. Chem.*, **266,** 490.

47. Komatsu, N., Adamson, J. W., Yamamoto, K., Altschuler, D., Torti, M., Marzocchini, R., *et al.* (1992). *Blood*, **80,** 53.

48. Brass, L. F., Manning, D. R., Williams, A. G., Woolkalis, M. J., and Poncz, M. (1991). *J. Biol. Chem.*, **266,** 958.
49. Vigon, I., Mornon, J.-P., Cocault, L., Mitjavila, M.-T., Tambourin, P., Gisselbrecht, S., *et al.* (1992). *Proc. Natl. Acad. Sci. USA*, **89,** 5640.
50. Vigon, I., Florindo, C., Fichelson, S., Guenet, J.-L., Mattei, M.-G., Souyri, M., *et al.* (1993). *Oncogene*, **8,** 2607.
51. Skoda, R. C., Seldin, D. C., Chiang, M.-K., Peichel, C. L., Vogt, T. F., and Leder, P. (1993). *EMBO J.*, **12,** 2645.
52. Methia, N., Louache, F., Vainchenker, W., and Wendling, F. (1993). *Blood*, **82,** 1395.
53. Bennett, B. D., Cowley, S., Jiang, S., London, R., Deng, B., Grabarek, J., *et al.* (1994). *J. Biol. Chem.*, **269,** 1068.
54. Visvader, J. E., Elefanty, A. G., Strasser, A., and Adams, J. M. (1992). *EMBO J.*, **11,** 4557.
55. Visvader, J. and Adams, J. M. (1993). *Blood*, **82,** 1493.
56. Tortolani, P. J., Johnston, J. A., Bacon, C. M., McVicar, D. W., Shimosaka, A., Linnekin, D., *et al.* (1995). *Blood*, **85,** 3444.
57. Drachman, J. G., Griffin, J. D., and Kaushansky, K. (1995). *J. Biol. Chem.*, **270,** 4979.
58. Gurney, A. I., Wong, S. C., Henzel, W. J., and de Sauvage, F. J. (1995). *Proc. Natl. Acad. Sci. USA*, **95,** 5292.
59. Pallard, C., Gouilleux, F., Benit, L., Cocault, L., Souyri, M., Levy, D., *et al.* (1995). *EMBO J.*, **14,** 2847.
60. Ezumi, Y., Takayama, H., and Okuma, M. (1995). *FEBS Lett.*, **374,** 48.

3

Preparation and uses of semi-permeabilized platelets

MICHAEL C. SCRUTTON, DEREK E. KNIGHT, and
KALWANT S. AUTHI

1. Introduction

Permeabilized cells have been widely used over many years to examine various aspects of cellular function which are not readily studied in the intact cell (1). Recently these preparations have been primarily employed to characterize cellular signal transduction mechanisms; and the current development of permeabilization methodology has occurred primarily in this context. The preparations can however be used for other purposes although less effort has been devoted to such aspects.

Table 1 summarizes the uses and limitations of the methods which have been employed in cellular permeabilization, and indicates which of these have been used to obtain permeabilized platelets. This article will focus primarily on these latter methods. In considering a potential permeabilization method the following aspects should be evaluated:

(a) Is the procedure capable of causing permeabilization of the plasma membrane and is this process reversible?

(b) Is the procedure selective for permeabilization of the plasma membrane, i.e. capable of producing a semi-permeabilized preparation? To what extent are the interior of the cell and membranes of intracellular organelles disrupted?

(c) How large are the lesions in the plasma membrane? What size of molecule can enter or leave the permeabilized cell and over what time course?

(d) Is the permeabilized preparation responsive to agonists?

Table 2 summarizes the situation for the two methods which have been primarily used to obtain semi-permeabilized preparations of platelets, namely electroporation and detergent-induced permeabilization. These two methods and suitable experimental protocols will form the basis of this chapter.

Table 1. Cellular permeabilization methods[a]

Permeabilizing method	Basis for permeabilization	Use for platelets	Reference
Organic solvent, e.g. toluene	Non-selective removal of membrane lipid.	?	2
Detergents, e.g. digitonin, saponin, filipin	Non-selective removal of cholesterol. Selectivity achieved for plasma membrane since cholesterol enriched in this membrane as compared with intracellular membranes.	+	3,4
Chelating agents, e.g. EDTA	Removal of surface (and ? subsurface) Ca^{2+} and Mg^{2+}.	(+)	5
ATP^{4-}	? For most cells apparently related to presence of an ATP receptor.	–	6
Sendai virus	Membrane fusion induced by virus.	–	7
Electroporation	Exposure to intense electric field causes localized membrane breakdown due to development of sufficient potential across membrane.	+	8

[a] Adapted from ref. 9.

Table 2. Properties of permeabilization regimes primarily used on platelets

Properties	Permeabilization regime	
	Detergents (saponin)	Electroporation
Reversibility	No	Yes (if voltage and/or number of applications of high density electric field restricted)
Size of lesions	Large, proteins of M_r < 125 000 released	Small, molecules of M_r 1000 equilibrated rapidly: restricted equilibrium of molecules up to M_r of 2000
Selectivity for plasma membrane	No	Yes, if applied voltage adjusted correctly
Responsiveness to an agonist, e.g. thrombin	Yes	Yes

2. Electroporation

When a cell or organelle is placed in an electric field a potential (V) develops across any membranes in the system. If the membrane bound particle is approximately spherical then the maximal potential develops across the membrane at the two points in line with the applied field. When the conductivity inside the membrane bound particle is approximately the same as that of the external fluid and is much greater than that of the membrane itself, the magnitude of the potential is given by the equation:

$$V = 1.5Er$$

where E is the magnitude of the applied field (in volts/cm) and r is the radius (cm) of the membrane bound particle (10,11). Hence the smaller the radius of the membrane bound particle the lower will be the potential difference (V) imposed across its limiting membrane when exposed to the electric field. The membrane breaks down and develops lesions permeable to solutes when the potential developed across it is approximately 1.1 V. However if such a voltage is applied briefly, in many cases only a transient lesion is created and the membrane reseals within a short time. Permanent lesions can be created in most instances by the application of a potential difference of 3 V or more across the membrane since the membrane appears not to be able to reseal after exposure to a field of this magnitude. Platelets are discoid cells which have an effective average diameter of approximately 2 μm. Hence an applied field strength of 20 kV/cm should induce a potential difference of 3 V across the platelet plasma membrane, but only 0.3 V across the boundary membranes of the lysosomes and of the protein and amine storage granules which are approximately 0.2 μm in diameter. As the developed potential is not sufficient to induce breakdown of the membranes of these intracellular organelles an applied field strength of 20 kV/cm should therefore allow selective permeabilization of the plasma membrane. Such selectivity has been directly demonstrated for the permeabilized platelet since significant release of the contents of the lysosomes and of the protein and amine storage granules does not occur on permeabilization by application of a field of 20 kV/cm in a medium which contains nanomolar Ca^{2+}, and is only induced in the absence of other additions if the Ca^{2+} concentration is increased into the micromolar range (12,13).

It is presumed, although less clearly established, that the mitochondria are not affected by the application of a field of this magnitude. The effect on the endoplasmic reticulum is less clearly defined since some (14), but not all (15,16), electroporated platelet preparations exhibit inositol 1,4,5-trisphosphate-driven Ca^{2+} release. The basis for the variable effect of electroporation on this latter response has not been defined and it is unclear whether in some studies application of the electric field causes permeabilization of the endoplasmic reticulum, or whether some other effect causes loss of the response to inositol 1,4,5-trisphosphate (15,16).

The principle of the electroporation method is to place the platelet suspension between two electrodes and discharge a capacitor through the system. The electric field imposed on the platelet suspension decays with a time course (in seconds) given by the product of the capacitance (in farads) and the electrical resistance of the platelet suspension (in ohms). The time course of decay of the field, and hence the period for which the potential difference is imposed across the membranes, can therefore be changed either by altering the capacitance, or by changing the composition of the suspending solution. A more detailed discussion of the theoretical basis of this method is given elsewhere (16). *Protocol 1* lists the apparatus and methodology for electroporation, and is designed to allow the flexibility needed to alter field decay. Presently the apparatus is also available commercially from Rank Bros (Cambridge, UK) and Bio-Rad (called Gene pulsar). The components of the apparatus are listed such that it may be constructed in any suitable workshop.

- 0–6 kV high voltage power supply
- one 2.5 µF plus two 1 µF capacitors
- switch
- electroporation cell consisting of two 5.2 × 3.6 cm stainless steel plates, each inlaid into an L-shaped piece of Perspex, and one U-shaped spacer 1 cm in thickness
- two large bulldog clips
- Perspex covers for the high voltage supply, the capacitors, the switch, and the electroporation cell—a picture of one form of this apparatus is shown in *Figure 1*

The design of the electroporation cell described (*Figure 1*) is simple but offers several valuable features. First, a field strength of for example 20 kV/cm can be obtained by a discharge of 2 kV across the 1 mm gap. Any increase in size of this gap requires imposition of a larger voltage difference between the electrodes to achieve the same applied field, and hence risks significant heating of the platelet suspension and the possibility of the suspension being blown out of the cell. Secondly, the cell can easily be dismantled to clean the electrodes which should be rubbed down with fine emery paper before the start of each series of runs.

The use of several capacitors as indicated allows a simple method for changing the applied capacitance, and hence altering the time course of decay of the applied field. This time course of decay can also be altered by changing the ionic strength of the suspending medium. The apparatus makes no provision for control of temperature since only minimal heating (2–3 °C increase in temperature) of the suspension occurs during ten exposures to a 2 kV field in the cell due to its contact with the large metal electrodes.

Both the commercially available equipment, like our original version, simply charges a selected capacitor to a chosen voltage and then discharges the capacitor through a cell chamber. The commercially available cell chambers that are provided with the Gene pulsar (Bio-Rad) suffer from the disadvantage that they are a sealed unit limiting access to the electrodes for cleaning. Multiple use of such a sealed unit may cause a deposit on the electrodes which will act as a high resistance between the cell suspension and the metal

CELL SUSPENSION CHAMBER

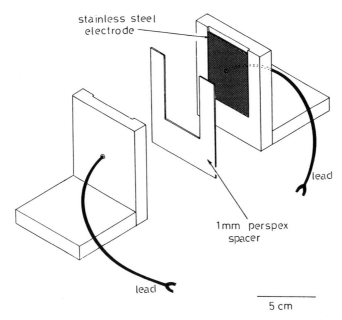

stainless steel
electrode

lead

1mm perspex
spacer

lead

5 cm

Figure 1. View of the disassembled electroporation chamber. Reproduced with permission from ref. 9.

electrode. The electric field strength imposed through the cell suspension will therefore be reduced and the effectiveness of the electroporation decreased. Such difficulties have not been encountered with the apparatus from Rank Bros when a controlled voltage can be applied across the electrodes and where the well chamber is easily dismantled for cleaning purposes (K. S. Authi, unpublished data, see also ref. 14).

Protocol 1. Electropermeabilization of platelets

Equipment and reagents

- Medium I: 0.15 M potassium glutamate, 0.02 M piperazine-N,N'-bis (2-ethanesulfonic acid (Pipes) or 4-(2-hydroxyethyl)-1-piperazine-ethanesulfonic acid (Hepes), 0.005 M disodium ATP, 0.007 M magnesium diacetate, 0.005 M D-glucose, 0.001 M ethylene glycol-bis (β-aminoethyl ether)-N,N,N',N'-tetraacetic acid (EGTA)[a]—adjust to pH 6.6 (Pipes) or 7.4 (Hepes) using KOH

- Anticoagulant ACD: 92 mM trisodium citrate, 72 mM citric acid, 100 mM D-glucose
- Acetylsalicylic acid (aspirin) 5 mM
- [^{3}H] or [^{14}C]5-hydroxytryptamine (Amersham)
- Electropermeabilization apparatus
- Medium II: as medium I but containing 0.28 M glycine and 0.01 M potassium glutamate in place of 0.15 M potassium glutamate

Protocol 1. *Continued*

- Medium III[b] (a modified Ca^{2+}-free Tyrode's solution): 0.154 M NaCl, 0.0027 M KCl, 0.001 M $MgCl_2$, 0.0056 M D-glucose, 0.007 M $NaHCO_3$, 0.0006 M NaH_2PO_4, 0.005 M sodium Pipes pH 6.5, 0.35% (w/v) bovine serum albumin (fraction V), 0.005 M potassium EGTA pH 6.5

- Medium IV[c]: 0.16 M potassium glutamate, 0.02 M Hepes, 0.0025 M ethylenedi- aminetetraacetic acid (EDTA), 0.0025 M EGTA, 0.00125 M $MgCl_2$—adjust pH to 7.4 with KOH

Method

1. Collect blood into 0.17 vol. of anticoagulant ACD (see Chapter 1).

2. Centrifuge the citrated blood for 20 min at 320 *g* room temperature and remove the supernatant (platelet-rich plasma) using a plastic transfer pipette.

3. Centrifuge the platelet-rich plasma at 8000 *g* for 30 sec to remove residual erythrocytes and leucocytes, and incubate at 37 °C for 60 min. At this stage the preparation may be incubated with radioisotopes as required, e.g. [^{14}C]5-hydroxytryptamine at 0.6 µM.

4. Centrifuge at 680 *g* for 25 min and suspend at 10^9 cells/ml in medium I.

5. Lightly grease the apposed faces of the stainless steel plate Perspex surrounds and the U-shaped spacer of the electroporation cell, taking care that no grease is left on the stainless steel plates.

6. Assemble the apparatus placing the jaws of the large bulldog clips 0.5–1.0 cm from the outside edge of the cell. Completely fill the cell with suspension medium and check for leakage.

7. Remove all this medium and load the cell with approx. 1.2 ml of the platelet suspension taking care that the level of fluid is adequate to cover the electrodes and that no air bubbles are introduced. These latter two precautions, and the cleanliness of the electrodes, are im- portant since they ensure that current will pass uniformly between the electrodes. Non-uniform passage of current can cause localized heat- ing, and hence rapid boiling, thus leading to explosive ejection of the platelet suspension from the cell. Air bubbles may be most simply removed by passing a fine piece of flexible tubing through the platelet suspension after it has been loaded into the cell.

8. Charge the capacitors to the desired voltage and discharge them through the platelet suspension by closing the switch. The design of the switch should be such that it ensures that the discharge occurs as a single event. The conditions required to obtain irreversible electro- poration are ten discharges of 2 kV.

9. Remove the platelet suspension from the cell using a 2 ml plastic syringe attached to a fine (0.5 mm) tube and without forming air bubbles

in the suspension. The permeabilized suspension can then either be used directly (17), or low molecular components released as a consequence of permeabilization may be removed by gel filtration or centrifugation (see Chapter 1) (18).

[a] The chelator biso-aminophenoxyethane-*N,N,N′,N′*-tetraacetic acid (BAPTA) may be used in place of EGTA to provide more effective control of Ca^{2+} concentration but care should be taken in the use of this alternative chelating agent since certain responses, e.g. lysosomal and amine storage granule secretion, are inhibited by BAPTA (20).

[b] If medium III is used the platelets, immediately after permeabilization, are transferred by gel filtration on Sepharose CL-4B at 4°C into medium IV which contains a high concentration of K^+, a low concentration of Na^+, and no added Cl^-.

[c] In respect to K^+, Na^+, and Cl^- concentration medium IV resembles media I and II and therefore mimics in these respects the intracellular environment. The absence of added Cl^- is particularly significant since in some cells, although not apparently in the platelet, certain responses, e.g. secretion, are irreversibly inhibited by the presence of a high concentration of Cl^- (22).

[d] Reversible electroporation can be achieved by the application of a lower voltage. For example transient breakdown of the plasma membrane can be achieved by application of seven discharges of 0.7 kV followed by incubation of the treated suspension for 60 min at 37°C (14). Multiple discharges are used to achieve the required degree of reversible or irreversible permeabilization since it is unlikely that any individual platelet will maintain the same orientation with respect to the applied field over the approx. 4 sec needed to complete the charge/discharge cycle. Unique lesions are therefore created by each application of the field. If a longer series (20 or more) of discharges is used the polarity of the electrodes should be reversed during the sequence in order to reduce the possibility of gas bubbles forming in the cell and hence inducing an explosive ejection of the platelet suspension.

3. Detergent-induced permeabilization

Detergents such as digitonin, saponin, and filipin are widely used in cellular permeabilization protocols. Their use depends on the higher cholesterol content of the plasma membrane (23) on the basis that under carefully controlled conditions selective removal of cholesterol from this membrane, and hence its permeabilization, can be achieved without significant damage to the intracellular membranes (24). Saponin is the most widely used of the detergents for this purpose. Filipin has been used in very few such studies. Although many earlier studies were performed using digitonin it appears that this detergent can fail to give a homogeneous permeabilized preparation in which the lesions are restricted to the plasma membrane (25).

A graded permeabilization of the plasma membrane can be obtained with increasing doses of saponin with low doses allowing full access to the cytosol for low molecular weight substances and higher doses giving access to proteins and antibodies but with most of the cytosolic proteins also released into the medium (26). At the lower doses (10–14 µg/ml) functional responses (such as aggregation, secretion) to agonists and intracellular messengers are maintained. These are principally lost at higher doses of the detergent, but a number of intracellular metabolic parameters can still be measured giving the technique wide application (see references).

Protocol 2. Saponin permeabilization of human platelets and its use in aggregation and secretion studies induced by the membrane impermeable messenger inositol trisphosphate

Equipment and reagents

- Bench centrifuge
- Aggregometer
- Citric acid wash buffer: 1 mM EDTA, 5 mM glucose, 5 mM KCl, 90 mM NaCl pH 6.5, 100 nM PGE₁
- Cytosolic-type KCl medium: 140 mM KCl, 1 mM glucose, 1 mM MgCl₂, 0.04 mM NaH₂PO₄, 6 mM NaHCO₃, 10 mM Hepes pH 7.4 in analytical grade water
- Inositol trisphosphate (IP₃) 1 mM

- Saponin: 5 mg/10 ml in analytical grade water
- [¹⁴C]5-hydroxytryptamine
- [³H]adenine
- [³H]arachidonic acid
- 0.3 M citric acid
- Stopping solution for 5-HT release experiments: 3% glutaraldehyde, 10 mM EDTA, 140 mM KCl pH 7.4

Method

1. Collect blood into 1/10 vol. 3.8% trisodium citrate.

2. Centrifuge at 200 g for 15 min at room temperature.

3. Recover platelet-rich plasma (PRP) carefully using a plastic pipette, leave buffy layer undisturbed.

4. Radiolabel the PRP with [¹⁴C]5-hydroxytryptamine (5-HT) (0.6 μM) to label the dense granule pool, or [³H]adenine (1 μM, 10 μCi/ml) to label the adenine nucleotide pool (mainly ATP) in the cytosol, or [³H]arachidonic acid to label phospholipids. These should be carried out for 15, 60, and 60 min respectively at 37 °C.

5. Cool to room temperature and add 0.3 M citric acid to bring the pH to 6.5 for centrifugation (this equates to 20 μl citric acid/1 ml PRP).

6. Spin at 1200 g for 15 min at room temperature in 12 ml polypropylene tubes.

7. Discard platelet-poor plasma and resuspend the pellet in citric acid wash buffer in equivalent amounts to the plasma removed.

8. Centrifuge at 1200 g for 15 min at room temperature.

9. Discard supernatant and resuspend pellet in KCl medium at 2–3 × 10⁸ cells/ml. Leave cells to equilibrate for 15 min before use.

10. Switch on aggregometer and allow the aggregation chamber to equilibrate at 37 °C. Add 480 μl platelet suspension to aggregometer tubes, switch on stirring, equilibrate for 5 min at 37 °C, and monitor aggregation trace.

11. Add 10–14 µg/ml (10–14 µl) saponin. Saponin gives less than 20% increase in light transmission over a 8 min incubation period.

12. Add stimulus, e.g. IP_3 after 45 sec, which is the time required for permeabilization to occur.

13. Measure release of [^{14}C]5-HT secretion as described in Chapter 1 using 500 µl glutaraldehyde.[a,b,c]

[a] After a 15 sec lag IP_3 should induce shape change (decrease in light transmission) followed by aggregation (60–70% over 4 min) and secretion (monitored by measuring release of [^{14}C]5-HT, see step 13). Similar responses are seen with GTPγ[S] after a slightly longer lag phase (see ref. 27).

[b] For measurement of lactate dehydrogenase (LDH), incubations are stopped with one-tenth volume 100 mM EDTA (cold) followed by rapid centrifugation at 12 000 g, for 3 min. Aliquots are removed and stored at –20 °C until assayed. LDH release into the medium is assayed as follows: incubations should contain 3 ml 50 mM sodium orthophosphate in 0.3 mM sodium pyruvate, 50 µl 9 mM NADH, to which 50 µl supernatant or cell lysate is added, and the change in OD at 366 nm measured/min for 5 min at room temperature.

[c] Similar treatment to that in step 13 is followed for measurement of release of cytosolic ATP pool in [^{3}H]adenine labelled platelets except that a fixative in the stopping solution is not required and stopping with cold 10 mM EDTA, 140 mM KCl is sufficient, followed by centrifugation at 12 000 g, and estimation of the release of [^{3}H] into the supernatant by liquid scintillation counting.

Protocol 3. Ca^{2+} sequestration and release in saponin permeabilized platelets

Equipment and reagents

- See *Protocol 2*
- Vacuum filtration apparatus
- 5 mM $CaCl_2$
- 5 mM EGTA
- 10 mM antimycin
- 10 mM oligomycin
- 1 mM A23187

- 1 mM IP_3
- 100 mM ATP
- [$^{45}Ca^{2+}$]
- Stop solution for [$^{45}Ca^{2+}$] uptake experiments: 5 mM EDTA, 140 mM KCl, 1 mM $MgCl_2$, 10 mM Hepes pH 7.4

Method

1. Prepare platelets as described in *Protocol 2*. Final resuspension should be in the KCl medium at 5×10^8 cells/ml. The cells are permeabilized with higher concentrations of saponin in the presence of ATP and [$^{45}Ca^{2+}$] such that sequestration into intracellular stores can take place.

2. Add 200 µl cytosolic buffer, 48 µl $CaCl_2$ (containing 2 µCi [$^{45}Ca^{2+}$]), 50 µl EGTA, 0.5 µl antimycin, 0.5 µl oligomycin, and 25 µl ATP (total volume

Protocol 3. *Continued*

500 µl). Add 20–25 µl saponin (0.5 mg/ml, to give 20–25 µg/ml final concentration) and 200 µl platelet suspension to start the reactions.

3. Incubate for 20 min at room temperature to allow uptake of [$^{45}Ca^{2+}$] into intracellular stores. Carry out triplicate incubations per experiment.

4. Stop reactions by rapid vacuum filtration of 450 µl mixture through 0.45 µm filters, wash with 2 × 10 ml ice-cold EDTA/KCl stop solution, and count the [$^{45}Ca^{2+}$] on filters by liquid scintillation.

The effect of any agent that alters Ca^{2+} homeostasis (e.g. A23187, thapsigargin, IP_3, antibodies to $Ca^{2+}ATPases$ or IP_3 receptors, etc.) can be tested either on uptake kinetics or release after equilibrium has been reached. Equilibrium of Ca^{2+} uptake is reached within 20 min incubation when any Ca^{2+} releasing agent (A23187, IP_3, thapsigargin, etc.) can be added and the reactions stopped after a measured time period. IP_3-induced Ca^{2+} release and aggregation are usually complete within 3 min (70% of maximal response within 30 sec) see *Figures 2* and *3*.

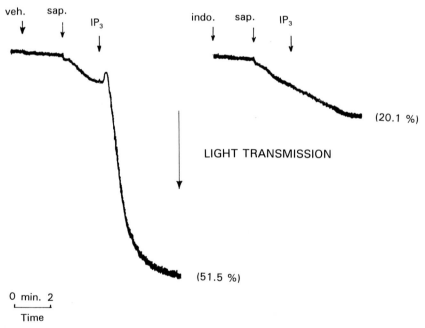

Figure 2. Typical aggregation responses of saponin permeabilized platelets stimulated by 20 µM IP_3 and the effect of indomethacin. Abbreviations: veh. vehicle; sap. saponin (12 µg/ml); indo. indomethacin (10 µM). Values in brackets represent secretion of [^{14}C]5-hydroxytryptamine. Adapted from ref. 24.

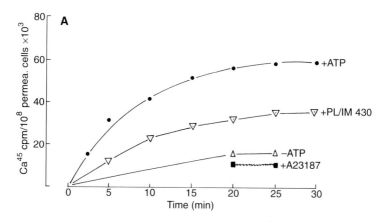

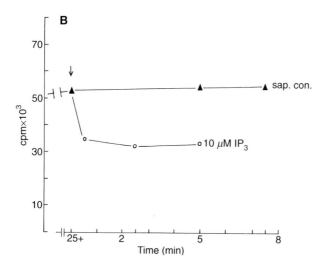

Figure 3. Kinetics of ^{45}Ca uptake and release from saponin permeabilized platelets. (A) Shown is uptake of ^{45}Ca in the presence of ATP (control), and effects of inclusion of the antibody PL/IM 430 (20 µg/ml), absence of ATP (–ATP), or presence of A23187 (10 µM). (B) Effect of addition of 10 µM IP_3 at equilibrium (25 min). Saponin (sap.) concentration used was 20 µg/ml.

4. Methods for assessing permeabilization

The criteria used to assess the permeabilized state should relate to the size of the species which are to gain access to the interior of the platelet. A variety of methods have been used in connection with studies on factors involved in responses such as secretion where uncontrolled access to molecules of molecular weight less than 1000 kDa is required (9). These methods are:

(a) Definition of the space accessible to Ca–EGTA—this method is particularly appropriate for studies on Ca^{2+}-driven responses, e.g. secretion. Aliquots of the platelet suspension are incubated for 5–10 min with ^3H_2O and ^{45}Ca–EGTA. On completion of the incubation the platelets are separated by centrifugation at 12 000 g through silicone oil. The space accessible to ^{45}Ca relative to the ^3H_2O space increases from approximately 20% in control cells to approximately 70% in irreversibly electroporated platelets within 5 min after suspension in medium I or II (see *Protocol 1*). The relatively high ^{45}Ca–EGTA space observed in control cells is likely to be due to trapping of extracellular fluid in the extensive invaginations of the plasma membrane which are characteristic of this cell.

(b) Immediate release of approximately 70% of the total cellular ATP from electroporated human platelets without any significant release of lactate dehydrogenase (or of [^{3}H] if the platelets had been pre-labelled by incubation with [^{3}H]adenine) when incubated in a medium containing less than 10 nM Ca^{2+}. The results described here apply specifically to electroporated human platelets since the total extent of ATP release will depend on the species from which the platelets are obtained due to differences in the fraction of cellular ATP which is sequestered in the amine storage granule (28). The selectivity of release will also depend on the permeabilizing regime used. Thus for permeabilization using higher concentrations of detergents, e.g. saponin or digitonin, immediate release of lactate dehydrogenase will accompany that of ATP (K. S. Authi, unpublished data).

(c) Electroporated platelets undergo an apparent increase in cellular volume as measured using a resistive particle (Coulter) counter (14). The apparent modal volume increases from 4–7 fl for untreated platelets to 10–15 fl after electroporation and transfer of an aliquot of the electroporated suspension into Isoton II. The change in apparent volume is reversible, and hence this method can be used to follow resealing. The effect is not observed if aliquots of the electroporated suspension are transferred either to Isoton III or to a high K^+ buffer, e.g. media I or II. The effect has been described as an apparent change in modal volume since direct measurement of this parameter by planimetry of scanning electron micrographs do not reveal a comparable significant increase in platelet area (14). This method applied to platelet preparations made using other permeabilizing regimes has not so far been reported.

(d) Reversible permeabilization can be monitored by uptake of the fluorescent dye Lucifer yellow (M_r 550) (14). If this method is used then it is necessary to expose the permeabilized platelets to 1 mM Lucifer yellow during resealing and then remove surface-associated fluorochrome by repeated (three times) centrifugation/resuspension.

5. Responses

Semi-permeabilized platelet preparations have been used to study a range of responses characteristic of this cell and to characterize the intracellular factor(s) involved in the promotion of the response. The following section gives some examples of responses which have been studied in this way. In all cases it is necessary to control the concentration of the factor to be added so that quantitative data are obtained on the relationship between the extent of response and the factor concentration. Since permeabilized preparations have primarily been used for the investigation of Ca^{2+}-driven responses most detail is available regarding systems for control of Ca^{2+} concentration. In order to define the Ca^{2+} concentration to which the system is exposed, typically in the micromole or nanomole range, a Ca^{2+} buffer must be employed. The Ca^{2+} buffers used most often in these studies are either Ca–EGTA or Ca–EGTA/EDTA, and the properties of these are illustrated in *Figure 4*. The Ca–EGTA system is the most effective buffer over the approximate physiological range of Ca^{2+} concentration (0.1–10 μM) (29) but only at pH 6.6. This buffer is pH-sensitive (30) and if used at a pH (7.4) more typical of the intracellular environment then control of Ca^{2+} concentration over the physiological range is not achieved (*Figure 4*). A decreased degree of pH sensitivity can be obtained using BAPTA rather than EGTA since the K_d for the Ca–BAPTA complex (approximately 0.1 μM) is not markedly altered by changes in pH. However the K_d for this complex means that the ligand is fully saturated with Ca^{2+} above 2 μM, and hence control is not obtained over the upper end of the physiological range (31). Ca^{2+} concentration can be buffered over the physiological range at pH 7.4 using a Ca^{2+}–EGTA/EDTA system in the presence of excess Mg^{2+} (32). However as shown in *Figure 4* this system is not as effective a Ca^{2+} buffer over the desired range as is Ca^{2+}–EGTA at pH 6.6 and should therefore be used with care. For example an increase from 2 mM to 3 mM in added total Ca^{2+} causes Ca^{2+} to increase from 0.2 to 17 μM. Furthermore unlike Ca^{2+}–EGTA or –BAPTA the use of the Ca^{2+}–EGTA/EDTA system is complicated by changes in Mg^{2+} concentration arising secondarily from an increase in added Ca^{2+}. This arises since the Ca^{2+}–EDTA and Mg–EDTA complexes have similar K_ds, and hence addition of Ca^{2+} displaces Mg^{2+} from EDTA. For example when the EGTA/EDTA system is titrated with Ca^{2+} the concentration of Mg^{2+} increases from 4 mM to greater than 7 mM. The possible effect of this change in Mg^{2+} concentration should not be ignored in relating any change in the extent of the response to the Ca^{2+} concentration.

A similar degree of consideration has not been given to maintenance of constant concentration in studies using other factors added to permeabilized preparations. Studies using cyclic 3',5'-AMP (cAMP) have in some, but not all, cases been performed in the presence of an inhibitor of cAMP phosphodiesterase to suppress cAMP breakdown (34). Measurements using saponin

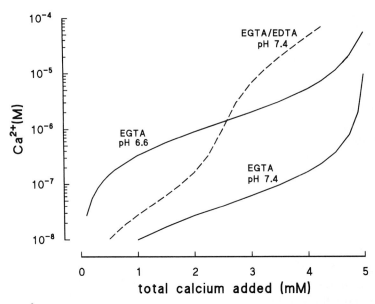

Figure 4. Ca^{2+} titration curves for a Ca–EGTA buffer at pH 6.6 and at pH 7.4, and for a Ca–EGTA/EDTA buffer at pH 7.4. Ca^{2+} concentrations were calculated using published dissociation constants (30,31) and for a total ligand concentration of 5 mM. The ordinate indicates the concentration of Ca^{2+} obtained when the total calcium concentration indicated on the abscissa is added to a buffer containing 5 mM EGTA, 7 mM Mg, and 5 mM ATP at pH 6.6 or 7.4, or one containing 2.5 mM EGTA, 2.5 mM EDTA, 12.5 mM Mg, and 5 mM ATP at pH 7.4. Modified from ref. 9.

permeabilized platelets (15) have however shown only a minimal (< 20%) extent of cAMP breakdown under the conditions used. Possible generation of cAMP from added ATP in for example the studies on secretion or arachidonate mobilization has not been evaluated. The importance of considering such possibilities is illustrated by experience with cGMP which was initially reported to stimulate the activation of Ca^{2+}-driven 5-HT secretion by thrombin (34). This effect was subsequently shown to result from the conversion of cGMP to GTP and the resultant enhancement of thrombin activation by this latter nucleotide (34).

Little consideration has been given to systems for the maintenance of the concentration of 1,2-diacylglycerol despite the importance of this factor in modulating Ca^{2+}-driven responses and the evidence that at least added 1,2-diacylglycerol is rapidly phosphorylated (35).

Access of semi-permeabilized platelets to antibodies has only been demonstrated for saponin treated preparations in which the lesions created are sufficiently large to allow entry of such proteins. Using saponin permeabilized platelets the role of a given protein in a response can be probed very selectively using a monoclonal antibody provided that the response is not affected by the detergent concentration required. An example of a study in which access of a monoclonal antibody (PL/IM 430) into saponin permeabilized platelets was used to interfere with [^{45}Ca^{2+}] uptake into this preparation is shown in *Figure 3* (see also ref. 26). The uptake of the ^{125}I-labelled monoclonal antibody occurs over the same range of saponin concentration (10–20 µg/ml) as the inhibition of [^{45}Ca] uptake and the release of lactate dehydrogenase.

Electroporated platelets neither release proteins nor appear to take them up (12) and the largest polypeptide which has been shown to enter this preparation is the pseudosubstrate for protein kinase C (M_r 2100 Da) (36). Although a similar system to that used for electroporation has been employed to cause the entry of DNA into cells it is likely that such entry of this large macromolecule involves the unwinding of the nucleotide polymer and the passage of the chain into the cell either by electroinjection and/or on a nucleotide by nucleotide basis (37).

5.1 Secretion

Markers from all three platelet secretory granules are released on exposure of electroporated platelets to micromolar Ca^{2+} (12,13,21). Half-maximal secretion occurs at 2–4 µM Ca^{2+} with a maximal response requiring the addition of approximately 10 µM Ca^{2+}. Other divalent cations other than Sr^{2+} are not effective. The Ca^{2+} dose–response relationship is similar at pH 6.6 and 7.4, and is not dependent on the Ca^{2+} buffering capacity of the system (38). Secretion also requires the presence of millimolar Mg–nucleotide triphosphate. MgATP^{2-} is the most effective species although other nucleotides, e.g. MgCTP^{2-}, will also support the response. Since non-hydrolysable ATP analogues are not effective either a Ca^{2+}-driven phosphorylation or dephosphorylation, or a Ca^{2+}ATPase, may be involved in these responses. The sensitivity of the secretory response to Ca^{2+} is increased in the presence of metabolically stable GTP analogues or of agonists especially on addition of GTP (13,32,34,39).

For secretion of the lysosomal markers a simple dose–response relationship for activation by Ca^{2+} is only observed in the presence of a protease inhibitor, e.g. leupeptin. In the absence of such an inhibitor a biphasic dose–response curve is obtained especially in the presence of GTP or GTP[S]. This suggests that in the permeabilized platelet a Ca^{2+}-dependent protease, e.g. calpain I, degrades a protein which facilitates this response (17). However there is no evidence that such an event occurs in the intact cell. Ca^{2+}-driven secretion does not appear to have been directly demonstrated for the saponin permeabilized preparation although secretion driven by inositol 1,4,5-trisphosphate has been shown, and may be mediated at least in part by release of Ca^{2+} from intracellular stores (24,40).

In contrast to the EC$_{50}$ (Ca^{2+}) for 5-HT secretion determined in the electroporated platelet (1.8 ± 0.2 µM) (21), agonist-driven 5-HT secretion from the intact platelet can occur at lower Ca^{2+} concentrations which in some cases, e.g. with thrombin as agonist, approximate those characteristic of the resting cell (0.05–0.1 µM) (41). This increase in the sensitivity of the system to Ca^{2+} is probably due to enhanced production of 1,2-diacylglycerol as a consequence of thrombin-induced activation of phosphoinositidase C, and resultant activation of protein kinase C. Thrombin-induced formation of 1,2-diacylglycerol has been shown in electroporated platelets (42) and addition of a synthetic 1,2-diacylglycerol (1-oleyl-2-acetylglycerol) enhances Ca^{2+}-driven secretion. Other structurally unrelated activators of protein kinase C, e.g. tetradecanyolphorbol acetate also mimic the enhancement by thrombin or by 1,2-diacylglycerol of Ca^{2+}-driven 5-HT secretion from the electroporated platelet (34,43). A central role for protein kinase C in this response is further indicated since 5-HT secretion induced by Ca^{2+} in the presence or absence of other factors is inhibited by addition of similar concentrations of selective protein kinase C inhibitors, e.g. the protein kinase C pseudosubstrate (36).

In the intact platelet secretion of 5-HT from the amine storage granule occurs selectively with some agonists, e.g. thromboxane A_2, and at lower agonist concentration with thrombin as agonist as compared to lysosomal secretion (12). The basis for such differential secretion has been defined using the electroporated platelet in which both secretory responses show a similar requirement for $MgATP^{2-}$ and occur over a similar range of Ca^{2+} concentration when this cation is used alone. However addition of thrombin increases the affinity for Ca^{2+} for 5-HT secretion but enhances the extent of lysosomal secretion over the same range of Ca^{2+} concentration (*Figure 5*). Similar effects are seen in the presence of GTPγ[S] or of activators of protein kinase C and can explain the differential response seen in the intact cell (17,44). Thus at low thrombin concentration the increase obtained in cytosolic $[Ca^{2+}]$ is only sufficient to cause 5-HT secretion due to the sensitization by 1,2-diacylglycerol. At higher thrombin concentration the greater increase in cytosolic $[Ca^{2+}]$ is sufficient also to cause lysosomal secretion.

5.2 Arachidonate release

This response has been measured only in the electroporated platelet (44) although less direct evidence makes clear that it underlies other responses in saponin treated platelets, e.g. thromboxane B_2 formation, secretion and aggregation induced by inositol 1,4,5-trisphosphate or an agonist such as thrombin (40,45).

At pH 7.4 Ca^{2+}-driven arachidonate release occurs over a somewhat lower range of Ca^{2+} concentration ($EC_{50} = 0.31 \pm 0.06$ µM) (*Figure 6*) than that required for other responses, e.g. secretion ($EC_{50} = 0.8 \pm 0.1$ µM) and is somewhat reduced by exposure of the electroporated preparation to millimolar Ca^{2+} (44). However this latter effect is less marked than that observed for lysosomal secretion (17). Ca^{2+}-driven arachidonate release absolutely

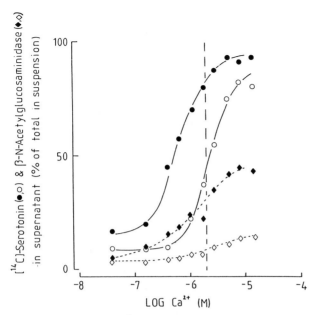

Figure 5. Effect of thrombin on the Ca^{2+} dependence of amine storage granule (●, ○) and lysosomal (◆, ◇) secretion from electroporated platelets. Data obtained in the absence (○, ◇) and presence (●, ◆) of thrombin. When added alone the Ca^{2+} concentration needed to achieve half-maximal activation of amine storage granule and lysosomal secretion as shown by the dashed line approximates 2 μM. Adapted from ref. 43.

requires $MgATP^{2-}$ (*Figure 6*). This effect is also given by non-hydrolysable ATP analogues, as well as other nucleotides, and does not therefore appear to be due to phosphate transfer to phospholipase A_2 (44). It may result from activation of this enzyme by a nucleotide binding protein as has been observed in heart (46).

5.3 Aggregation

This response, as well as the exposure of competent fibrinogen receptors detected using the monoclonal antibody PAC-1, has only been shown for saponin permeabilized platelets (24,40,47). Attempts to demonstrate aggregation of electropermeabilized platelets induced by agonists such as thrombin have thus far been unsuccessful (16). It is not clear whether this failure is inherent to some property of the electropermeabilized preparation or is due to the use of incorrect experimental conditions. Saponin permeabilized platelets aggregate on stimulation by agonists such as thrombin and collagen, and as indicated in *Figure 6* also show an aggregation response to inositol 1,4,5-trisphosphate (24,40). This latter response, which is prevented by blockade of cyclo-oxygenase and accompanied by thromboxane B_2 production, is likely to be due to activation of phospholipase A_2 due to localized Ca^{2+}

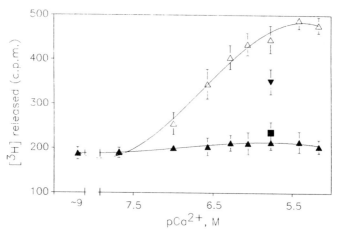

Figure 6. Release of [³H]arachidonate and its metabolites from electroporated platelets measured as a function of Ca^{2+} concentration in the presence (△) and absence (▲) of 5 mM $MgATP^{2-}$. The additional data points indicate results obtained in the presence of 5 mM ATP[S] (▼) and p[NH]ppA (■). Adapted from ref. 44.

release, and hence increased arachidonate availability (24,40,45). Similar conclusions have been drawn in regard to the inositol 1,4,5-trisphosphate induced increase in competent fibrinogen receptors as detected by PAC-1 (47).

References

1. Baker, P. F. and Knight, D. E. (1987). In *In vitro methods for studying secretion* (ed. A. Poisner and E. Trifaro), p. 223. Elsevier, New York.
2. Hilderman, R. H. and Deutscher, M. P. (1974). *J. Biol. Chem.*, **249**, 5346.
3. Zuurendonk, P. F. and Tager, J. M. (1974). *Biochim. Biophys. Acta*, **333**, 393.
4. Gogelein, H. and Huby, A. (1984). *Biochim. Biophys. Acta*, **773**, 32.
5. McClellan, G. B. and Winegrad, S. (1978). *J. Gen. Physiol.*, **72**, 737.
6. Gomperts, B. D. (1983). *Nature*, **306**, 64.
7. Impraim, C. C., Foster, K. A., Micklem, K. J., and Pasternack, C. A. (1980). *Biochem. J.*, **186**, 847.
8. Knight, D. E. (1981). *Techniques in cellular physical* (ed. P. F. Baker), p. 113. Elsevier/North Holland, Amsterdam.
9. Knight, D. E. and Scrutton, M. C. (1993). In *Methods in enzymology*, Vol. 221, p. 123.
10. Zimmerman, U., Pilwat, G., and Riemann, F. (1974). *Biophys. J.*, **14**, 881.
11. Baker, P. F. and Knight, D. E. (1981). In *Methods in enzymology*, Vol. 171, p. 817.
12. Knight, D. E., Hallam, T. J., and Scrutton, M. C. (1982). *Nature*, **296**, 256.
13. Peltola, K. and Scrutton, M. C. (1990). *Biochem. Soc. Trans.*, **18**, 466.
14. Hughes, K. and Crawford, N. (1989). *Biochim. Biophys. Acta*, **981**, 227.

15. Moos, M. and Goldberg, N. D. (1988). *Second Messengers and Phosphoproteins*, **12,** 163.
16. Scrutton, M. C. and Knight, D. E. Unpublished observations.
17. Knight, D. E. and Scrutton, M. C. (1981). *Thromb. Res.*, **20,** 437.
18. Haslam, R. J. and Davidson, M. M. L. (1984). *Biochem. J.*, **222,** 351.
19. Neumann, E., Sowers, A. E., and Jordan, C. A. (ed.) (1989*). Electroporation and electrofusion in cell biology*. Plenum, New York.
20. Athayde, C. M. and Scrutton, M. C. (1990). *Eur. J. Biochem.*, **189,** 647.
21. Haslam, R. J. and Coorssen, J. R. (1994). In *Mechanisms of platelet activation and control* (ed. K. S. Authi, S. P. Watson, and V. V. Kakkar). *Adv. Exp. Med. Biol.*, **344,** 149.
22. Knight, D. E. and Baker, P. F. (1982). *J. Membr. Biol.*, **68,** 107.
23. Menashi, S., Weintroub, H., and Crawford, N. V. (1981). *J. Biol. Chem.*, **256,** 4095.
24. Authi, K., Evenden, B. J., and Crawford, N. (1986). *Biochem. J.*, **233,** 709.
25. Purdon, A. D., Daniel, J. L., Stewart, G. J., and Holmsen, H. (1984). *Biochim. Biophys. Acta*, **800,** 178.
26. Hack, N., Authi, K., and Crawford, N. (1988). *Biosci. Rep.*, **8,** 379.
27. Authi, K. S., Rao, G. H. R., Evenden, B. J., and Crawford, N. (1988). *Biochem. J.*, **255,** 885.
28. Ugurbil, K. and Holmsen, H. (1981). In *Platelets in biology and pathology II* (ed. J. L. Gordon), p. 147. Elsevier/North Holland, Amsterdam.
29. Rink, T. J. and Hallam, T. J. (1984). *Trends Biochem. Sci.*, **12,** 215.
30. Martell, A. E. and Sillen, L. G. (1964). *Chem. Soc. Spec. Publ.*, **17,** 634.
31. Tsien, R. Y. (1980). *Biochemistry*, **19,** 2396.
32. Haslam, R. J. and Davidson, M. M. L. (1984). *Biochem. J.*, **222,** 351.
33. Knight, D. E. and Scrutton, M. C. (1984). *Nature*, **309,** 66.
34. Haslam, R. J., Davidson, M. M. L., Knight, D. E., and Scrutton, M. C. (1985). *Nature*, **313,** 822.
35. Nishizuka, Y. (1983). *Phil. Trans. R. Soc. London Ser. B*, **302,** 101.
36. Knight, D. E. and Athayde, C. M. (1990*). J. Physiol.*, **426,** 78P.
37. Winterbourne, D. J., Thomas, S., Hermon-Taylor, J., Hussain, T., and Johnstone, A. P. (1988). *Biochem. J.*, **251,** 427.
38. Knight, D. E. and Scrutton, M. C. (1987). *FEBS Lett.*, **223,** 47.
39. Haslam, R. J. and Davidson, M. M. L. (1984). *FEBS Lett.*, **174,** 90.
40. Watson, S. P., Ruggiero, M., Abrahams, S. L., and Lapetina, E. G. (1986). *J. Biol. Chem.*, **261,** 5368.
41. Rink, T. J. and Hallam, T. J. (1984). *Trends Biochem. Sci.*, **12,** 215.
42. Haslam, R. J. and Davidson, M. M. L. (1984). *J. Recep. Res.*, **4,** 605.
43. Knight, D. E., Niggli, V., and Scrutton, M. C. (1985). In *Mechanisms of stimulus response coupling in platelets* (ed. J. Westwick, M. F. Scully, D. E. MacIntyre, and V. V. Kakkar). *Adv. Exp. Biol. Med. Biol.*, **192,** 171.
44. Patel, S. and Scrutton, M. C. (1991). *Biochem. J.*, **273,** 561.
45. Authi, K. S., Hornby, E. J., Evenden, B. J., and Crawford, N. (1987). *FEBS Lett.*, **213,** 95.
46. Hazen, S. L. and Gross, R. W. (1991). *Biochem. J.*, **280,** 581.
47. Shattil, S. J. and Brass, L. F. (1987). *J. Biol. Chem.*, **262,** 992.

4

Use of fluorescent indicators to measure intracellular Ca^{2+} and other ions

STEWART O. SAGE

1. Introduction

Changes in cytosolic calcium ion concentration ($[Ca^{2+}]_i$) play a major rôle in platelet activation. Elevation of $[Ca^{2+}]_i$ alone can stimulate shape change, aggregation, and secretion, although physiologically other second messengers such as diacylglycerol may contribute to these events. As with other non-excitable cells, platelet agonists stimulate a rise in $[Ca^{2+}]_i$ by promoting the entry of Ca^{2+} into the cytosol from two sources. Ca^{2+} is released from intra-cellular stores in the dense tubular system, a structure analogous to the endo-plasmic reticulum of other cells, and Ca^{2+} enters the platelet across the plasma membrane.

Agonists release Ca^{2+} from internal stores by binding to surface receptors and activating phospholipase C via a GTP binding protein. Phospholipase C cleaves the membrane phospholipid, phosphatidylinositol 4,5-bisphosphate, to produce two second messengers, diacylglycerol and inositol 1,4,5-trisphos-phate. The diffusible messenger, inositol 1,4,5-trisphosphate, then binds to receptors on the intracellular Ca^{2+} store, opening a Ca^{2+}-release channel.

The mechanisms by which agonists stimulate Ca^{2+} entry across the plasma membrane are poorly understood and this is an intensive area of investiga-tion in platelets and other non-excitable cells, which are generally agreed to lack voltage-operated Ca^{2+} channels. Three types of so-called receptor-medi-ated Ca^{2+} entry (RMCE) are envisaged:

(a) Receptor-operated channels (ROCs), where agonist–receptor binding is closely coupled to channel opening, either through subunits of the recep-tor protein, or via a GTP binding protein.

(b) Second messenger-operated channels (SMOCs), where agonist–receptor binding results in the formation of a diffusible second messenger, which in turn binds to a receptor on the cytosolic face of the plasma membrane to open a channel.

(c) Store-regulated Ca^{2+} entry, where depletion of the intracellular Ca^{2+} store is somehow signalled to the plasma membrane to activate Ca^{2+} entry.

In platelets, ADP has been shown to activate a receptor-operated, non-selective cation channel which can conduct Ca^{2+} into the cells. It is still uncertain whether other agonists can generate Ca^{2+} entry directly via ROCs or SMOCs. Depletion of the platelet intracellular Ca^{2+} store, for example by using inhibitors of the store Ca^{2+}ATPase such as thapsigargin, stimulates Ca^{2+} entry in the absence of changes in other second messengers. Hence store-regulated Ca^{2+} entry appears to occur in platelets and any agonist which discharges stored Ca^{2+} is likely to promote Ca^{2+} influx by this route.

This chapter describes the use of fluorescent Ca^{2+}-sensitive indicators to measure or monitor platelet $[Ca^{2+}]_i$. Fluorescent indicators for cytosolic pH (pH_i) and cytosolic sodium concentration ($[Na^+]_i$) are also briefly considered. The use of radioisotopes to investigate platelet Ca^{2+} fluxes is described in Chapter 5.

Ca^{2+} entry mechanisms may also be studied electrophysiologically using the patch clamp technique. However, only one laboratory has reported this type of work with stimulated platelets (1,2) and patch clamping is not considered here.

2. Use of Ca^{2+}-sensitive fluorescent indicators in platelets

2.1 Principles of indicator function

2.1.1 Chemical structure

The most widely used fluorescent Ca^{2+} indicators are derivatives of the Ca^{2+} chelator BAPTA, itself a double aromatic analogue of the common Ca^{2+} chelator, EGTA. The four carboxyl groups of BAPTA provide the Ca^{2+} binding site or 'chelation claw' of the probes and occupation of this site by Ca^{2+} alters the fluorescent properties of the indicator. The particular spectral characteristics of the probes are determined by the fluorophores added to the basic BAPTA backbone.

2.1.2 Available indicators

The preferred indicator in most laboratories working with platelets is fura-2. Some use is also made of indo-1. Quin2, the precursor of these probes, has largely fallen from use because it is much less fluorescent than the newer indicators. Consequently, quin2 must be loaded into cells at much higher concentrations than fura-2 or indo-1 (0.5 mM cf. 30 µM) to overcome cellular autofluorescence. This has a number of drawbacks, particularly increased cytosolic Ca^{2+} buffering which may distort the change in $[Ca^{2+}]_i$ being measured. If however, increased Ca^{2+} buffering is desired experimentally, quin2 may be the indicator of choice (3). However, in cases where Ca^{2+}

buffering is required, but $[Ca^{2+}]_i$ measurement is not, it is preferable to use BAPTA as this is a more rapid chelator.

There has been a large proliferation of fluorescent indicators over recent years, providing a range of spectral properties (particularly optimal excitation wavelengths) and various Ca^{2+} affinities to suit different experimental requirements and conditions (4). As yet, however, there are few or no reports of the use of most of these new probes in platelets. This section will therefore concentrate of the use of fura-2 and indo-1.

2.1.3 Spectral properties and calibration principles

i. Fura-2

Ca^{2+} binding to fura-2 results in a shift in absorbance, and so in fluorescence excitation spectrum, to shorter wavelengths (*Figure 1A*). This is accompanied by a modest increase in the magnitude of the maximum emission . It is possible to record and calibrate fura-2 fluorescence by exciting the indicator at a single wavelength (e.g. 340 nm, at which a rise in $[Ca^{2+}]_i$ increases fluorescence), if the maximum and minimum fluorescences are determined at the end of the experiment (see Section 2.4.4). The preferred method of calibration, however, is to use a *ratio* of fluorescence excited at two excitation wavelengths. The ratio signal is independent of the intracellular indicator concentration, and so is relatively unaffected by photobleaching and indicator leakage. Similarly, instrumental fluctuations, particularly in the excitation light, are not a problem since both raw signals are affected and the ratio unaltered. Usually wavelengths of 340 and 380 nm are employed. Fluorescence emission excited at 340 nm increases with $[Ca^{2+}]$ whilst that at 380 nm

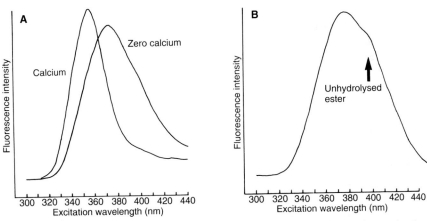

Figure 1. Excitation spectra of fura-2. (A) Spectra of intracellular fura-2 from platelets loaded as in *Protocol 1*. The cells were permeabilized with 50 µM digitonin in the presence of 1 mM $CaCl_2$ or 1 mM EGTA (zero calcium). (B) Spectrum from platelets prepared as in (A) but with 20 µM fura-2/AM rather than 3 µM. The presence of unhydrolysed ester is apparent.

decreases, giving a large range of ratio changes. Ratiometric calibration requires determination of maximum and minimum ratio and other parameters (see *Protocol 5*).

ii. Indo-1

Indo-1 shows a shift in both excitation and emission spectra to shorter wavelengths with Ca^{2+} binding. As with fura-2, single wavelength calibration is possible but ratiometric calibration is preferable. A ratio of fluorescence at two different emission wavelengths (405 and 490 nm) with fixed excitation (350 nm) is used.

Apparatus for recording and processing fluorescence signals is considered in Section 2.3.

2.2 Loading platelets with fura-2 or indo-1

2.2.1 Indicator esters

The functional forms of fura-2, indo-1, and other fluorescent indicators are polyvalent anions and as such are not membrane permeant. Although microinjection provides a means of introducing indicators into the cytosol of large cells, this is not technically feasible in platelets. Instead, the usual approach in platelets as in other cells is to load the indicator using an esterified form of the probe. The esters of the indicators are lipid soluble and so membrane permeant. Once inside the cell, cytosolic esterases hydrolyse the ester to re-form the polyvalent anionic form of the indicator, which should then be trapped in the cytosol. Since hydrolysis maintains the gradient for entry of the ester, quite large cytosolic indicator concentrations can be acheived by incubating cells with low concentrations of ester. Fura-2, indo-1, and many other indicators are loaded from their acetoxymethyl esters (fura-2/AM, indo-1/AM, etc.).

Although simple in principle, loading cells with indicators from the esterified form can lead to a number of problems in practice which can catch out the unwary. Fortunately, platelets are less temperamental in this respect than many cells. Problems with ester loading and possible solutions are discussed in Section 2.7.

2.2.2 Loading platelets in platelet-rich plasma or washed suspensions

i. Choice of PRP or washed suspension

Human platelets load with most fluorescent indicators from the esterified form very satisfactorily in citrated platelet-rich plasma. There may even be advantages in that potential difficulties can arise from poor dispersal of the ester during loading, and dispersal is aided by plasma proteins. Nevertheless, some workers load human platelets using indicator esters in washed suspensions. Since there is some deterioration of the cells with handling and certain responses such as the ADP ROC are rapidly lost after washing, loading in

PRP would seem preferable. However, circumstances may dictate that loading be carried out in washed suspensions and this will often be satisfactory.

Difficulties have been experienced when attempting to load platelets of some species other than man when using indicator esters in PRP. For example, rat and horse plasma have a high esterase activity such that most of the ester added to PRP from these species is hydrolysed outside the cells and consequently little is accumulated intracellularly. Washed suspensions therefore have to be used. Species variations are considered in Chapter 17.

ii. Preparation of platelet-rich plasma or washed suspensions for indicator loading

Detailed protocols for platelet preparation are given in Chapter 1. For human platelets, loading using indicator esters is commonly done using PRP prepared from fresh blood anticoagulated by mixing with one-sixth volume acid–citrate–dextrose (ACD) (see Chapter 1). Washed suspensions may be prepared by centrifugation of this PRP and resuspension in a similar volume of Hepes-buffered saline (145 mM NaCl, 5 mM KCl, 10 mM Na Hepes, 1 mM MgSO$_4$, 10 mM D-glucose pH 7.4 at 37°C). The addition of 0.1% (w/v) bovine serum albumin may be beneficial. Other PRPs and washed suspensions should be satisfactory.

iii. Loading procedures and subsequent handling

Protocol 1. Loading platelets with indicators in PRP

Equipment and reagents

- Screw-top plastic tubes
- Fura-2/AM or indo-1/AM dissolved in dry DMSO at 5 mM (store desiccated at –20°C)
- Water-bath at 37°C
- Bench-top centrifuge
- Buffer for resuspension (e.g. see Section 2.2.2.*ii*)
- Plastic transfer pipettes

Method

1. Add fura-2/AM or indo-1/AM (2 μM)[a] to PRP in a plastic tube.

2. Mix gently by inverting the tube a few times.

3. Incubate tube in water-bath at 37°C for 45 min.

4. Collect platelets by centrifugation at 700 *g* for 20 min.

5. Resuspend in buffer by dispersing pellet gently using a plastic transfer pipette.

[a] The concentration required to give a satisfactory signal may vary between batches of ester and will be influenced by problems which may arise (see Section 2.7). Concentrations between 0.5 and 5 μM may be needed.

The procedure for loading platelets in washed suspensions is similar to that used with PRP. However, lower ester concentrations may be needed. The risk of partial platelet activation during handling and so lower quality platelets is increased when washed cells are used. The cells may clump or aggregate when pelleted the second time, making satisfactory resuspension impossible. It helps to acidify the medium prior to centrifugation of the washed suspension. Apyrase should be added to the suspension to remove traces of ADP. See Chapter 1 for further discussion of this.

Protocol 2. Loading platelets with indicators in washed suspensions

Equipment and reagents

- See *Protocol 1*
- Apyrase (20 mg/ml stock in resuspension buffer)

- Acid–citrate–dextrose (ACD) solution: 2.0 g D-glucose, 2.5 g sodium citrate, 1.5 g citric acid in 100 ml distilled water

Method

1. Add fura-2/AM or indo-1/AM (0.5 μM)[a] to washed platelet suspension (density about 2×10^8/ml) containing 20 μg/ml apyrase and 200 μM $CaCl_2$.

2. Mix gently by inverting tube.

3. Incubate tube in water-bath at 37 °C for 45 min.

4. Add 12 μl/ml ACD and mix well by inversion.[b]

5. Collect platelets by centrifugation at 700 *g* for 20 min.

6. Resuspend in buffer by dispersing pellet gently using plastic transfer pipette.

[a] The concentration required to give a satisfactory signal may vary between batches of ester and will be influenced by problems which may arise (see Section 2.7). Concentrations between 0.1 and 3 μM may be needed.
[b] If platelets tend to clump or aggregate and not resuspend well, 0.2–0.5 μM PGE_1 could be added at this stage. However, inhibition of responses due to elevated cAMP may persist when the cells are first resuspended.

Once indicator loaded platelets have been resuspended, they should be stored at room temperature and used rapidly. Optimal results will be obtained if the cells are used within 60–90 min of resuspension. Slow leakage of the dye from the cells occurs at room temperature and this is more rapid at higher temperatures. Extracellular indicator can make calibration and interpretation of fluorescence signals difficult (see Section 2.7.2). Apyrase (20 μg/ml) should be added to suspensions to remove traces of ADP and prevent activation until use. The platelets should be stored in the absence of added Ca^{2+} and the external $[Ca^{2+}]$ adjusted for each aliquot just before use by adding 1 mM CaCl$_2$ or 1 mM EGTA as required. Storage in the presence of Ca^{2+} may assist premature activation whilst storage with EGTA will tend to Ca^{2+} deplete the cells. An adequate fluorescent signal should be obtained from platelets at a final density of about 1.5×10^8/ml.

2.3 Recording fluorescent signals

2.3.1 Cell suspensions

A sizeable range of fluorimeters or spectrophotometers suitable for recording from platelet suspensions is available. It is essential that there is provision for stirring the suspension by means of a plastic-coated magnetic stir bar and that the temperature can be controlled. If glass cuvettes are used these should be siliconized (e.g. using Sigmacote). Plastic cuvettes may be preferable but check that these have suitable optical properties (some may be excessively fluorescent).

Given the desirability of ratiometric monitoring and recording, the apparatus should ideally be capable of providing at least two excitation wavelengths (for fura-2) or recording at two emission wavelengths (for indo-1). Some machines may offer both possibilities. The light source is usually a xenon lamp.

For dual excitation, the fluorimeter may have two monochromators to supply the chosen wavelengths, which are directed through the sample alternatively by a rotating mirror. An alternative is to provide dual or multiple excitation wavelengths by means of a filter wheel rotating in the excitation light path. Cairn Research make a relatively inexpensive modular fluorimeter system which can include a stirred cuvette module and is based on a rotating filter wheel. This can be used for dual emission or multiple excitation work. Multiple excitation allows the simultaneous use of fura-2 with indicators for other ions such as H$^+$.

Fluorescence from the cell suspension is usually collected at right angles to the excitation light. For dual excitation (fura-2) work, the emission light is filtered and passed to a photomultiplier tube (PMT). For dual emission (indo-1) work, the emission beam is split and filtered before reaching two PMTs. A dichroic mirror, which reflects light below a particular wavelength and transmits light above this wavelength, may be used to divide the beam before further filtering. A PMT consists of an evacuated glass tube containing a series of electrodes and a phosphor-coated surface. It functions as follows:

(a) A photon strikes the phosphor-coated surface and electrons are displaced.

(b) The photoelectrons are accelerated by high voltages applied to the chain of electrodes.

(c) As the accelerated electrons strike successive electrodes, more electrons are displaced amplifying the signal.

(d) The PMT produces a pulse of current for each photon striking the phosphor-coated surface.

The output from the PMT may be handled in one of two ways. Either the current is integrated and converted to a voltage signal or the current pulses resulting from individual photons are counted over defined periods (photon counting). Photon counting may be preferable at low light levels, such as with single cell work, but is unnecessary in fluorimeter systems designed for suspension work.

Dual or multiple wavelength fluorimeters are usually computer controlled with ratioing and calibration carried out by the software.

2.3.2 Single platelets

Work on single platelets is in its infancy, mainly because of the difficulty or anticipated difficulty of getting an adequate fluorescent signal from such a small cell. This approach is important however, since it is now known that many excitable cells show complex temporal and spatial arrangements in their Ca^{2+} signals. Agonists have been shown to evoke oscillations or spikes in $[Ca^{2+}]_i$, which may or may not be dependent on agonist concentration. Similarly, Ca^{2+} signals may not be uniform throughout a cell. Gradients in $[Ca^{2+}]_i$ may be created and propagating waves of elevated $[Ca^{2+}]_i$ may sweep across cells. Early work indicates that these types of phenomena are features of platelet Ca^{2+} signalling.

Single cell fluorescence work requires an inverted microscope adapted for epifluorescence use. The excitation light is delivered to the cell through the microscope optics which are also used to collect the fluorescence from the indicator. A dichroic mirror which reflects at the excitation wavelength(s) and transmits at the emission wavelength(s) is included in the light path.

Two approaches for recording the signal are possible. Photometric recording directs the fluorescent signal from a single platelet to a photomultiplier. An alternative is to use a sensitive camera to form an image of the fluorescence from one or more platelets and then to process the signal by digital video imaging. For a comparison of photometric and imaging systems, see ref. 5.

i. Photometric recording from single platelets
This technique is being developed in a laboratory which routinely patch clamps platelets with the aim of making combined electrophysiological and fluorescence recordings from the same cell. A small volume of a suspension of indicator loaded platelets is placed in a siliconized bath on the microscope stage and a patch pipette is lowered into the suspension. Using normal illumination to visualize the cells, a single platelet is drawn on to the tip of the patch pipette by applying gentle suction. A seal forms between the glass and the membrane, immobilizing the platelet. Other cells are then washed away by perfusing the bath with the buffer used to resuspend the platelets. A diaphragm in the emission path is adjusted to restrict the field to the immobi-

lized platelet. Ultraviolet illumination is then used and the patch pipette moved using micromanipulators so as to position the platelet optimally in the light path. The microscope is then focused to give the maximal signal. Agonists etc. may be applied to the bath, through the perfusion system or from a pressure injection pipette placed in the bath (2).

The photometric system used for work with single fura-2-loaded platelets in our laboratory consists of:

- a xenon light source (Photon Technology Inc)
- rotating filter wheel (Cairn Research)
- liquid light guide (Cairn Research)
- inverted microscope (Nikon Diaphot, modified for epifluorescence use)
- photomultiplier tube (Thorn-EMI)
- basic elements of a modular spectrofluorimeter with personal computer for rotor control and data recording (Cairn Research)

ii. Digital video imaging

The requirements for a digital video imaging system on the excitation side are similar to those for a photometric system such as that described above. However, on the emission side a sensitive video camera replaces the photomultiplier(s). Most systems for fluorescent indicator work use an intensified CCD (charge coupled device) camera.

In an intensified CCD camera, the image is intensified prior to reaching the CCD target, conferring high sensitivity. Photoelectrons are displaced from a photocathode (as in a PMT) and the photocurrent amplified within the intensifier. The electrons then hit a phosphor which emits photons to re-form the intensified image. The image falls on the CDD target which consists of a silicon semiconductor material. Photons of sufficient energy penetrate the silicon and break bonds between the atoms, creating electron-hole pairs. This photoelectric effect creates electrical charge at specific locations on the target, which will give rise to pixels (light points) in the final image. The charge is stored in potential wells created by the application of potential differences to electrodes near the surface of the silicon. The charge is then passed through the silicon by changing the potentials on a series of electrodes. A spatially coded signal is thus delivered to the output amplifier. The analogue output from the camera is passed to a high speed video converter (the 'frame grabber') which digitizes the signal. The signal is then passed to an averager and on to the image processor.

With a dual excitation system, several images may be captured at each excitation wavelength and be averaged before further processing. The background signal from an area free of cells is subtracted from the images at each wavelength and then a ratio image produced. The image is typically composed of 256×256 pixels, although higher resolution is possible. Each pixel is assigned one of (usually) 256 grey levels according to its ratio value. Most software then converts the value assigned to give a coloured output, producing the final 'pseudo-coloured' image. Calibration parameters can be supplied so that an estimated $[Ca^{2+}]_i$ can be assigned to each pixel of the image. The software then allows the data to be processed and presented in various ways. For example, the temporal details of changes in $[Ca^{2+}]_i$ in defined areas of the image (single cells or parts of single cells) may be abstracted, or the spatial details of $[Ca^{2+}]_i$ at particular times may be presented as 'contour' maps. Data may be stored on tape or optical disc (CD–ROM).

For more technical details on fluorescence detection and imaging, see ref. 5.

iii. Immobilizing cells for imaging work

Ratio imaging indicator loaded cells requires that they be immobilized on glass coverslips, so that the same parts of the cells are represented by the same pixels in the images to be ratioed. This is a problem with platelets, which are naturally in suspension and activate on contact with glass. Early attempts at platelet imaging have used coverslips coated with adhesion molecules such as fibrinogen, fibronectin, or collagen. Fibrinogen has proved successful in immobilizing platelets which both $[Ca^{2+}]_i$ measurement and electron microscopy indicate are unactivated. Single cell responses evoked by collagen have been studied by allowing fura-2 loaded platelets to settle on collagen-coated coverslips. Siliconized glass or glass with other coatings may reduce activation if this proves a problem.

Protocol 3. Immobilization of indicator loaded platelets for imaging on fibrinogen-coated coverslips

Equipment and reagents

- Glass coverslips (thickness 1.0)
- Ethanol/2 M HCl (3 : 1, v/v)
- Fibrinogen (10 mg/ml in saline)
- Resuspension buffer with 0.5% bovine serum albumin and 10 μM H–Arg–Gly–Asp–Ser–OH

- Suspension of indicator loaded platelets containing 5% (w/v) bovine serum albumin (fraction V; Sigma), 20 μg/ml apyrase, 10 μM H–Arg–Gly–Asp–Ser–OH (Bachem, Bubendorf, Switzerland), and 1 μM prostaglandin E$_1$

Method

1. Wash coverslips in ethanol/2 M HCl, then deionized distilled water.
2. Cover coverslips with fibrinogen solution and leave for 10 min.
3. Wash coverslips in resuspension buffer.
4. Mount a coverslip in the microscope perfusion chamber.
5. Add platelet suspension and leave for a few minutes.[a]
6. Wash away unattached cells with resuspension buffer containing CaCl$_2$, EGTA, etc., as required.

[a] Vary settling time to achieve a suitable platelet density.

The movement or total loss of the cells from the image is a frustrating feature of platelet imaging. Some software allows tracking of cells so that temporal changes in $[Ca^{2+}]_i$ in single cells can still be resolved if there is moderate movement during the experiment.

2.4 Calibration of fluorescence signals

2.4.1 Theory of calibration

Ratio signals from fura-2 are generated using two excitation wavelengths and recording at one emission wavelength. Usually excitation is at 340 and 380 nm with emission collected at 500 nm. Some workers excite at 360 and 380 nm, particularly for single cell work with microscopes not equipped with quartz optics, since transmission at 340 nm may be poor. With indo-1, a ratio of two emission wavelengths is produced using a single excitation wavelength. Excitation is usually at 350 nm and emission collected at 405 and 490 nm. Indicators should be calibrated under intracellular conditions since their fluorescence is affected by factors such as viscosity.

The $[Ca^{2+}]_i$ indicated by a ratio value R is given by the expression:

$$[Ca^{2+}]_i = \frac{K_d \cdot S_f \cdot (R - R_{min})}{S_b \cdot (R_{max} - R)}$$

where K_d is the dissociation constant of the indicator under intracellular conditions, S_f and S_b are the maximum and minimum values of fluorescence at one excitation wavelength (380 nm; fura-2) or one emission wavelength (490 nm; indo-1) under Ca^{2+}-saturating and Ca^{2+}-free conditions respectively. R_{max} and R_{min} are the maximum and minimum values of the ratio under Ca^{2+}-saturating and Ca^{2+}-free conditions. All raw signals should be corrected by subtraction of autofluorescence.

The dissociation constants (K_ds) of the indicators are affected by temperature and other factors such as total ionic strength and viscosity. Ideally, the K_d of the probe should be determined intracellularly at the appropriate temperature. In practice, most workers use published values which will give a reasonable approximation in most cases. The K_ds of quin2, fura-2, and indo-1 at 37°C under intracellular conditions are usually taken as 115 nM, 224 nM, and 250 nM. At 20°C the K_d of fura-2 is 135 nM.

Ca^{2+}-saturated signals are obtained by adding digitonin to permeabilize the plasma membrane, or using the Ca^{2+} ionophore ionomycin, in the presence of millimolar external Ca^{2+}. The Ca^{2+}-free signals are then obtained by chelating external Ca^{2+} using EGTA. Autofluorescence is determined by adding digitonin or ionomycin in the presence of external Mn^{2+}. Mn^{2+} quenches the fluorescence of fura-2 and indo-1, revealing the autofluorescence of the cells and components in the light path.

2.4.2 Platelet suspensions

Calibrations must be performed on each platelet preparation. The usual practice is to calibrate at the beginning and end of the experiment. The autofluorescence should be determined each time a calibration is performed and the values determined for both excitation wavelengths (fura-2) or both emission wavelengths (indo-1) should then be subtracted from all raw signals, including those from calibrations.

Protocol 4. Measuring autofluorescence from platelet suspensions

Equipment and reagents

- 500 mM $MnCl_2$
- 50 mM digitonin in DMSO

Method

1. Equilibrate an aliquot of platelet suspension to 37 °C.
2. Add $MnCl_2$ by 1 : 100 dilution to give a final concentration of 5 mM.
3. Add digitonin by 1 : 1000 dilution to a final concentration of 50 μM.[a]
4. Wait for signal to become steady, if uncertain that the autofluorescence has been reached, repeat steps 2 and 3.
5. Note signal at both excitation wavelengths (fura-2) or both emission wavelengths (indo-1).
6. Set instrumental offsets at these autofluorescence values or subsequently subtract from all raw signals of appropriate wavelength to correct for autofluorescence.

[a] 0.5–1 μM ionomycin may be used in place of digitonin. Add by 1 : 1000 dilution from a stock in DMSO.

Protocol 5. Calibrating ratiometric signals from platelet suspensions

Equipment and reagents

- 100 mM $CaCl_2$[a]
- 500 mM EGTA containing 10 mM Hepes and brought to pH 7.4 using KOH
- 50 mM digitonin (in DMSO)
- 500 mM Tris base[b]
- Autofluorescence values (*Protocol 4*)

Method

1. Equilibrate an aliquot of platelet suspension to 37 °C.
2. Add $CaCl_2$ by 1 : 100 dilution to give a final concentration of 1 mM.

3. Add digitonin by 1 : 1000 dilution to a final concentration of 50 µM.

4. Wait (about 30 sec) for signal to become steady to report R_{max} and S_b.[c]

5. Add 10 mM EGTA and 10 mM Tris base by 1 : 500 dilutions.

6. If uncertain that R_{min} has been reached, repeat step 5.

7. Wait (about 1 min) for signal to become steady to report R_{min} and S_f.

[a] It is recommended to purchase $CaCl_2$ as a solution (BDH) rather than preparing from the solid salt since this is hygroscopic.

[b] Since H^+ ions are displaced from EGTA when Ca^{2+} binds, Tris base is also added to maintain an alkaline pH. A large pH change affects the fluorescence of the indicator and can lead to erroneous calibration.

[c] For fura-2, S_b is the minimum value of the signal excited at 380 nm. For indo-1, S_b is the minimum value of the signal emitted at 490 nm. Likewise, S_f is the maximum value of these signals for the respective indicators at the two wavelengths.

2.4.3 Single platelets

As discussed above, ideally fluorescent probes should be calibrated intracellularly. To date however, there have been no published reports where this has been achieved in single platelets. Although in principle, calibration should be possible by perfusing the immobilized platelets with high and low Ca^{2+} media in the presence of a Ca^{2+} ionophore, difficulties arise in practice.

(a) The small platelet volume means that there is relatively little indicator present, so that bleaching limits the time that measurements can be made.

(b) Long equilibration times (5–15 min) may be needed to reach R_{min}/S_f after application of ionophore and EGTA.

(c) Platelets are easily detached and lost from the image when the bath is perfused or solutions added.

However, qualitative data from single platelets contain much information and conversion of ratio values to estimated $[Ca^{2+}]_i$ is not essential to the study of temporal or spatial aspects of Ca^{2+} signalling. Some calibrated data from single platelet studies have been published. Such work has either used calibration parameters determined on the same apparatus using other cell types (6) or has used solutions of fura-2 (free acid) in different Ca^{2+} buffers to determine the calibration parameters. The simplest approach for the latter is to prepare two solutions of 50 µM fura-2 free acid in 150 mM KCl, one with 5 mM $CaCl_2$ (to give R_{max} and S_b) and another with 10 mM EGTA (to give R_{min} and S_f). These approaches give a *rough estimate* of $[Ca^{2+}]_i$, but are really no more useful than uncalibrated ratio data.

2.4.4 Single wavelength calibration

Although ratiometric calibration of fura-2 and indo-1 fluorescence is preferred, single wavelength calibration is also possible. This is the normal way of working with quin2.

The $[Ca^{2+}]_i$ indicated by a fluorescence value F is given by the expression:

$$[Ca^{2+}]_i = \frac{K_d \cdot (F - F_{min})}{(F_{max} - F)}$$

where K_d is the dissociation constant of the indicator under intracellular conditions, and F_{max} and F_{min} are the maximum and minimum values of the fluorescence under Ca^{2+}-saturating and Ca^{2+}-free conditions. All raw signals should be corrected by subtraction of autofluorescence.

F_{max}, F_{min}, and autofluorescence values are found in the same way as described for ratiometric calibration in *Protocol 4* and *Protocol 5*. With fura-2, single wavelength measurements are usually made with excitation at 340 nm and emission at 500 nm. For quin2, excitation is set at 338 nm and emission at 500 nm, and for indo-1, 350 nm and 405 nm are used.

2.4.5 Accuracy of calibration

The literature is full of values for $[Ca^{2+}]_i$ cited to the nearest 1 nM or even less. This suggests a degree of accuracy which is simply not possible using fluorescent indicators. The best that can be achieved is an *estimate* of $[Ca^{2+}]_i$. It will soon become apparent to anyone entering the field that calibration parameters are seldom if ever completely reproducible, even using samples of the same cell preparation. The calculated values of $[Ca^{2+}]_i$ will thus depend on the parameters chosen and there will therefore often be an inevitable subjective element to this type of work. The main thing to hope for is that adoption of a consistent approach to calibration gives reasonably reproducible results, particularly reproducible estimates of basal $[Ca^{2+}]_i$, such that other values can be relied upon.

In practice, the obsession with calibration is often unjustified. Many experiments do not require accurate calibration or even calibration at all. Often, one only requires a *comparison* of Ca^{2+} signals under different conditions, or details of temporal or spatial organization, and there is nothing that a calibrated trace can indicate that an uncalibrated ratio cannot.

2.5 Using Mn²⁺ as a tracer for Ca²⁺ entry

Changes in $[Ca^{2+}]_i$ may result from both Ca^{2+} entry across the plasma membrane and the release of Ca^{2+} from intracellular stores. The measuring or monitoring of $[Ca^{2+}]_i$ under physiological conditions with external Ca^{2+} present can give no information as to the source of Ca^{2+}. Internal release can be studied by preventing entry (removing external Ca^{2+} with EGTA or blocking entry with Ni^{2+}), but monitoring influx requires the use of a surrogate for Ca^{2+}. Mn^{2+} is the ion most frequently used and can permeate at least some Ca^{2+} entry pathways in most cell types. Remember, however, that not all Ca^{2+} entry pathways are Mn^{2+} permeable and that the Mn^{2+} permeability of different pathways may vary.

Mn^{2+} binds to indicators such as fura-2 and quenches their fluorescence (the indicator ceases to fluoresce with Mn^{2+} bound). If fluorescence is excited at the isoemissive (isobestic) wavelength, at which the fluorescence of the indicator is Ca^{2+}-insensitive, any fall in fluorescence when Mn^{2+} is present externally can be ascribed to Mn^{2+} entry since there is normally none present intracellularly. If multiple wavelength excitation is available, Mn^{2+} quench at the isoemissive wavelength can be monitored simultaneously with a ratio to give an estimate of $[Ca^{2+}]_i$, as long as some unquenched dye is present throughout the experiment.

Protocol 6. Mn^{2+} tracing of Ca^{2+} entry in fura-2 loaded platelet suspensions

Equipment and reagents

- 50 mM $MnCl_2$
- 100 mM $CaCl_2$
- 50 mM digitonin in DMSO

- Excitation light at the isoemissive wavelength (360 nm for fura-2)

Method

1. Equilibrate an aliquot of fura-2 loaded platelet suspension to 37°C.

2. Add 1 mM $CaCl_2$ by 1 : 100 dilution.[a]

3. Add 50 μM $MnCl_2$ by 1 : 1000 dilution.[b]

4. Add agonists, etc., as required.

5. End experiment by adding 50 μM digitonin to check availability of unquenched dye.

[a] It is advisable to include external Ca^{2+} to ensure events which may be influenced by Ca^{2+} entry proceed as physiologically as possible (7).
[b] It may be necessary to vary the $[Mn^{2+}]$ to get a suitable quench of signal. Be aware that Mn^{2+} may block some entry pathways, particularly at higher concentrations.

2.6 Stopped-flow fluorimetry

Stopped-flow fluorimetry may be used to study the early stages of Ca^{2+} signals in platelets with a high degree of temporal accuracy (i.e. on a millisecond time-scale). This is not possible in stirred cuvette experiments due to uncertainty as to the time of addition of agonists and a relatively long and unknown mixing time. Good temporal resolution is also impossible in imaging experiments for the above reasons and because the data capture rate is relatively slow. Single platelet photometry can give good temporal resolution if the pressure injection system used to apply the agonist can be calibrated (see ref. 2).

Stopped-flow fluorimeters are commercially available, but a simple stopped-flow attachment which can be mounted in a conventional fluorimeter is entirely satisfactory. Indeed, a hand-operated stopped-flow attachment may be preferable to a compressed gas-driven specialist machine. The latter is really designed for chemical or biochemical use rather than intact cell work, and the very high pressures and flow rates generated can cause some cell lysis or activation. Both types of apparatus are available from High-Tech Scientific Ltd.

To use a stopped-flow attachment in a standard fluorimeter:

(a) Mount the mixing chamber of the stopped-flow attachment in the fluorimeter cuvette holder and shield from external light.

(b) Thermostat both cuvette holder and stopped-flow apparatus at 37 °C.

(c) Trigger fluorimeter recording from a microswitch activated by the stopping syringe of the stopped-flow apparatus.

The precise requirements for stopped-flow experiments with indicator loaded platelet suspensions will vary, but the following points may be helpful:

(a) Prepare platelet suspensions at twice the density that would be used in cuvette work (i.e. about 3×10^8/ml).

(b) Prepare agonist solutions in resuspension buffer at twice desired final concentration.

(c) $CaCl_2$ or EGTA should be added to both cell suspension and agonist solution.

(d) $MnCl_2$ should be added mostly to the agonist solution to avoid excessive leakage into the cells prior to experimentation, but some should be included with the cells to avoid a quenching artefact from external indicator upon mixing (e.g. if a final $[Mn^{2+}]$ of 200 nM is required, add 350 nM to the agonist and 50 nM to the cells).

(e) Fill one injection syringe with cells and the other with agonist solution, always keep these the same so that cells never pass through tubes which may be contaminated with agonist.

(f) Before starting recordings, flush apparatus through with cells and agonist to ensure that the tubes and mixing chamber are filled and that all air is displaced.

(g) If changing conditions (e.g. to a different agonist) and at the end of experiments, wash the syringes and tubes well by flushing with 1 M NaOH, ethanol, distilled water, and finally resuspension buffer.

(h) Check that platelets prepared using your protocol are not activated or lysed during the injection process (injecting indicator loaded cells to mix with buffer containing 1 mM $CaCl_2$ and 100 μM $MnCl_2$ should result in no fluorescence change).

(i) If lysis is a problem, arrange to subtract control traces from experimental runs to reveal the effects of agonists.

(j) Stopped-flow records are usually noisy, but are highly reproducible and so can be averaged to overcome this.

(k) Measure the mixing time of the apparatus and check that it is consistent (trigger a recording manually and inject 1 µM fura-2 free acid in buffer to mix with buffer containing 1 mM $MnCl_2$, pre-fill mixing chamber with fura-2 solution only).

2.7 Problems and possible solutions in fluorescent Ca²⁺ indicator work

2.7.1 Loading difficulties

i. No intracellular indicator

If there is no signal above background:

(a) Check instrument is functioning by placing a piece of paper (which is fluorescent) or a solution of indicator free acid in the light path.

(b) Check cells are being incubated with the membrane permeant indicator ester (fura-2/AM, indo-1/AM) not the indicator free acid.

(c) For species other than human, try loading in washed suspensions rather than PRP in case there is significant plasma esterase activity.

ii. Poor loading

If the signal is too weak to be usable (increasing instrument gain results in excessive noise):

• increase indicator ester concentration used for loading

• vary loading time

• increase platelet density if using suspensions

It is a good idea to get an estimate of the intracellular indicator concentration (8).

2.7.2 Calibration problems

A number of problems can distort the parameters determined during calibration such that the resulting calculated estimates of $[Ca^{2+}]_i$ are not believable. Be guided by resting $[Ca^{2+}]_i$. This should be reasonably consistent within and between experiments. Different workers report values between about 30 nM and 100 nM.

i. Unhydrolysed ester

The presence of unhydrolysed or incompletely hydrolysed indicator ester intracellularly or in the suspension makes calibration difficult since fura-2/AM and indo-1/AM are fluorescent but not Ca^{2+}-sensitive.

The best way to to test for the presence of unhydrolysed ester is to examine the excitation spectrum of indicator loaded cells in a scanning fluorimeter.

Fura-2 free acid should give a single peak with a maximum around 360 nm in unstimulated cells. Ester contamination shows up as a 'shoulder' around 400 nm (*Figure 1B*).

(a) Reduce ester concentration used for loading.

(b) Stand platelet suspension after resuspension to allow further hydrolysis of ester.

(c) If loading in washed suspensions, add 0.1% bovine serum albumin or pre-mix stock ester solution with an equal volume of pluronic solution (25% w/v in DMSO) to improve dispersal of ester (see *Protocol 7*).

ii. Compartmentalization

A complication of loading indicators from their ester forms is that the esters may enter organelles and accumulate, either as ester or hydrolysed product. In some cells fura-2 (free acid) has been observed to gradually accumulate in organelles after an apparently satisfactory cytosolic loading. Organelles such as the endoplasmic reticulum have a high lumenal $[Ca^{2+}]$ which will result in a high average $[Ca^{2+}]_i$ for the whole cell if indicator is compartmentalized.

Compartmentalized indicator will not be subjected to changes in $[Ca^{2+}]_i$ such as those imposed during calibration, leading to errors.

(a) Reduce ester concentration used for loading.

(b) If loading in washed suspensions, add 0.1% bovine serum albumin or pre-mix stock ester solution with an equal volume of pluronic solution (25% w/v in DMSO) to improve dispersal of ester.

(c) Try loading at room temperature rather than 37°C.

iii. Indicator leakage

Indicators gradually leak from cells. With single cells where the bath is per-fused this is not a problem as long as ratioing is employed, since the external indicator is washed away. In suspensions, leakage may be a problem since the external indicator will contribute to the measured signal giving an overesti-mate of $[Ca^{2+}]_i$ in medium containing physiological $[Ca^{2+}]$ and an underesti-mate in medium with EGTA. An apparent drift in estimated basal $[Ca^{2+}]_i$ during an experiment is likely to be caused by leakage.

To check the contribution of external indicator to the fluorescence of a suspension either:

(a) Centrifuge a sample of the suspension and examine the fluorescence of the supernatant.

(b) Or add 100 µM $MnCl_2$ to the suspension. A biphasic quench in fluor-escence will occur: a rapid drop due to quenching of external indicator, and a slower fall as Mn^{2+} leaks into the cells and quenches intracellular dye.

A small amount of leakage is inevitable and usually ignored. To reduce leakage:

- store suspensions of loaded platelets at room temperature
- limit duration of experiments on a given preparation

If leakage is severe, or particularly accurate calibration is required, the signals can be corrected for the contribution of external indicator. The fluorescence of the supernatant after centrifugation can be determined at the required wavelengths after experiments and subtracted from the raw signals before ratioing. An alternative is to add 100 μM $MnCl_2$ to quench external indicator and then rapidly follow this with 0.5 mM Ca–DTPA (Ca diethylenetriaminepentaacetic acid) (Sigma) to chelate the Mn^{2+} before significant amounts leak into the cells. The magnitude of the quench at appropriate wavelengths can then be subtracted as above.

2.7.3 Noisy signals

If signals are unacceptably noisy, the amount of signal averaging prior to recording may be increased although this is obviously at the expense of temporal resolution.

Extremely noisy records from platelet suspensions may be caused by the presence of small aggregates. These may be visable to the naked eye, but certainly will be under the light microscope.

- store platelets in nominally Ca^{2+}-free suspension (i.e. without added Ca^{2+})
- add 20 μg/ml apyrase to suspensions
- limit duration of experiments using a particular suspension

Aggregates may result from poor resuspension, particularly if loading is done in washed suspensions. See *Protocol 2* for hints.

2.7.4 Photobleaching

Indicators may be photobleached (cease to fluoresce) after the absorption and emission of relatively few photons. Modest bleaching is not a problem in ratio work with suspensions, but can be a problem in single platelet work where relatively little dye is available because of the small cell volume.

(a) Use the lowest intensity excitation light that gives an adequate fluorescent signal by introducing neutral density filters, etc., into the excitation light path.

(b) Only expose cells to excitation light when essential by closing shutter in excitation light path when not recording.

(c) Increase indicator loading.

3. Indicators for ions other than Ca^{2+}

Fluorescent indicators are now available for many ions of biological interest, including H^+, Na^+, K^+, Cl^-, and Mg^{2+} (4). Many of these indicators have as yet been little used, particularly in platelets. Only indicators for Na^+ and H^+ are briefly considered here.

3.1 Cytosolic Na^+

3.1.1 SBFI

SBFI (sodium-binding benzofuran isophthalate) is the only $[Na^+]_i$ indicator in general use. SBFI can be used for ratio work and be loaded from its acetoxymethyl ester, SBFI/AM. The preferred excitation wavelengths are 340 and 385 nm, with emission collected at 500 nm.

Loading SBFI in most cells, including platelets, is more difficult than loading fura-2 or indo-1. SBFI also leaks from platelets quite rapidly, making correction for external dye necessary. To date, there are only reports of the use of SBFI in platelet suspensions. Calibration in suspension is rather complicated. SBFI should be satisfactory for monitoring $[Na^+]_i$ qualitatively in single platelets, but calibration is likely to be very difficult since many solution changes would be required. Only suspension work is considered here.

3.1.2 Loading platelets with SBFI

It is difficult to get a satisfactory loading of platelets with SBFI using SBFI/AM. This appears at least in part to be due to difficulties with dispersal of the ester. It is therefore best to load in PRP (plasma proteins aid dispersal) and to add the detergent, pluronic.

Protocol 7. Loading platelets with SBFI

Equipment and reagents

- Screw-top plastic tubes
- SBFI/AM dissolved in dry DMSO at 5 mM (store desiccated at –20°C)
- A solution of pluronic F-127 (Molecular Probes) (25% w/v in DMSO)
- Water-bath at 37°C
- Centrifuge
- Vortex mixer
- Buffer for resuspension
- Plastic transfer pipettes

Method

1. Measure out SBFI/AM required to give final concentration of 10 μM when added to PRP.
2. Mix SBFI/AM with an equal volume of pluronic solution in a plastic tube by vortexing.
3. Add PRP to SBFI/AM–pluronic mixture.
4. Mix well by inverting the tube a few times.

---

5. Incubate tube in water-bath at 37 °C for 1 h.

6. Collect platelets by centrifugation at 700 *g* for 20 min.[a]

7. Resuspend in buffer by dispersing pellet vigorously using a plastic transfer pipette.

---

[a] If calibration is required, some PRP should be reserved so that cells can be resuspended in calibration buffers. See *Protocol 8*.

When using SBFI loaded platelets, each aliquot should be centrifuged in a microcentrifuge after use and the fluorescence of the supernatant be determined at both excitation wavelengths. These values should then be subtracted from raw signals before ratioing.

3.1.3 Calibrating SBFI in platelets

SBFI fluorescence is considerably greater in the intracellular environment even compared with cell lysates, so the indicator must be calibrated intracellularly. The aim is to set $[Na^+]_i = [Na^+]_o$ using the Na^+–K^+ ionophore gramicidin and to do this at several different $[Na^+]_o$. This is difficult with platelets in suspension which are likely to activate if subjected to repeated centrifugation and resuspension. The method given in *Protocol 8* has been sucessfully used to get around this difficulty, centrifuging many aliquots of PRP separately so that some can be resuspended in calibration media.

When gramicidin is used to collapse the transmembrane gradients of monovalent cations, Cl^- fluxes may occur and cause changes in cell volume. To minimize this effect, the external $[Cl^-]$ should be set to equal internal $[Cl^-]$, which is approximately 30 mM.

Protocol 8. Calibration of SBFI in platelet suspensions

Equipment and reagents

- Calibration solutions containing 1, 5, 10, 20, 50, and 150 mM Na^+ prepared by appropriate mixing of a solution containing (in mM): 30 NaCl, 120 Na gluconate, 1 $MgCl_2$, 1 $CaCl_2$, 10 Na Hepes pH 7.4 at 37 °C, and a similar solution in which K^+ completely replaces Na^+
- Gramicidin (Sigma) (5 mM in DMSO)
- Small (1.5 ml) plastic tubes (Eppendorf)
- Microcentrifuge
- Plastic transfer pipettes
- PRP with SBFI loaded platelets (*Protocol 7*)

Method

1. Pipette six 0.6 ml aliquots of the PRP into small plastic tubes.

2. Centrifuge in microcentrifuge at 2900 *g* for 45 sec.

3. Pipette away as much supernatant as possible.

4. Resuspend one aliquot in 1 ml of each calibration solution.

5. Equilibrate an aliquot to 37 °C.

Protocol 8. *Continued*

  6. Add 5 µM gramicidin.

  7. Wait for signal to become steady then record raw signals at both excitation wavelengths.

  8. Centrifuge suspension in microcentrifuge and determine fluorescence of supernatant at both excitation wavelengths.

  9. Subtract external signals from raw data before calculating ratio.

 10. Repeat steps 5–9 until all calibration aliquots are used.

 11. Determine and use calibration parameters as described in *Protocol 9*.

Protocol 9. Calculating $[Na^+]_i$ from SBFI signals

1. Determine fluorescence ratios at six known $[Na^+]_i$ as described in *Protocol 8*.

2. Let R_1 be ratio at 1 mM $[Na^+]_i$, R_2 be that at 10 mM, and R_3 that at 150 mM.

3. Solve the simultaneous equations:[a]

- $R_o = [1490R_1R_3 - 140R_2R_3 - 1350R_1R_2] / [140R_1 + 1350R_3 - 1490R_2]$

- $R_\infty = [9R_1R_2 + 140R_2R_3 - 149R_1R_3] / [149R_2 - 9R_3 - 140R_1]$

- $(K_d \cdot S_{f2} \cdot S_{b2}) = [(R_\infty - R_1) / (R_1 - R_\infty) + 10(R_\infty - R_2) / (R_2 - R_\infty \cdot \text{lm3} + 150(R_\infty - R_3 - R_3 - R_\infty)] / 3$

4. Use the parameters determined in step 3 to check that the ratios (R) determined at $[Na^+]_i$ of 5, 20, and 50 mM give acceptable estimates of these values when substituted into the equation:

$$[Na^+]_i = (K_d \cdot S_{f2} \cdot S_{b2})(R - R_o) / (R_\infty - R).$$

5. If estimates of known $[Na^+]_i$ are acceptable use equation in step 4 to calculate unknown $[Na^+]_i$.

---

[a] In these equations, R_o is the fluorescence ratio at 0 Na^+, R_∞ that at saturating $[Na^+]$, K_d the dissociation constant of the indicator, and S_{f2}/S_{b2} the ratio of excitation efficiencies at the longer excitation wavelength. For more details see ref. 9.

3.2 Cytosolic pH
3.2.1 Indicators for pH

Several fluorescent indicators for cytosolic pH (pH_i) are available, including the SNARF and SNAFL series, and BCECF. Only BCECF has been used extensively in platelets, and only in suspension work. BCECF alone is considered briefly here.

3.2.2 Loading BCECF

BCECF loads readily into platelets from its acetoxymethyl ester, BCECF/AM. The ester should be prepared and used in exactly the same way as fura-2/AM or indo-1/AM (*Protocols 1* or *2*). An ester concentration of 3 μM should give satisfactory loading, although the concentration may need to be varied.

3.2.3 Using BCECF loaded platelets

BCECF is usually used ratiometrically, with excitation wavelengths of 430 and 490 nm and emission collected at 530 nm. BCECF leaks quite rapidly from platelets, which should therefore be stored at room temperature and used rapidly. Correction for the contribution of external dye is advisable and should be done in the manner described for SBFI loaded platelets (Section 3.1).

3.2.4 Calibrating BCECF signals

Calibration must be carried out intracellularly and is achieved using the H^+–K^+ exchanger, nigericin, which sets $[H^+]_i/[H^+]_o = [K^+]_i/[K^+]_o$. Suspension work requires aliquots of the loaded platelets to be suspended in different buffers of known pH and containing K^+ at the intracellular concentration so that $[H^+]_i = [H^+]_o$. For ratiometric calibration, the indicator must be exposed to acid (pH 4.3) and alkaline (pH 9.2) extremes. The pH_i is calculated using the equation:

$$pH_i = pK + \log \frac{(R - R_{min})}{(R_{max} - R)} + \log (S_b/S_f)$$

where R is the ratio at pH_i, R_{max} and R_{min} are the ratios at extreme alkaline and acid pH respectively, and S_b and S_f the fluorescence values at the shorter excitation wavelength (430 nm) under extreme acid and alkaline conditions. The pK for BCECF under intracellular conditions can be calculated from calibration experiments. A value of 6.97 has been reported in several cell types.

Protocol 10. Calibrating $[H^+]_i$ from BCECF signals

Equipment and reagents
- Calibration solutions containing 135 mM KCl, 15 mM NaCl, 1 mM MgCl₂, 10 mM D-glucose, 10 mM Hepes set to pH values of 4.3, 7.4, and 9.2 using NaOH
- Nigericin (Sigma) (0.2 mg/ml in DMSO)
- Small (1.5 ml) plastic tubes
- Microcentrifuge
- Plastic transfer pipettes
- PRP with BCECF loaded platelets (*Protocol 9*)

Method
1. Pipette three 0.7 ml aliquots of the PRP into small plastic tubes.
2. Centrifuge in microcentrifuge at 2900 *g* for 45 sec.

89

Protocol 10. *Continued*

3. Pipette away as much supernatant as possible.

4. Resuspend one aliquot in 1 ml of each calibration solution.

5. Equilibrate aliquot at pH 4.3 to 37 °C.

6. Add 0.2 µg/ml nigericin by 1 : 1000 dilution.

7. When fluorescence becomes steady, determine R_{min} and S_b.[a]

8. Equilibrate aliquot at pH 9.2 to 37 °C.

9. Add 0.2 µg/ml nigericin by 1 : 1000 dilution.

10. When fluorescence becomes steady, determine R_{max} and S_f.

11. Equilibrate aliquot at pH 7.4 to 37 °C.

12. Add 0.2 µg/ml nigericin by 1 : 1000 dilution.

13. When fluorescence becomes steady, determine R.

14. Substitute into the above equation to determine pK.

[a] This protocol assumes rapid work after resuspension such that there is negligible external indicator. If leakage is a problem, centrifuge each aliquot and correct raw fluorescences for the external signal.

Acknowledgements

Drs M. P. Mahaut-Smith and J. W. M. Heemskerk are greatly thanked for their comments and advice on this chapter, particularly regarding single platelet work. S. O. S. held a Royal Society 1983 University Research Fellowship. This work is partly supported by the BBSRC.

References

1. Mahaut-Smith, M. P., Sage, S. O., and Rink, T. J. (1990). *J. Biol. Chem.*, **265**, 10479.
2. Mahaut-Smith, M. P., Sage, S. O., and Rink, T. J. (1992). *J. Biol. Chem.*, **267**, 3060.
3. Cobbold, P. H. and Rink, T. J. (1987). *Biochem. J.*, **248**, 313.
4. Haughland, R. P. (1993). *Handbook of fluorescent probes and research chemicals*. Molecular Probes, Eugene, Oregon, USA.
5. Mason, W. T. (ed.) (1993). *Fluorescent and luminescent probes for biological activity*. Academic Press, London.
6. Heemskerk, J. W. M., Hoyland, J., Mason, W. T., and Sage, S. O. (1992). *Biochem. J.*, **283**, 379.
7. Sage, S. O., Reast, R., and Rink, T. J. (1990). *Biochem. J.*, **265**, 675.
8. Rink, T. J. and Pozzan, T. (1985). *Cell Calcium*, **6**, 133.
9. Sage, S. O., Rink, T. J., and Mahaut-Smith, M. P. (1991). *J. Physiol.*, **441**, 559.

5

Preparation of highly purified human platelet plasma and intracellular membranes using high voltage free flow electrophoresis and methods to study Ca^{2+} regulation

KALWANT S. AUTHI

1. Introduction

The ability of experimentalists to harvest and study purified fractions of plasma and intracellular membranes and organelles has contributed tremendously to our knowledge of platelet structure and to our understanding of the mechanisms associated with platelet activation and its control. The platelet is a delicately poised cell capable of rapid activation upon contact with a stimulus. The ease with which a *relatively homogeneous* population of platelets can be obtained, its importance in the cardiovascular system, and the surprising magnitude of signalling mechanisms that are present has made this cell one of the most thoroughly studied within the body. Its size (being one of the smallest of mammalian cells) and rapid excitability has prompted the development of new strategies in both its handling and disruption. Indeed, these techniques have allowed a study of platelet structure and membrane organization at a level of sophistication that in some respects has not been possible for other cell types.

The resting platelet is a discoid cell whose plasma membrane contains numerous invaginations into the interior of the cell (open canalicular system) that are known to be important in many functions including granule exocytosis (for a review on platelet ultrastructure see ref. 1). The plasma membrane in addition to the presence of surface receptors for agonists, is rich in glycoproteins that mediate cell–extracellular matrix (adhesion) and cell–cell (aggregation) interactions (2). The most prominent of these is the GPIIb–IIIa (αIIbβ_3) complex which is the major integrin responsible for aggregation and adhesion of activated platelets. Other glycoproteins that participate in these interactions include; $\alpha_v\beta_3$, GPIb–IX, GPIa–IIa ($\alpha_2\beta_1$), GPIc–IIa ($\alpha_5\beta_1$), GPIć–IIa ($\alpha_6\beta_1$), and GPV. Within the platelet there is a characteristic abundance of dense and α granules in addition to the lysosomal granules present in most other cell types. The energy requirements of this highly activatable cell are satisfied by the mitochondria and also glycogen storage granules. An important intracellular membrane system that extends throughout the cytoplasm but prominent at sites adjacent to membranes of the open canalicular system is the dense tubular system. This membrane system exhibits some features similar to those of the endoplasmic reticulum and is rich in enzymes associated with prostanoid synthesis and Ca^{2+} sequestration (see later). Prominently observed in transverse sections from the electron microscope are rings of microtubules arranged circumferentially within the cytoplasm which together with a system of microfilaments (composed mainly of actin) and the membrane skeleton regulate the shape of the platelet.

The purpose of this chapter is to provide the reader with an extensive experimental protocol that yields highly purified fractions of human platelet plasma and intracellular membranes and some of their characteristics. The method combines a number of approaches from gentle 'massaging' of the plasma membrane at the whole cell stage by neuraminidase treatment in order to reduce its net negative charge, to density gradient centrifugation and high voltage free flow electrophoresis. While the procedure is extensive, time-consuming, and requires specialist apparatus, it represents the only procedure to date that is able to best satisfy the three major criteria used in membrane fractionation, namely:

- the membrane fraction be relatively free from cross-contamination by other organelles

- the procedure should compromise as little as possible the functional and analytical properties of the membrane

- recoveries should be sufficient to allow the initial goals to be attained reproducibly

This procedure was first described in 1981 by Crawford's group (3) when three protein peaks (NI, NII, and NIII in decreasing order of electronegativity) were described from which one (NI) was characterized as intracellular membranes and the others (NII and NIII) were thought to represent two fractions of plasma (or surface) membranes. The separation of plasma membranes into two peaks (NII and NIII) though itself very interesting as it separated a myosin-rich membrane fraction, was subsequently found to be due to the presence of EDTA in the sorbitol density gradients and the procedure modified (through the removal of EDTA) (4) to yield only two discrete peaks representing intracellular and plasma membranes (reviewed in ref. 5).

2. Methods available for the preparation of platelet membranes

It is outside the scope of this chapter to provide a review of the current methods available for the preparation of platelet membranes and the reader is advised to consult an earlier review by Crawford (6) and Sixma and Lips (7), and references therein of the methods developed to study platelet membranes. However, because the procedure described here requires a specialist piece of apparatus, an outline of methods known which provide measurable success in purification will be mentioned and the reader is advised to consult appropriate references for further experimental details. The most straightforward preparation of membranes is to obtain a particulate preparation by centrifugation in excess of 40 000 g for 60 min of platelet homogenates obtained by any one of many methods (e.g. sonication, freeze–thawing, nitrogen cavitation, glycerol loading followed by osmotic lysis, etc.). The resulting pellet can be used to address the question of whether the protein or functional parameter of interest, associates with the membrane fraction (albeit to membranes from plasma, intracellular, granular, or lysosomal constituents). Differential centrifugation alone is unable to separate, to an acceptable degree, membrane fractions from any of the secretory granules present in platelets. Such a separation however can be achieved through the use of sucrose density gradients (8). Sucrose (or in our case, sorbitol) density gradients provide a population of mixed membranes containing elements from plasma and intracellular origin in good yields with little or no alteration of either functional or structural integrity and essentially free from contamination by granular constituents. The method has been widely used and has contributed tremendously to our understanding of membrane structure and function. However there appear to be insufficient differences in size or density of human platelet plasma and intracellular membranes to allow a *clear* separation of the two by conventional density gradients, although (and exceptionally) such a separation has been reported from pig platelet homogenates (9,10). Fractions rich in plasma membranes have been reported to be obtained using sucrose step gradients particularly after lysis of platelets by glycerol loading followed by osmotic lysis (11). Additionally, considerable success in separating plasma and intracellular membranes from mixed membranes of human platelets has been reported with the use of Percoll gradients spun at alkaline pH (12–15). In this procedure a population of mixed membranes is first separated from granule constituents with Percoll gradients run at neutral pH, followed by a further separation of the mixed membranes by centrifugation at alkaline pH (13). For unknown reasons, the intracellular membranes in Percoll exhibit higher densities at alkaline pH allowing their separation from plasma membranes. The properties of the membrane fractions obtained using this procedure with respect to polypeptide profiles, lipid composition, distribution of marker enzymes, and Ca^{2+} sequestration properties compared favourably with those obtained using free flow electrophoresis (see later). It is surprising therefore that this membrane preparation has not seen widespread usage.

In the quest to definitively localize important proteins a number of authors have devised ingenious methods of obtaining purified fractions of plasma membranes free from contamination by intracellular organelles. Kinoshita *et al.* (16) reported a plasma membrane fraction prepared by binding platelets to polylysine beads, followed by sonication to release intracellular constituents, and then recovery of plasma membranes from the polylysine beads. An 'affinity' column-type approach using wheat germ agglutinin–Sepharose 4B (WGA–S4B) was used to prepare plasma membranes of high purity from a 40 000 *g* membrane pellet (17). Plasma membranes bind to the WGA–S4B column through an interaction of glycoproteins rich in *N*-acetylglucosamine after which they are eluted with addition of *N*-acetylglucosamine. This procedure however does not allow for recovery of intracellular membranes. It is likely that in the future we will see further developments of affinity-type approaches using a particular property of a protein present in abundance in plasma and intracellular membranes. GPIIb, GPIIIa, and GPIb are good candidates for this approach in the purification of plasma membranes because of their concentrations. The Ca^{2+}ATPases belonging to the sarco–endoplasmic reticulum Ca^{2+}ATPase (SERCA) family are perhaps the best candidate proteins for the preparation of intracellular membranes using this approach.

Protocol 1. Preparation of human platelet membranes using high voltage free flow electrophoresis

Equipment and reagents

- High voltage free flow electrophoresis apparatus (Dr Weber GmbH)
- Ultracentrifuge with a swing-out rotor (e.g. Beckman XL-90)
- Refrigerated bench centrifuge
- Six packs of fresh human blood buffy coats or three units of blood
- Sonicator (Ultrasonics Ltd.)
- Gradient maker suitable for 20–30 ml gradients (e.g. Bio-Rad Model 385)
- Electrophoresis chamber buffer: 10 mM triethanolamine (TEA), 0.4 M sorbitol—dissolve in 4 litres of water, take to pH 6.8 via acetic acid, and then back to 7.2 via 2 M NaOH (this slightly increases the ionic strength of the solution)
- Electrode buffer: 100 mM TEA in 2 litres H_2O—adjust to pH 7.2 via acetic acid
- Electrophoresis chamber coated with 3% bovine serum albumin (BSA)
- Sorbitol gradients: prepare 200 ml solutions of 1 M sorbitol, 10 mM Hepes pH 7.2, and 3.5 M sorbitol, 10 mM Hepes pH 7.2
- Hepes washing buffer pH 7.2: prepare 400 ml solution containing 152 mM NaCl, 4.17 mM KCl, 10 mM Hepes, 3 mM EDTA pH 7.2—take an aliquot (50 ml) and adjust the pH to 6.2 for neuraminidase treatment
- Hepes enriched buffer pH 7.5: 50 ml 500 mM Hepes, 152 mM NaCl, 3 mM EDTA
- Sonication buffer pH 7.2: 0.34 M sorbitol, 10 mM Hepes pH 7.2. Prepare 200 ml and cool on ice. To 50 ml add the following proteolytic inhibitors: 1 mM dithiothreitol (DTT), 0.3 U/ml aprotinin, 200 µM phenyl methyl sulfonyl fluoride (PMSF), 5 µg/ml pepstatin A, 1 µM E64, and 1 mg/ml soybean trypsin inhibitor.
- 0.3 M citric acid
- Neuraminidase type X (Sigma)

Method

1. Check group of blood. Groups must not be mixed.

2. Transfer to suitable polycarbonate or polypropylene centrifuge tubes (50 or 100 ml volume).

3. Spin at 200 *g* for 20 min at 25°C to separate platelet-rich plasma (PRP) from the red cell fraction.

4. Take off PRP with plastic syringe into plastic beaker, taking care not to disturb the buffy layer containing white cells.

5. Respin PRP again at 200 *g* for 5 min to remove more red cells.

6. Remove PRP as previously and if overnight storage is to be made add 1/10 vol. Hepes enriched buffer pH 7.5. (Cover with Nescofilm, with holes to allow gaseous exchange, and stand at room temperature overnight) *or better*, carry on to next step.

7. Adjust pH of PRP to pH 6.4 with citric acid (0.3 M).

8. Spin at 1200 *g* for 20 min at 25°C.

9. Pour off top layer (plasma) from pellet (platelets) in each tube. Resuspend platelets in Hepes washing buffer pH 6.2, so that total volume including platelets is approx. 20 ml (i.e. all platelets from six packs of blood).

10. Equilibrate at 37°C for 5 min. Add neuraminidase, reconstituted in Hepes washing buffer pH 6.2, dropwise whilst mixing. Incubate for 20 min at 37°C, swirling occasionally. Final concentration of neuraminidase is 0.05 U/ml.

11. At the end of the incubation dilute fourfold using Hepes washing buffer pH 7.2. This will stop the reaction of the neuraminidase and restore platelets to a neutral pH. Split into two 50 ml tubes and spin for 15 min at 1200 *g* at room temperature.

12. Pour off supernatant and resuspend platelets in Hepes washing buffer pH 7.2. Fill tubes. Respin under same conditions.

13. Resuspend platelets in ice-cold sonication buffer containing proteolytic inhibitors (see reagents) at 4 ml buffer/g wet wt of cells. Leave to equilibrate on ice for 15 min, keep in ice throughout the remaining procedure, and keep all centrifugations at 4°C.

14. Sonicate at position 7 (maximum scale, 10) with tuning at maximum. Sonicate the platelet suspension for 15 sec. Centrifuge for 10 min at 1200 *g* (4°C) to separate homogenate from unbroken cells. Remove supernatant (homogenate) and store in another tube. Resuspend remaining cells in 15 ml of cold sonication buffer and resonicate. Respin and remove homogenate. Continue until all cells are lysed reducing the volume of sonication buffer used for resuspension appropriately (requires three to six sonications).

Protocol 1. *Continued*

15. When homogenates are all pooled, spin for a further 10 min at 1500 g 4°C to deposit the few remaining cells and aggregates.

16. Prepare linear (1–3.5 M) sorbitol density gradients using a gradient maker in ultracentrifuge tubes suitable for swing-out rotors. For the Beckman XL-90 this corresponds to six 30 ml tubes. For each 30 ml tube prepare 20 ml sorbitol gradients.

17. Carefully layer homogenates on to gradients, weigh tubes to balance, and carefully load in the swing-out rotor.

18. Centrifuge at 42 000 g for 90 min at 4°C.

19. Remove tubes from rotor and locate membrane and granule layers (this is facilitated by a black background). The membranes will locate as a diffuse layer extending from within the top soluble fraction to approximating 1.7 M in the gradient fraction. Platelet granules will locate as a discrete band at greater than 2.0 M sorbitol with the remaining unbroken cells and aggregates sedimenting at the bottom (3.5 M). Discard the top of the cytosol that is clear. Take rest of cytosol containing membranes and all of the membrane layer into another tube. Take granule layer if required into another tube.

20. Fill tubes with sonication buffer, balance, and spin at 100 000 g for 60 min at 4°C.

21. After centrifugation pour off supernatant, resuspend mixed membranes in approx. 10 ml chamber buffer until the suspension is near homogeneous.

22. Set-up the free flow apparatus (see below) to run at 750–1100 V, 100–150 mA, at 6.5°C. The flow rate of the chamber buffer or suction should be approx. 2–3 ml/h per individual fraction (about 180 ml/h total) at setting 80–100. Dosage for the mixed membranes should also be the same ($\approx$ 100). The setting should be stable for at least 6 h.

23. Collect membrane fractions using the fraction collector, determine OD 280 nm to establish protein peaks using chamber buffer as blank. Pool the tops of the peaks avoiding any cross-contamination and spin at 100 000 g for 60 min to concentrate the membranes. Resuspend in small volumes (0.5–2.0 ml) of chamber buffer or as desired.[a]

---

[a] If ATP-dependent [$^{45}Ca^{2+}$] uptake is to be studied in the purified membranes then it is necessary to harvest the purified intracellular membranes on a 3.5 M sorbitol cushion (3–5 ml depending on tube size). In this case, carefully layer the pooled fractions on top of the 3.5 M sorbitol cushion, spin at 100 000 g for 60 min at 4°C, and recover the membranes from the top of the cushion using a long fine pipette avoiding as much dilution as possible.

2.1 Preparation of free flow electrophoresis (FFE) apparatus

The author currently uses a VAP 5 apparatus manufactured by Benden Hobein (Germany). This version is no longer manufactured but an updated version (Octopus) is available from Dr Weber GmbH (Germany). The reader is advised to follow the apparatus manual closely as the instrument preparation is complex. The apparatus consists of an electrophoresis chamber measuring 500 cm high and 10 cm wide with platinum electrodes along the vertical length. The top of the chamber is connected to a reservoir for chamber buffer and the bottom to 90 collecting tubes which pass over a suction pump with which the flow rate of the chamber buffer can be controlled. When in operation, the mixed membranes are injected through an inlet port near the top at the same rate as the chamber buffer and the membranes migrate according to their relative electrophoretic mobilities. Most biological membranes exhibit a net negative charge and thus migration in an electrophoretic field occurs to the positive electrode. The net migration depends upon the field strength applied, the electronegative charge of the biological membranes, and the transit time in the chamber (controlled by the flow rate of the buffer).

Before use the glass chamber should be cleaned with a mild detergent, thoroughly rinsed, and coated with 3% BSA for 1 h. Chamber buffer is then introduced and the flow rate set at ≈ 2 ml/h/fraction (equating to approx. 180 ml/h). The cooling is then switched on and when the temperature approaches 6.5 °C, the voltage is gradually increased to between 750 and 1000 V. The apparatus is sufficiently temperature and voltage stable and will run for many hours (routinely used in author's laboratory for up to 6 h). The mixed membranes are applied to the chamber at the same rate as the chamber buffer flow and protein peaks determined by measuring their absorbance at 280 nm. *Figure 1* shows a typical platelet mixed membrane preparation separated into intracellular and plasma membranes using this procedure. Two discrete protein peaks are resolved of which the smaller, most electronegative peak has been extensively characterized to be intracellular membranes with the larger least electronegative peak as plasma membranes (see characteristics later). The tops of the peaks are pooled and centrifuged at 100 000 g for 60 min to pellet the membrane.

2.2 Modifications to the procedure

If a free flow electrophoresis apparatus is not available then the mixed membrane fraction obtained from the sorbitol density gradient represents an excellent preparation that is essentially free from granular constituents. If this is to be the end-point of the preparation then the steps involving neuraminidase treatment should be left out as they become redundant.

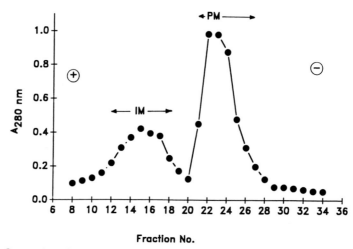

Figure 1. Separation of platelet intracellular and plasma membranes by free flow electrophoresis. A typical protein profile (measuring absorbance at 280 nm) of free flow electrophoresis fractions is shown. Fractions at the tops of the peaks are pooled and centrifuged at 100 000 *g* to concentrate. IM, intracellular membranes; PM, plasma membranes; + and – indicate the polarity of the chamber.

3. Characterization of purified platelet membrane fractions

Most membrane fractionation regimes employ extensive use of marker enzymes with which the purification is followed and the end-points assessed. However the value of many commonly used marker enzymes (such as 5′ nucleotidase and alkaline phosphatase) with platelet membranes is limited because of their low activities and in some cases association with both membrane systems (3). An exception is the endoplasmic reticulum marker enzyme NADH cytochrome *c* reductase, which is found almost exclusively in intracellular membranes prepared by free flow electrophoresis. An experimental protocol for its measurement is provided in *Protocol 2*. However since their first description, these membrane fractions have been extensively characterized and found to have a well defined protein and lipid composition (see ref. 5). In many cases this information has been used to redefine the criteria used to assess plasma and intracellular membrane purity. Examination of one-dimensional sodium dodecyl sulfate–polyacrylamide gel electrophoresis (SDS–PAGE) reveals very distinctive polypeptide profiles with few components found in both membrane systems (*Figure 2*). Particularly striking is that the plasma membrane contains all of the complement of actin, myosin, and actin binding protein present in the parent mixed membranes. Thus their near total depletion in intracellular membrane fractions represents an easily measurable index of the purity of this membrane system. As stated in the

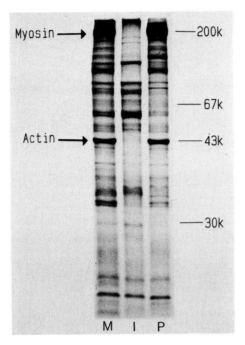

Figure 2. Protein profile of IM and PM fractions prepared using free flow electrophoresis. Coomassie brilliant blue staining pattern of platelet membrane polypeptides separated by 10% (acrylamide) SDS–PAGE. M, mixed membranes; P, plasma membranes; I, intracellular membranes. The molecular weight markers in kDa (k) are shown on the *right*. The positions of myosin and actin present almost exclusively in plasma membranes are indicated.

Introduction, the plasma membranes are rich in surface glycoproteins that mediate the interactions of the cell with other platelets and extracellular matrix constituents. Thus detection of these glycoproteins (especially GPIb, GPIIb, or GPIIIa, which are absent in intracellular membranes) by chemical staining (e.g. using periodic acid/Schiff's reagent) (18) or immunostaining (using antibodies to the glycoproteins) represents an important method of characterizing plasma membranes. *Figure 3* show the distribution of GPIb with membrane fractions prepared by free flow electrophoresis using standard methods of SDS–PAGE followed by Western blotting using an antibody to GPIb. Descriptions of the procedures used for SDS–PAGE and Western blotting are given in Chapter 2 and in Chapter 7. The enrichment of GPIb in the plasma membrane and near total absence in intracellular membranes exemplifies its use as a plasma membrane marker.

Characterization of key enzymes and receptors involved in signal transduction mechanisms have also demonstrated the distinctive properties exhibited by plasma and intracellular membranes. The intracellular membranes have been found to be rich in enzymes that release and metabolize arachidonic

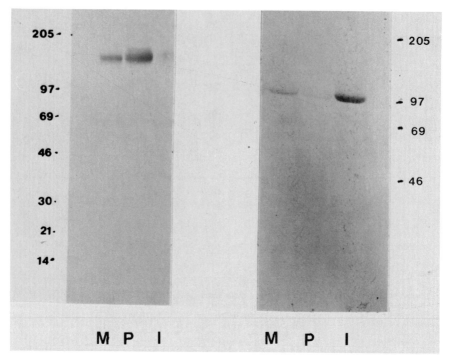

Figure 3. Distribution of GPIb and Ca^{2+}ATPase in platelet membranes. Membranes are separated by SDS–PAGE (5–15% acrylamide gradient) followed by transfer to nitrocellulose and Western blotting with an antibody to GPIb (A) and the antibody PLIM 430 to Ca^{2+}ATPase (B). Full details of the conditions used are given in ref. 36 for GPIb and refs 29 and 43 for PLIM 430.

acid. These include; phospholipase A$_2$, diacylglycerol lipase, cyclo-oxygenase, thromboxane synthase, fatty acyl CoA transferase (12–22), that are either absent or poorly expressed in plasma membranes. Additionally the intracellular membranes are rich in Ca^{2+}ATPases that sequester Ca^{2+} into rapidly releasable Ca^{2+} stores, and are the predominant location for the inositol 1,4,5-trisphosphate (IP$_3$) receptor involved in Ca^{2+} release (4,23–25). The receptor for inositol 1,3,4,5-tetrakisphosphate (IP$_4$), whose function is still to be characterized, has been found to be predominantly located with the plasma membrane (26). Recent studies have now identified the Ca^{2+}ATPases by biochemical and immunological methods as belonging to the SERCA 2b and SERCA 3 isoforms (27–29). There is also evidence that these two isoforms serve distinct rather than a common Ca^{2+} pool (30). Both of these two SERCA isoforms are inhibited by thapsigargin (Tg) and 2,5 di-*t*-butyl-1,4-benzohydroquinone (tuBUBHQ) (31) although there is evidence for relative selectivity of Tg towards the SERCA 2b and of tuBuBHQ towards the SERCA 3 isoforms (32). However total inhibition of both types by maximal concentrations of Tg (29) can be used as a good marker to identify a SERCA class $Ca^{2+}ATPase$. The presence of a plasma membrane $Ca^{2+}ATPase$ (PMCA) had been controversial for many years (see ref. 30) and only recently has its identification by both biochemical and immunological methods been made (29,33). In our studies plasma membranes prepared by free flow electrophoresis have been shown to contain a $Ca^{2+}ATPase$ activity that is insensitive to Tg and can be immunologically identified using an antibody raised to the red cell $Ca^{2+}ATPase$ (29). Additionally a Na^+/Ca^{2+} exchange activity which is readily demonstrable in both intact platelets (34) and plasma membrane preparations (15,35), is important in Ca^{2+} removal across the plasma membrane. However the relative contributions of these activities to Ca^{2+} extrusion remain to be fully evaluated along with their biochemical characterization and possible effects upon cell activation. *Protocols 3, 4*, and *5* describe methods used to determine Ca^{2+} sequestration, $Ca^{2+}ATPase$, and Na^+/Ca^{2+} exchange activities. We have recently characterized the particulate localization of cAMP- and cGMP-dependent protein kinases and their substrates (36). Both cyclic nucleotide kinases have been found to be located almost exclusively with the plasma membranes using both *in vitro* activation by cyclic nucleotide analogues and Western blotting with antibodies to the respective proteins. These studies have additionally revealed a number of newly detected substrates for cAMP-dependent protein kinase on intracellular membranes that await identification (36).

Protocol 2. Estimation of NADH cytochrome *c* reductase—intracellular membrane marker

The method is taken from the procedures described by Tolbert (37) and Mackler (38).

Equipment and reagents
- Spectrophotometer to measure OD at 550 nm, linked to a chart recorder
- 0.2 M KH_2PO_4 pH 7.0
- 5 mg/ml cytochrome *c* (oxidized) in H_2O
- 19 mM KCN
- 2 mg/ml antimycin A in ethanol
- 30 mg/ml NADH in H_2O

Method

1. Allow spectrophotometer to equilibrate, set slit width at 0.4 cm, temperature of the cuvette holder to 30°C.

2. Pipette 0.4 ml of 0.2 M KCN, 0.2 ml cytochrome *c*, 20 µl 10 mM KCN, 10 µl antimycin A. Allow to equilibrate for 5 min.

3. Add 20 µl NADH, and either 0.3 ml fractions from free flow electrophoresis collections, or 30–50 µg protein from concentrated membrane fractions (total volume in reaction is 10 ml). Measure OD at 550 nm for 5 min.

Protocol 2. *Continued*

4. Repeat in triplicate for each concentrated membrane fraction to be tested.

5. Results can be expressed as rate of change of OD 550 nm/min/mg protein or nmoles/min/mg protein using an extinction coefficient of 21.1/mol/cm for cytochrome *c* at 550 nm.

3.1 Contamination of membranes by granule constituents

An important issue that should be considered is where the boundary membranes of granules (α, dense, or lysosomes) migrate if, during the platelet cell disruption procedure (sonication, freeze–thawing, N_2 cavitation, etc.), a small level of granule lysis occurs. Until relatively recently the protein constituents of the granule boundary membranes were largely obscure. However a number of important glycoproteins have been identified which in the resting platelet are integral boundary membrane proteins and are varyingly expressed on the platelet surface as the granules fuse with the plasma membrane after stimulation by platelets agonists. These include; for α granules, GMP140 (or P-selectin, CD62) which is important in mediating platelet–neutrophil interactions (39); granulophysin (CD63) that is thought to be present on the boundary membranes of lysosomes (40), and dense granules (41), and is expressed on the surface after stimulation; and LAMP-1 and LAMP-2 that are lysosomal granule membrane proteins and appear to be expressed after stimulation by strong agonists such as thrombin (42). It will be important to determine the presence of these proteins in membrane (plasma and intracellular) preparations as they will provide an estimate of whether cell activation has occurred or if granule integrity has been lost.

4. Regulation of Ca^{2+} in platelet plasma and intracellular membranes

4.1 ATP-dependent Ca^{2+} sequestration in platelet membranes

ATP-dependent Ca^{2+} sequestration is rich in platelet mixed and intracellular membranes and poor in plasma membranes. In addition to estimation of the SERCA-type Ca^{2+}ATPase activity (see *Protocol 4*) it provides an excellent determination of intracellular membrane functional activity. To demonstrate Ca^{2+} sequestration in purified intracellular membranes it is necessary for the intracellular membranes to be harvested on a 3.5 M sorbitol cushion for adequate resealing of vesicles. This is not necessary for the activity to be demonstrated in mixed membranes taken from the sorbitol density gradient.

Protocol 3. ATP-dependent Ca^{2+} sequestration in platelet membranes

Equipment and reagents

All reagents should be in analytical grade water.

- Liquid scintillation counter (β)
- Membrane filtration apparatus (Millipore)
- Incubation buffer: 120 mM KCl, 5 mM MgCl$_2$, 20 mM Hepes pH 7.2
- 100 mM K$^+$ATP pH 7.2 (store on ice)
- 5 mM CaCl$_2$
- 5 mM EGTA
- 0.45 μm filters (Millipore)

- Platelet membranes (MM or IM, 0.5–4 mg/ml)
- [$^{45}Ca^{2+}$]Cl$_2$ 5–50 mCi/mg Ca^{2+} (Amersham International, ICN etc.)
- A23187 (10 mM in DMSO)
- Stop buffer: 120 mM KCl, 5 mM MgCl$_2$, 20 mM Hepes, 5 mM EGTA pH 7.2

Method

1. To incubation tubes add 0.8 ml incubation buffer containing approx. 2 μCi [$^{45}Ca^{2+}$] per incubation.

2. Add in final concentrations 5 mM ATP, 40 μM Ca^{2+}, and 50 μM EGTA, mix well.

3. Add platelet membranes (50–150 μg protein) to start the reaction, incubate for 15 min at room temperature to allow equilibrium to be attained.

4. Stop reaction by taking 0.9 ml reaction mixture and applying to a 0.45 μm filter under vacuum in a filtration apparatus. Wash the filter with 2 × 10 ml application of stop buffer.

5. When semi-dry take the 0.45 μm filter, place in scintillation vials, add 4 ml scintillation liquid, allow to dissolve, and count the radioactivity using a β-scintillation counter.

6. Run appropriate controls, e.g. samples without platelet membranes, without ATP, construct a time course, and also incubations with a cation ionophore such as A23187 or ionomycin (1 μM final concentration), to determine non-specific binding of [$^{45}Ca^{2+}$] that is not sequestered. The rapidly releasable [$^{45}Ca^{2+}$] uptake is determined after subtraction of the value in the presence of A23187, and should be approx. 85–95% of the total if the membrane vesicles have completely sealed. Results can be expressed simply as d.p.m. [^{45}Ca] uptake or as nmol [$^{45}Ca^{2+}$]/mg protein (4,24,30). *Figure 4* represents a typical Ca^{2+} uptake and release profile measured with intracellular membranes.

4.1.1 Modifications to the procedure

A number of investigators frequently use a precipitating anion such as phosphate or oxalate (at 1–10 mM) to increase uptake of [$^{45}Ca^{2+}$] into the

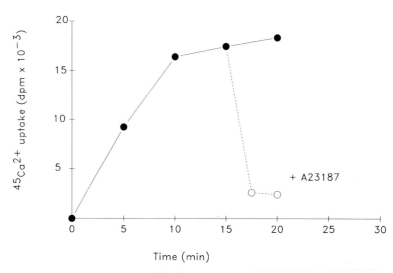

ATP dependent $^{45}Ca^{2+}$ uptake into platelet IM vesicles

Figure 4. ATP-dependent uptake of [$^{45}Ca^{2+}$] in platelet intracellular membranes. The figure shows a typical time course of [$^{45}Ca^{2+}$] uptake into IM using 33 µg protein, representing at equilibrium an uptake of 7.4 nmol/mg protein. The addition of 10 µM A23187 (or ionomycin) at equilibrium causes approx. 85% release of sequestered [$^{45}Ca^{2+}$] within 2 min.

organelles. This is effective but has the disadvantage that both uptake and release kinetics (by any Ca^{2+} mobilizing agent) are decreased and if the amount of the precipitating anion used is high (10 mM), equilibrium for uptake is not achieved (24). We recommended that if required they only be used at 1 mM. A variety of agents have been described that affect the Ca^{2+} uptake process including agents that inhibit Ca^{2+}ATPases (e.g. Tg, tuBuBHQ) (31), a monoclonal antibody to Ca^{2+}ATPase that inhibits Ca^{2+} uptake (43,44), and agents that cause release of sequestered Ca^{2+} via an action on Ca^{2+} channels (e.g. IP$_3$ (4,44), neomycin (30), etc.). Most of these agents can be added either at the start of the reaction (to test the effect on uptake) or at equilibrium (usually at 15 min) to determine release kinetics.

Protocol 4. Determination of Ca^{2+}ATPase activities of purified platelet membranes

Equipment and reagents

- Bench centrifuge
- Liquid scintillation counter (β)
- Incubation buffer (2 ×): 240 mM KCl, 10 mM MgSO$_4$, 40 mM Hepes pH 7.2
- 50 mM CaCl$_2$
- 500 mM EGTA
- [γ-^{32}P]ATP > 3000 Ci/mmol (e.g. Amersham or ICN)

104

- 100 mM ATP pH 7.2
- Platelet membranes (1–4 mg/ml)
- Thapsigargin (Tg) 10 mM (in DMSO)

- Stop solution: activated charcoal (Norit A, Sigma) 25 mg/ml in 0.1 M H_3PO_4

Method

1. Carry out the reactions in 12 ml polypropylene tubes with caps (or equivalent tubes that can be centrifuged at 1500 g for 15 min).

2. Reaction mixture total should be 500 µl; add 250 µl incubation buffer and ATP and $CaCl_2$ to give 1 mM and 50 µM final concentrations respectively. Add [γ-^{32}P]ATP to approx. 2 µCi per incubation. This will not affect significantly the final concentration of ATP.

3. Incubate mixture at 37 °C for 5 min to equilibrate.

4. Add platelet membranes (50–150 µg protein) to start the reaction. Incubate for 15 min at 37 °C.

5. Stop reaction by adding 2.5 ml cold activated charcoal that is kept under a stirrer (or the reagant bottle should be shaken to maintain a uniform suspension).

6. Mix well, allow to stand for 30 min at 4 °C, centrifuge 1500 g for 15 min, and take 1 ml of the supernatant for liquid scintillation counting to estimate released [^{32}P]P$_i$.

7. Count also the total [γ-^{32}P]ATP added to the reaction mixture. Express results as nmoles P$_i$ released/min/mg protein. The above provides an estimation of the total Ca^{2+} plus Mg^{2+}ATPase activity present in platelet membranes. The Mg^{2+}ATPase activity can be estimated using 1 mM EGTA (final concentration) in the reaction mixture and subtracted from the total to give Ca^{2+}ATPase activity. Reaction mixtures containing Ca^{2+} should also be carried out with the inclusion of 3 µM Tg which inhibits all SERCA-type Ca^{2+}ATPases that are associated with intracellular membranes. The Ca^{2+}ATPase activity in the presence of 3 µM Tg provides the contribution of the Ca^{2+}ATPase activity that is of the PMCA-type (29), and thus detects the presence of plasma membranes.

4.2 Measurement of Ca^{2+} flux in plasma membranes using the Na^+/Ca^{2+} exchanger

This protocol is based on the method described by Rengasamy and Feinberg (15,35) and is rich in mixed and plasma membranes but poorly expressed in intracellular membranes. This method allows the effects of agents that influence Ca^{2+} influx across plasma membranes without interference of activities present in intracellular organelles. The platelet Na^+/Ca^{2+} exchange activity has been shown to be K^+-dependent (45).

Protocol 5. [^{45}Ca^{2+}] uptake into plasma membranes using the Na$^+$/Ca^{2+} exchange activity

Equipment and reagents

All reagants should use analytical grade water.

- Membrane filtration apparatus
- Liquid scintillation counter (β)
- 0.45 μm filters
- Exchange buffer: 150 mM KCl, 10 mM Mopes–Tris pH 7.4, to contain 2 μCi [^{45}Ca^{2+}] per 300 μl buffer

- Membrane buffer: 150 mM NaCl, 10 mM Tris–HCl pH 7.4
- Stop buffer: 5 mM Mopes–Tris pH 7.4, 150 mM KCl, 5 mM LaCl$_3$
- 10 mM ionomycin (in DMSO)

Method

1. Incubate plasma membranes in membrane buffer (approx. 40 μg protein, 4 μl) at 37°C for 30 min. This allows sodium to equilibrate inside the membrane vesicle.

2. Dilute membranes 60-fold into exchange buffer (300 μl) containing high K$^+$ and [^{45}Ca^{2+}] and incubate for 10 min. The dilution causes a Na$^+$ gradient to occur across the membranes, which then exchanges for [^{45}Ca^{2+}] rapidly as equilibrium is reached. [^{45}Ca^{2+}] uptake reaches a maximum within 5 min and equilibrium is maintained up to 30 min (*Figure 5*). Add any agent that influences Ca^{2+} flux (e.g. A23187, iono-mycin) at 10 min and incubate for a further 5 min.

3. Stop reactions by adding 200 μl ice-cold stop buffer.

4. Rapidly place the mixture on 0.45 μm filters under vacuum, wash the filter with 2 × 10 ml cold stop buffer, and after semi-drying the filter count the radioactivity by liquid scintillation spectrometry. Express results as nmol [^{45}Ca^{2+}] retained/mg protein; typical values are approx. 2 nmol/mg protein.

[^{45}Ca^{2+}] uptake via a Na$^+$/Ca^{2+} exchange mechanism is not ATP-dependent, and the studies can be carried out using 100 μM vanadate which is a known inhibitor of Ca^{2+}ATPases. If dilution of the membranes is made into a high Na$^+$ medium (150 mM) exchange buffer, the [^{45}Ca^{2+}] uptake is low and little different from non-specific binding. The reader is referred to a recent review for a further discussion on the mechanisms of Ca^{2+} homeostasis in human platelets (30).

Na$^+$/Ca^{2+} exchange in platelet PM vesicles

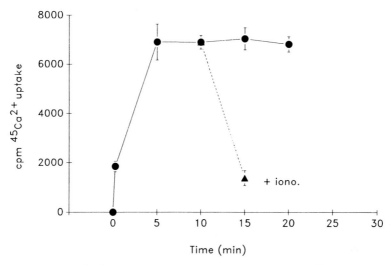

Figure 5. Uptake of [^{45}Ca^{2+}] into plasma membranes using the Na$^+$/Ca^{2+} exchange activity. Concentrated plasma membrane vesicles are incubated with high Na$^+$, after which they are diluted 60-fold into high K$^+$ medium containing [^{45}Ca^{2+}]. Exchange reaches equilibrium rapidly and the addition of 10 μM ionomycin at 10 min releases approx. 80% vesicle loaded [^{45}Ca^{2+}].

Acknowledgements

The work of the author is supported by grants from the Thrombosis Research Trust and the British Heart Foundation. Drs Y. Patel, S. S. El-Daher, and S. Bokkala are acknowledged for many fruitful discussions.

References

1. White, J. G. (1994). In *Haemostasis and thrombosis* (ed. A. L. Bloom, C. D. Forbes, D. P. Thomas, and E. G. D. Tuddenham), pp. 49–87. Churchill Livingstone, Edinburgh.
2. Nurden, A. T. (1994). In *Haemostasis and thrombosis* (ed. A. L. Bloom, C. D. Forbes, D. P. Thomas, and E. G. D. Tuddenham), pp. 115–65. Churchill Livingstone, Edinburgh.
3. Menashi, S., Weintroub, H., and Crawford, N. (1981). *J. Biol. Chem.*, **256**, 4095.
4. Authi, K. S. and Crawford, N. (1985). *Biochem. J.*, **230**, 247.
5. Crawford, N., Hack, N., and Authi, K. S. (1992). In *Methods in enzymology* (ed. J. J. Hawiger), Vol. 245, pp. 5–20. Academic Press Inc., Orlando, Florida, USA.
6. Crawford, N. (1986). In *Platelet membrane glycoproteins* (ed. J. N. George, A. T. Nurden, and D. R. Phillips), pp. 13–49. Plenum Press, New York and London.

7. Sixma, J. J. and Lips, J. P. N. (1978). *Thromb. Haemost.*, **39,** 328.
8. Marcus, A. J., Zucker-Franklin, D., Safier, L.-B., and Ullman, M. L. (1966). *J. Clin. Invest.*, **45,** 14.
9. Taylor, D. G. and Crawford, N. (1974). *FEBS Lett.*, **41,** 317.
10. Taylor, D. G. and Crawford, N. (1974). In *Methodological developments in biochemistry*, Vol. 4 (ed. E. Reid), pp. 319–26. Longmans Press Ltd., Essex, UK.
11. Harmon, J. T., Greco, N. J., and Jamieson, G. A. (1992). In *Methods in enzymology* (ed. J. J. Hawiger), Vol. 215, pp. 32–6. Academic Press Inc., Orlando, Florida, USA.
12. Mauco, G., Fauvel, J., Chap, H., and Douste-Blazy, L. (1984). *Biochim. Biophys. Acta*, **796,** 169.
13. Fauvel, J., Chap, H., Rogues, V., Levy-Toledano, S., and Douste-Blazy, L. (1986). *Biochim. Biophys. Acta*, **856,** 155.
14 Mauco, G., Dajeans, P., Chap, H., and Douste-Blazy, L. (1987). *Biochem. J.*, **244,** 757.
15. Rengasamy, A., Soura, S., and Feinberg, H. (1987). *Thromb. Haemost.*, **57,** 337.
16. Kinoshita, T., Nachman, R.-L., and Minick, R. (1979). *J. Cell Biol.*, **82,** 688.
17. Steiner, B. and Lusher, L. F. (1985). *Biochim. Biophys. Acta*, **818,** 299.
18. Hack, N. and Crawford, N. (1984). *Biochem. J.*, **222,** 235.
19. Lagarde, M., Menashi, S., and Crawford, N. (1981). *FEBS Lett.*, **124,** 23.
20. Authi, K. S., Lagarde, M., and Crawford, N. (1985). *FEBS Lett.*, **180,** 95.
21. Carey, F., Menashi, S., and Crawford, N. (1982). *Biochem. J.*, **204,** 847.
22. McKean, M. L., Silver, M. J., Authi, K. S., and Crawford, N. (1986). *FEBS Lett.*, **195,** 38.
23. Hack, N., Croset, M., and Crawford, N. (1986). *Biochem. J.*, **233,** 661.
24. Menashi, S., Authi, K. S., Carey, F., and Crawford, N. (1984). *Biochem. J.*, **222,** 413.
25. Authi, K. S. (1992). *FEBS Lett.*, **298,** 173.
26. Cullen, P. J., Patel, Y., Kakkar, V. V., Irvine, R. F., and Authi, K. S. (1994). *Biochem. J.*, **298,** 739.
27. Enouf, J., Bredoux, R., Papp, B., Djaffar, I., Lompre, A. M., Kieffer, N., *et al.* (1992). *Biochem. J.*, **286,** 135.
28. Wuytack, F., Papp, B., Verboomen, H., Raeymaekers, L., Dode, L., Bobe, R., *et al.* (1994). *J. Biol. Chem.*, **269,** 1410.
29. Bokkala, S., El-Daher, S. S., Kakkar, V. V., Wuytack, F., and Authi, K. S. (1995). *Biochem. J.*, **306,** 837.
30. Authi, K. S. (1993). In *Mechanisms of platelet activation and control* (ed. K. S. Authi, S. P. Watson, and V. V. Kakkar), in *Adv. Exp. Med. Biol.*, Vol. 344, 83–104.
31. Authi, K. S., Bokkala, S., Patel, Y., Kakkar, V. V., and Munkonge, F. (1993). *Biochem. J.*, **294,** 119.
32. Papp, B., Enyedi, A., Paszty, K., Kovacs, T., Sarkadi, B., Gardos, G., *et al.* (1992). *Biochem. J.*, **288,** 297.
33. Cheng, H. Y., Magocsi, M., Cooper, R. S., Penniston, J. T., and Borke, J. L. (1993). *Cell Physiol. Biochem.*, **4,** 31.
34. Brass, L. F. (1984). *J. Biol. Chem.*, **259,** 12571.
35. Rengasamy, A. and Feinberg, H. (1988). *Biochem. Biophys. Res. Commun.*, **150,** 1021.
36. El-Daher, S. S., Eigenthaler, M., Walter, U., Furuichi, T., Miyawaki, A., Mikoshiba, K., *et al.* (1996). *Biochem. J.*, submitted.

37. Tolbert, N. E. (1974). In *Methods in enzymology* (ed. S. Fleischer and L. Packer), Vol. 31, pp. 734–46. Academic Press Inc., Orlando, Florida, USA.
38. Mackler, B. (1961). *Biochim. Biophys. Acta*, **50,** 141.
39. McEver, R. P. (1991). *Thromb. Haemost.*, **66,** 80.
40. Nieuwenhuis, H. K., Van Dosterhout, J. G., Rozemuller, E., Van Iwaardes, F., and Sixma, J. J. (1987). *Blood*, **70,** 838.
41. Nishibori, M., Cham, B., McNicol, A., Shaleu, A., Jain, N., and Gerrard, J. M. (1993). *J. Clin. Invest.*, **91,** 1775.
42. Febbraio, M. and Silverstein, R. L. (1992). *Blood*, **80,** 1470.
43. Hack, N., Wilkinson, J. M., and Crawford, N. (1988). *Biochem. J.*, **250,** 355.
44. Hack, N., Authi, K. S., and Crawford, N. (1988). *Biosci. Rep.*, **8,** 379.
45. Kimura, M., Asiv, A., and Reeves, J. P. (1983). *J. Biol. Chem.*, **268,** 6874.

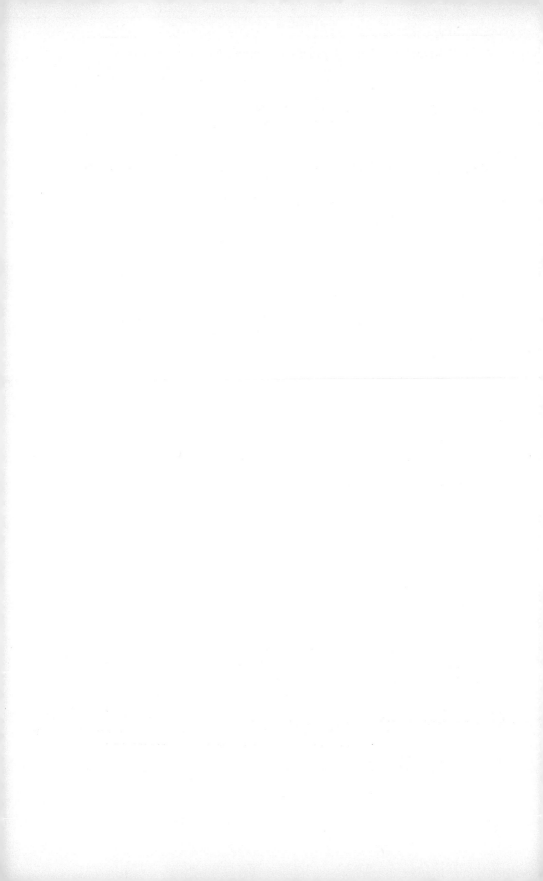

6

The use of flow cytometry to study platelet activation

ALAN D. MICHELSON and SANFORD J. SHATTIL

1. Introduction

Many common clinical conditions have been reported to be associated with platelet hyperreactivity and/or circulating activated platelets:

- coronary artery disease (angina pectoris, acute myocardial infarction)
- diabetes mellitus
- stroke
- exercise
- emotional stress
- cigarette smoking
- pregnancy and pre-eclampsia
- blood bank storage of platelets for transfusion
- cardiopulmonary bypass
- angioplasty
- deep vein thrombosis
- hyperlipoproteinaemia
- essential thrombocythemia
- adult respiratory distress syndrome

However, the role of platelet activation in clinical settings is controversial, in part because the methods used to detect platelet activation (e.g. platelet aggregation and radioimmunoassays of plasma β-thromboglobulin (βTG) and/or platelet factor 4 (PF4) have major methodologic problems (1–6)). Platelet aggregometry may show whether a particular clinical condition results in changes in platelet reactivity, but cannot determine whether the condition directly activates platelets. In contrast, radioimmunoassays of plasma βTG and PF4 concentrations may indirectly determine that a clinical condition activates platelets, but cannot measure changes in platelet reactivity associated with the condition. None of these assays can measure the extent of activation of individual platelets nor can they detect distinct subpopulations of platelets. Platelet aggregation studies are semi-quantitative and subject to standardization problems (1,4). As a result of the plasma separation procedures required, radioimmunoassays of plasma βTG and PF4 concentrations are particularly vulnerable to artefactual *in vitro* platelet activation (2,3). Clinical studies that utilize flow cytometric assays of washed platelets (7,8) are also susceptible to artefactual *in vitro* platelet activation as a result of the washing procedures.

We have described a whole blood flow cytometric assay that circumvents many of the problems associated with assays of βTG, PF4, and platelet aggregation. In this assay (5), platelets are directly analysed in their physiological milieu of whole blood (including red cells and white cells, both of which affect platelet activation) (9,10). The minimal manipulation of the samples limits artefactual *in vitro* activation and potential loss of platelet subpopulations (5,6,11). Both the activation state of circulating platelets and the reactivity of circulating platelets can be determined. The flow cytometric method permits the detection of a spectrum of specific activation-dependent modifications in the platelet membrane surface. A subpopulation of as few as 1% of partially activated platelets can be detected in whole blood by this method (5,12). Only minuscule volumes (~ 2 μl) of whole blood are required (5,11), making whole blood flow cytometry particularly advantageous for neonatal studies (13). The platelets of patients with profound thrombocytopenia can also be accurately analysed.

Addition to whole blood of thrombin, one of the most physiologically important platelet activators (14–16), results in a fibrin clot, thereby precluding the use of thrombin as an agonist in the whole blood assay. Furthermore, thrombin is a potent inducer of platelet to platelet aggregation, which precludes analysis by flow cytometry of activation-dependent changes in individual platelets. However, one of us (A. D. M.) has recently described a flow cytometric assay that enables platelet activation by thrombin to be directly measured in whole blood (11,12,17). In this method, the synthetic tetrapeptide glycyl-L-prolyl-L-arginyl-L-proline (GPRP) is used to inhibit both fibrin polymerization and platelet to platelet aggregation (11,12,17). GPRP corresponds in part to the amino terminal sequence of the α chain of fibrin and is an analogue of the polymerization sites involved in fibrin polymer formation (18). GPRP therefore competitively inhibits fibrin polymerization (18) (*Figure 1*). In addition, GPRP inhibits fibrinogen binding to its platelet receptor, thereby partially inhibiting platelet aggregation (19,20) (*Figure 1*). However, GPRP does not block platelet activation (11) (*Figure 1*). GPRP is stable, resistant to proteolytic agents (including thrombin), and does not suppress thrombin activity (18).

An alternative to the use of thrombin and GPRP in the whole blood flow

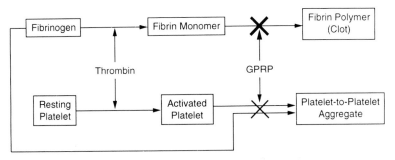

Figure 1. The synthetic peptide GPRP competitively inhibits fibrin polymerization and, via inhibition of fibrinogen binding to its receptor, partially inhibits platelet aggregation. Reproduced with permission from Michelson (17).

cytometric assay is the use of a thrombin receptor agonist peptide (TRAP)—a peptide fragment of the 'tethered ligand' receptor for thrombin (21). TRAP directly activates platelets, without resulting in a fibrin clot. The advantage of TRAP is that it can be used in the absence of GPRP. The disadvantage of TRAP is that it may not reflect all aspects of thrombin-induced platelet activation, because the 'tethered ligand' receptor may not be the only platelet receptor for thrombin (22).

The advantages of whole blood flow cytometry are:

(a) Platelet activation can be studied in the more physiological milieu of whole blood.

(b) Activation-dependent changes in multiple surface receptors can be detected.

(c) High degree of sensitivity for the detection of platelet subpopulations.

(d) Both the activation state of circulating platelets and the reactivity of circulating platelets can be determined.

(e) Minimal manipulation of samples prevents artefactual *in vitro* platelet activation and potential loss of platelet subpopulations.

(f) Only ~ 2 μl of blood is required for the assay.

(g) The platelets of patients with profound thrombocytopenia can be accurately analysed.

2. Monoclonal antibodies

Monoclonal antibodies can be used to measure the expression of any platelet surface antigen. However, there has been particular interest in the use of monoclonal antibodies that are 'activation-dependent', i.e. antibodies that bind only to activated platelets not to resting platelets (*Table 1*).

The two most widely studied activation-dependent antigens are P-selectin

Table 1. Activation-dependent monoclonal antibodies (i.e. antibodies that bind to activated but not resting platelets)

Activation-related surface change	Prototypic antibodies	Reference
Changes in GPIIb–IIIa		
Conformational change in GPIIb–IIIa resulting in exposure of the fibrinogen binding site	PAC1	25
Receptor-induced conformational change in ligand (fibrinogen)	2G5; 9F9	38,63
Ligand-induced conformational change in GPIIb–IIIa	PM 1.1; LIBS1; LIBS6	40,64,65
Exposure of granule membrane proteins		
P-selectin (from α granule)	S12; AC1.2	66,67
CD63 (from lysosomes)	CLB-gran/12	68
LAMP-1 (from lysosomes)	H5G11	69
Binding of secreted platelet proteins		
Thrombospondin	P8; TSP-1	70,71
Development of a procoagulant surface		
Factor Va binding	V237	43
Factor VIII binding	1B3	46

and the GPIIb–IIIa complex. P-selectin, also referred to as GMP-140, PADGEM protein, and CD62P, is a component of the α granule membrane of resting platelets that is only expressed on the platelet surface membrane after α granule secretion (23). Therefore a P-selectin-specific IgG monoclonal antibody such as S12 (developed by Dr Rodger P. McEver, University of Oklahoma, Oklahoma City, OK) only binds to degranulated platelets, not to resting platelets (*Figures 2* and *3B*). P-selectin mediates adhesion of activated platelets to neutrophils and monocytes. The GPIIb–IIIa complex is a receptor for fibrinogen, von Willebrand factor, fibronectin, and vitronectin that is critical for platelet aggregation (24). Whereas most monoclonal antibodies directed against the GPIIb–IIIa complex bind to resting platelets, PAC1 is directed against the fibrinogen binding site exposed by a conformational change in the GPIIb–IIIa complex of activated platelets (25). Thus, PAC1 only binds to activated platelets, not to resting platelets (*Figures 2* and *3B*). While native PAC1 is an IgM, a recombinant Fab fragment of PAC1 produced in a baculovirus expression system also binds to platelets in an activation-dependent manner (26).

In addition to monoclonal antibodies that bind only to activated, not resting, platelets (*Table 1*), some investigators have used monoclonal antibodies that bind to resting platelets but have increased binding to activated platelets, e.g. GPIV-specific monoclonal antibodies (*Figure 2*) (12).

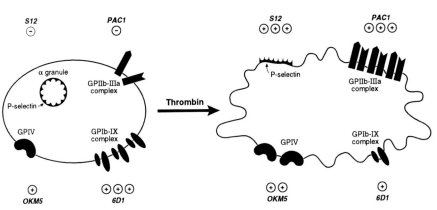

RESTING PLATELET **ACTIVATED PLATELET**

Figure 2. Effect of platelet activation on monoclonal antibody binding. The cartoon depicts the binding of monoclonal antibodies (in italics) to resting platelets and the relative change in the binding of these antibodies after thrombin activation. *S12* is directed at the α granule membrane protein P-selectin. P-selectin is not detectable on the surface of resting platelets. After thrombin activation, P-selectin is translocated to the platelet plasma membrane. Thus, *S12* only binds to the surface of activated platelets. *PAC1* is directed at the fibrinogen binding site on the glycoprotein (GP) IIb–IIIa complex. The fibrinogen binding site is not exposed on resting platelets. Thrombin stimulation results in a conformational change in the GPIIb–IIIa complex that exposes the fibrinogen binding site. Thus, *PAC1* only binds to the surface of activated platelets. *OKM5* is directed at an epitope on GPIV which may be a thrombospondin binding site. *OKM5* binds to resting platelets but binding is increased following thrombin stimulation. *6D1* is directed at the von Willebrand factor binding site on GPIb. In contrast to the other monoclonal antibodies, the binding of *6D1* is markedly reduced following thrombin stimulation. Reproduced with permission from Kestin *et al.* (12).

In contrast to the 'activation-dependent' monoclonal antibodies (*Table 1*) and the monoclonal antibodies that bind resting platelets but have increased binding to activated platelets, the binding of GPIb–IX-specific monoclonal antibodies to activated platelets is markedly *decreased* compared to resting platelets (*Figures 2* and *3A*) (11,27,28). The activation-induced decrease in the platelet surface expression of the GPIb–IX complex appears to be the result of a translocation of GPIb–IX complexes to the membranes of the open surface canalicular system (29). The GPIb–IX complex is a receptor for von Willebrand factor that is critical for platelet adhesion to damaged blood vessel walls (30). The activation-dependent decrease in the binding of monoclonal antibodies to the platelet GPIb–IX complex may be a very sensitive marker of platelet activation *in vivo*. For example, using a whole blood flow cytometric assay, we recently demonstrated that strenuous exercise in sedentary subjects, but not physically active subjects, resulted in both platelet activation and platelet hyperreactivity (12). However, these changes were more

115

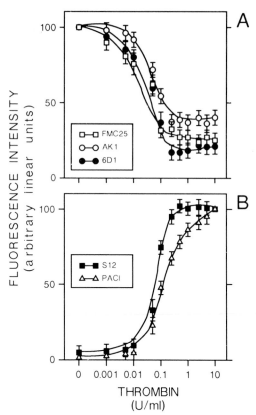

Figure 3. Effect of thrombin on the binding of monoclonal antibodies to the platelet sur-face, as determined by whole blood flow cytometry. (A) Monoclonal antibodies 6D1, FMC25, and AK1 are directed against GPIb, GPIX, and the GPIb–IX complex, respectively. For each antibody in panel A, the fluorescence intensity of resting platelets was assigned 100 units. (B) Monoclonal antibodies S12 and PAC1 are directed against P-selectin and the GPIIb–IIIa complex, respectively. For each antibody in panel B, the fluorescence intensity of maximally activated platelets was assigned 100 units. Data from panels A and B were obtained from the same three experiments (mean ± S.E.M.). Reproduced with permission from Michelson *et al.* (11).

readily detected with monoclonal antibodies directed against GPIb (6D1, developed by Dr Barry S. Coller, Mount Sinai Medical Center, New York, NY) and, to a lesser extent, GPIV (OKM5, Ortho Diagnostic Systems) rather than with monoclonal antibodies directed against the GPIIb–IIIa complex and P-selectin (12). This study (12) also illustrates the importance of analysing activation-dependent alterations by use of a panel of monoclonal antibodies directed against different platelet surface antigens.

Platelet-specific monoclonal antibodies are now available from a number of commercial sources. These antibodies can often be purchased conjugated to either biotin or fluorescein isothiocyanate (FITC). Alternately, antibodies can be FITC-conjugated by the method of Rinderknecht (31) or (easier and more rapidly) by a kit method (e.g. QuickTag FITC conjugation kit, Boehringer Mannheim). Antibodies can be biotinylated as described by Shattil *et al.* (5) or by following the biotin manufacturer's directions.

The saturating concentration of each antibody for platelet binding must be specifically determined by each laboratory. This concentration is typically between 0.5 and 40 µg/ml. In addition, when two monoclonal antibodies are used in the same assay (see below), it is necessary to determine that they do not interfere with each other for platelet binding.

3. Practical aspects of flow cytometric analysis of platelet activation state and platelet reactivity in whole blood

---

Protocol 1. Sample preparation

Equipment and reagents

- Sodium citrate Vacutainer (Becton Dickinson)
- Tyrode's buffer: 137 mM NaCl, 2.8 mM KCl, 1 mM MgCl$_2$, 12 mM NaHCO$_3$, 0.4 mM Na$_2$HPO$_4$, 0.35% bovine serum albumin, 10 mM Hepes, 5.5 mM glucose pH 7.4
- Polypropylene tubes (Costar)
- Thrombin (Sigma)
- U46619 (Cayman Chemical Company)
- ADP (Sigma)
- Adrenaline (Sigma)

- FITC-conjugated 'platelet identifier' monoclonal antibody (e.g. GPIIIa-specific or GPIb-specific)
- Phycoerythrin–streptavidin (e.g. Jackson ImmunoResearch)
- Methanol-free formaldehyde in modified Tyrode's buffer pH 7.4 (final concentration of paraformaldehyde: 1%)
- Biotinylated test antibody (e.g. S12, PAC1, or 6D1)

Method

1. Use no tourniquet, or tourniquet with only light pressure.

2. Discard the first 2 ml of blood drawn.

3. Draw blood into a sodium citrate Vacutainer.[a]

4. Within 15 min of drawing, dilute 10 µl of the blood with 50 µl modified Tyrode's buffer resulting in a final pH of 7.3.

5. Aliquot diluted whole blood (12 µl) into polypropylene tubes containing 4 µl of a saturating concentration of biotinylated test antibody (e.g. S12, PAC1, or 6D1).

6. Add 8 µl of an agonist at three times desired final concentration (e.g. final concentration of either thrombin[b] 0.001–10 U/ml, the stable thromboxane A$_2$ analogue U46619 0.1–10 µM, or a combination of adenosine diphosphate (ADP) 0.01–10 µM, and adrenaline 1–10 µM,

---

117

Protocol 1. *Continued*

then mix gently (e.g. three or four flicks of a finger against a conical-bottom tube).

7. Incubate undisturbed at 22 °C for 15 min or at 37 °C for 10 min.

8. Add 4 µl of a near saturating concentration of FITC-conjugated 'platelet identifier' monoclonal antibody (e.g. GPIIIa-specific or GPIb-specific) and a saturating concentration of phycoerythrin–streptavidin.

9. Incubate at 22 °C for 15 min.

10. Fix for 30 min at 22 °C with an equal volume of methanol-free formaldehyde in modified Tyrode's buffer pH 7.4.

11. Dilute approx. 20-fold in modified Tyrode's buffer pH 7.4. Final platelet concentration should be > 200/µl.

12. Store at 4 °C, ideally for no longer than 72 h prior to flow cytometric analysis.

[a] A plastic syringe containing 0.38% sodium citrate (final concentration) could also be used or, if calcium depletion needs to be avoided, hirudin 40 U/ml (final concentration) can be used as the anticoagulant (32).
[b] For assays with thrombin, include the peptide GPRP (Calbiochem) (final concentration at this step of 4 mM) in the modified Tyrode's buffer.

3.1 Flow cytometric analysis

Samples prepared as described in *Protocol 1* are analysed in a flow cytometer, e.g. an EPICS Profile (Coulter Cytometry) or a FACScan (Becton Dickinson). The fluorescence of FITC and phycoerythrin are detected using band pass filters (e.g. 525 nm for FITC and 575 nm for phycoerythrin in a Coulter EPICS Profile).

Platelets are identified in the diluted whole blood samples by:

- setting the discriminator (Coulter) or threshold (Becton Dickinson) on the identifying FITC-conjugated monoclonal antibody
- setting a gate on the platelet light scatter region

The binding of the biotinylated activation-sensitive antibody is determined by analysing 5000–10000 individual platelets for phycoerythrin fluorescence. A typical example is illustrated in *Figure 4*. Background binding, obtained from parallel samples with purified biotinylated mouse IgM (e.g. for PAC1 assays) or IgG (most other antibody assays), is subtracted from each test sample. Alternately, the platelet binding of irrelevant, isotypic-identical monoclonal antibodies can be subtracted. The assay can also be performed with a biotinylated monoclonal antibody as the platelet identifier and a FITC-conjugated monoclonal antibody as the test antibody.

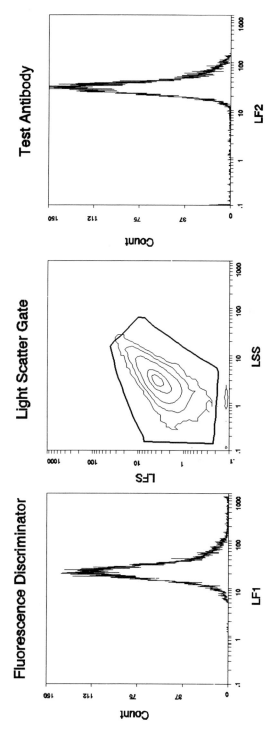

Figure 4. Identification of platelets by whole blood flow cytometry. Platelets were first identified in diluted whole blood samples by setting the discriminator on an identifying FITC-conjugated monoclonal antibody (Y2/51; GPIIIa-specific) (*left* panel). A light scatter gate was set on the platelet light scatter region of these particles (*middle* panel). The binding of a biotinylated antibody (TM60; GPIb-specific) was determined by analysing 10 000 of these particles for phycoerythrin fluorescence (*right* panel). The illustrated data were obtained with a Coulter EPICS Profile II flow cytometer. Abbreviations: count, cell number; LF1, log fluorescence 1 (FITC); LF2, log fluorescence 2 (phycoerythrin), LFS, log forward light scatter; LSS, log side light scatter.

Platelets can be identified in whole blood by light scatter only. However, under certain experimental conditions, some of the particles falling within the light scatter gate for platelets may not bind any platelet-specific monoclonal antibody. Each laboratory should therefore confirm the validity of this method with their specific experimental conditions.

3.2 Methodological issues

3.2.1 Expression of antibody binding

Antibody binding should not be reported as mean channel number, because this is a log scale. Antibody binding can be expressed as mean particle fluorescence intensity (in linear units) or as the per cent of particles staining positive for a particular antibody (based on an analysis marker placed to the right of the negative control fluorescence histogram).

It is very important to realize that 'antibody positive' platelets may have very little antigen expressed on their surface. For example, in a given clinical setting, the data may be reported as 20% circulating activated platelets, based on P-selectin positivity. However, if each P-selectin positive platelet expresses only 10% of maximal platelet surface P-selectin, then the overall average increase in platelet surface P-selectin is only 2%.

Mean fluorescence intensity is therefore the preferred method of data presentation if the goal is to determine the total amount of platelet surface antigen. For activation-dependent antibodies, inclusion of a control of platelets maximally activated by thrombin, TRAP, or phorbol myristate acetate, assists in the quantification of the amount of surface antigen per platelet.

3.2.2 Number of antibody binding sites

Although flow cytometry does not result in a measure of the absolute number of binding sites, Shattil *et al.* (5) and Johnston *et al.* (33) used monoclonal antibodies double labelled with ^{125}I and biotin to demonstrate a direct linear relationship between the number of antibody binding sites per platelet as determined by ^{125}I-labelled and (after incubation with phycoerythrin–streptavidin) fluorescent labelled antibody. Once this relationship is known for a given monoclonal antibody, it is possible to use subsequent batches of the biotinylated or FITC-conjugated antibody for binding site quantitation, provided that the molar ratio of fluorescein to antibody is known. The lower limit of detection of antibody binding by flow cytometry is approximately 500 antibody molecules per platelet.

3.2.3 Minimizing platelet aggregates

Fluorescence, or the number of molecules of an antigen, *per platelet* cannot be determined by flow cytometry if the platelets are aggregated. This is because flow cytometry measures the amount of fluorescence per individual particle, irrespective of whether the particle is a single platelet or an aggregate of an unknown number of platelets. Platelet aggregates can be minimized in the preparation of platelets for whole blood flow cytometry by a combination of the methods shown below:

(a) Most important:
- smooth, easy flow from blood draw
- discard the first 2 ml of blood
- polypropylene (or siliconized glass) tubes or syringes
- immediate mixture with anticoagulant
- no washing, centrifugation, gel filtration, vortexing, or stirring steps
- mix gently after addition of agonist, then incubate undisturbed
- reduce the platelet count by dilution of the samples

(b) Other measures:
- prepare reagents in advance and avoid delays in procedure
- use a light tourniquet and a 19 gauge needle to collect blood
- fixation prevents any further platelet aggregation

(c) Optional:
- if thrombin is the agonist, inclusion in the assay of the peptide GPRP

3.2.4 Giant platelet syndromes

Because light scatter (especially forward light scatter) reflects platelet size, light scatter gates may need to be adjusted in giant platelet syndromes (e.g. Bernard–Soulier syndrome; see Chapter 16).

3.2.5 Sample collection

Collection of blood into a Vacutainer does not result in platelet activation in our hands (*Figure 5*). Because other investigators have argued against the use of Vacutainers (see Chapter 1), each investigator should determine whether their method of collection results in artefactual *in vitro* platelet activation.

An important internal control for the whole blood flow cytometric assay is the lack of binding of activation-dependent monoclonal antibodies (e.g. S12 or PAC1) to normal donor samples in the absence of an added agonist. Under these conditions, the binding of S12 and PAC1 should be almost as low as that of the isotypic control. This internal control confirms that the platelets are in a resting state, i.e. that neither the sampling, the preparation, nor the analysis introduced artefactual *in vitro* platelet activation.

3.2.6 Fixation

The above described 'antibody labelling before fixation' method results in no significant differences in fluorescence intensity between samples analysed immediately and samples analysed within 24 hours (5).

A 'fixation before antibody labelling' method (34) (which is very advantageous in a clinical setting) also results in no significant differences in fluorescence intensity between samples analysed immediately and samples

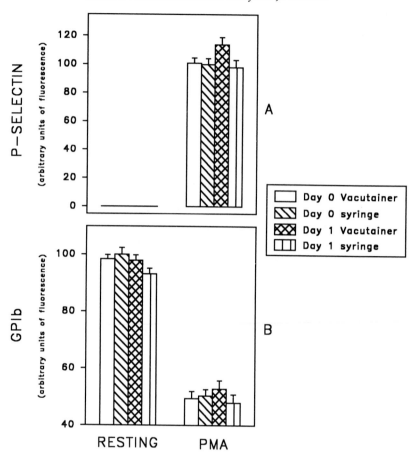

Figure 5. Stability of antibody binding. Peripheral blood samples were collected into either a Vacutainer or a polypropylene syringe that contained the same citrate anticoagulant. Whole blood samples were incubated with or without 10 μM phorbol myristate acetate (PMA), fixed in 1% formaldehyde, stained with a FITC-conjugated platelet identifying monoclonal antibody (Y2/51; GPIIIa-specific) and a biotinylated test monoclonal antibody, and then incubated with phycoerythrin–streptavidin. The samples were analysed by whole blood flow cytometry immediately (day 0) and then again after 24 h at 4°C (day 1). (A) Platelet binding of monoclonal antibody S12 (P-selectin-specific). The fluorescence intensity of platelets collected into a syringe, incubated with PMA, and analysed immediately were assigned a value of 100 units. (B) Platelet binding of monoclonal antibody 6D1 (GPIb-specific). The fluorescence intensity of platelets collected into a syringe, incubated without PMA, and analysed immediately were assigned a value of 100 units. Data are mean ± S.E.M., n = 4. Reproduced with permission from Kestin *et al.* (34).

analysed within 24 hours of antibody tagging (*Figure 5*). However, fixation is an important variable to be controlled for, especially in a 'fixation before antibody labelling' method, because the binding of activation-dependent monoclonal antibodies to fixed platelets is often markedly decreased compared to unfixed platelets. The optimal fixation method for each new mono-clonal antibody must be defined.

3.2.7 Detection of the activation-dependent decrease in the platelet surface expression of the GPIb–IX complex

(a) Whole blood flow cytometric assays frequently employ a GPIb-specific monoclonal antibody to identify platelets. Because GPIb is not present on any circulating blood cell except platelets (35,36), the activation-induced decrease in the platelet surface expression of GPIb (11,27,28) generally does not result in fluorescence below the threshold used to dis-tinguish platelets from other cells (5,12). Thus, no subpopulations of platelets are excluded. However, the use of EDTA as an anticoagulant should be avoided, because this augments the activation-induced decrease in the platelet surface expression of the GPIb–IX complex (29). A method of avoiding the activation-induced decrease in binding of a GPIb-specific monoclonal antibody is to add a direct conjugate of the GPIb-specific antibody before addition of the agonist (37) (see Section 3.2.7(c)).

(b) To analyse the activation-induced decrease in the platelet surface expression of the GPIb–IX complex in whole blood, a GPIIb–IIIa-specific mono-clonal antibody can be employed as the platelet identifying reagent (34).

(c) There is an important methodologic point with regard to the detection of the activation-induced decrease in the platelet surface expression of the GPIb–IX complex (37). In these assays, GPIb–IX-specific antibodies that are directly conjugated (e.g. with FITC) must be added to the assay *after* the addition of the agonist (37). In contrast, GPIb–IX-specific antibodies that require an additional (indirect) detection reagent (e.g. phycoery-thrin–streptavidin (11,12) or FITC-conjugated polyclonal goat anti-mouse antibody (27)) can be added to the assay before or after the addition of thrombin, provided the additional detection reagent is added to the assay after the addition of thrombin. (See ref. 37 for rationale and details.)

3.2.8 Calibration of the flow cytometer

To ensure day to day sample reproducibility, the flow cytometer should be calibrated daily using commercially available fluorescent beads. As per the instructions of the manufacturer of the flow cytometer, daily confirmation of satisfactory fluidics and alignment should also be performed.

Because of spectral emission overlap, the proper electronic colour com-pensation must be set for each combination of antibodies (fluorophores) per the instructions of the manufacturer of the flow cytometer and confirmed by the investigator.

4. Other flow cytometric assays of platelets

4.1 Whole blood flow cytometric assay of platelet activation in shed blood

Because of the minuscule volumes of blood required, whole blood flow cytometry can be used to analyse the shed blood that emerges from a standardized bleeding time wound (38). The time-dependent increase in the platelet surface expression of P-selectin in this shed blood reflects *in vivo* activation of platelets (38). The assay can be used to demonstrate deficient platelet reactivity in response to an *in vivo* wound. An example of the utility of this method is the clinical setting of cardiopulmonary bypass (34). Cardiopulmonary bypass results in normal platelet reactivity *in vitro* but, as determined by the time-dependent exposure of platelet surface P-selectin in the shed blood emerging from a bleeding time wound, markedly deficient platelet reactivity *in vivo* (34).

Protocol 2. Sample preparation from bleeding time wounds

Equipment and reagents

- Micropipette
- FITC-conjugated platelet-specific monoclonal antibody (e.g. GPIIIa-specific)
- Biotinylated activation-dependent monoclonal antibody (e.g. P-selectin-specific)
- Biotinylated mouse IgG in control samples
- Tyrode's buffer pH 7.4 (see *Protocol 1*)
- Phycoerythrin–streptavidin (1 : 30)
- Formaldehyde (2%)
- Microcentrifuge tubes

Method

1. Perform a standardized bleeding time test.

2. Collect the blood emerging from the bleeding time wound with a micropipette at 1 min intervals until the bleeding stops. After each pipetting, remove any residual blood at the bleeding time wound site with filter paper. Do not touch the wound with the pipette tip or filter paper.

3. Add the pipetted blood (2 μl per antibody tested) to a microcentrifuge tube containing sodium citrate, immediately fix by incubation (30 min, 22°C) with an equal volume of 2% formaldehyde, and dilute 1 : 6 by volume in modified Tyrode's buffer pH 7.4.

4. Incubate at 22°C for 15 min with a near saturating concentration of a FITC-conjugated platelet-specific monoclonal antibody (e.g. GPIIIa-specific) and a saturating concentration of a biotinylated activation-dependent monoclonal antibody (e.g. P-selectin-specific). Use biotinylated mouse IgG in control samples.

5. Incubate at 22°C for 15 min with 1 : 30 phycoerythrin–streptavidin.

6. Dilute approx. tenfold in modified Tyrode's buffer pH 7.4.

7. Store at 4°C, ideally for no longer than 72 h prior to flow cytometric analysis.

8. Analyse samples by flow cytometry as described above.

Note: immediately before the bleeding time, prepare control samples of peripheral blood drawn from the antecubital vein of the opposite arm of the same subject. After discarding the first 2 ml, place one drop of non-anticoagulated blood from the butterfly tubing on a piece of Parafilm and process the aliquots for flow cytometry exactly as described for the bleeding time samples. As a positive control, incubate a peripheral blood sample with a maximal concentration of thrombin, as in *Protocol 1*.

4.2 Flow cytometry of washed platelets

The ability of a reagent to directly affect platelets in the absence of plasma, white cells, and red cells can be evaluated by flow cytometric analysis of washed platelets. However, the disadvantages of analysing washed platelets are referred to in the Introduction.

Washed or gel filtered platelets are processed and analysed in a similar way to whole blood samples. The platelets can be identified solely on the basis of their characteristic forward and orthogonal light scattering profile. However, as for whole blood assays, depending on the experimental conditions, a proportion of the particles falling within the light scatter gate for platelets may not bind a platelet-specific monoclonal antibody. Each investigator should therefore confirm that a fluorescent labelled monoclonal antibody as a 'platelet identifier' is unnecessary for the specific experimental conditions.

The methods of sample preparation shown above for the minimization of platelet aggregate formation should be used. Dilution of the platelets to $< 50\,000/\mu l$ prior to activation is the most important of these methods.

4.3 Diagnosis of inherited platelet disorders

Flow cytometry provides a rapid and simple means for the diagnosis of the homozygous and heterozygous states of platelet membrane glycoprotein deficiencies, such as Bernard–Soulier syndrome and Glanzmann's thrombasthenia (39). In addition, a panel of activation-dependent monoclonal antibodies can be used to evaluate patients with defects in platelet aggregation (40), secretion (41), or procoagulant activity (42).

4.4 Platelet-derived microparticles

Platelets that are activated *in vitro* by thrombin, collagen, thrombin plus collagen, or C5b–9 (the membrane attack complex of complement) undergo a vesiculation reaction that correlates temporally with the development of a procoagulant platelet surface. The latter is defined operationally by:

(a) An increased transbilayer movement of negatively charged, anionic phospholipids from the inner leaflet to the outer leaflet of the plasma membrane.

(b) Vesiculation from the platelet surface membrane of 'microparticles' with an average diameter of 0.1 μm.

(c) An increase in the number of membrane binding sites for coagulation factors VIIIa and Va on platelets and microparticles.

The binding of factors VIIIa and Va is required for optimal assembly of the intrinsic 'tenase' and 'prothrombinase' enzyme complexes, respectively. Thus, development of a procoagulant surface on activated platelets and microparticles enables the efficient catalysis of factor X to factor Xa and prothrombin to thrombin (43–46) (also see Chapter 15).

The molecular basis for the agonist-induced exposure of anionic phospholipids and platelet vesiculation is unclear, although calcium influx is required (47). Platelet aggregation is not essential, but it can potentiate the process in a manner that appears dependent on activation of platelet calpain (48). Although granule secretion supplies factor Va for the prothrombinase reaction, platelet secretion is not required for reorientation of phospholipids or microparticle formation (47). Under certain experimental conditions, platelet procoagulant activity can be induced while microparticle formation is inhibited, indicating that, while the two processes are usually linked, vesiculation is not required for the initial development of the procoagulant surface (49).

Although the development of procoagulant on activated platelets and perturbed endothelial cells appears essential for normal haemostasis (50), the significance of microparticles for haemostasis and/or thrombosis *in vivo* remains unclear (42,51–53). Flow cytometry may be useful in further studies of both the biochemical basis and clinical significance of microparticle formation. This technique can:

(a) Discriminate between single platelets and platelet-derived microparticles on the basis of particle light scatter (43,54).

(b) Measure the binding of factors Va and VIIIa to platelets and microparticles through the use of fluorophore labelled monoclonal antibodies specific for these cofactors (43,46).

(c) Measure the amount of externally oriented anionic phospholipids through the use of fluorophore labelled annexin V (55).

(d) Monitor transbilayer movement of phosphatidylserine and other phospholipids across the plasma membrane through the use of NBD labelled phospholipids (56).

The reader is referred to the primary references for specific methods.

4.5 Intracellular signalling

Other chapters in this book contain detailed methods for the study of the biochemical basis of platelet activation. Flow cytometry is finding increasing use in such studies due to the availability of specific fluorescent probes and the ability to discriminate among subpopulations of platelets with respect to size and/or function. Examples include studies of:

- cytoplasmic free Ca^{2+} using indo-1 (57,58)
- F-actin content using NBD- or bodipy-phallicidin (59–61)
- the effects of membrane impermeable bioactive peptides and other mediators on the activation state of permeabilized platelets (62)

Primary references and other chapters in this book should be consulted for more information pertaining to these very specialized applications of flow cytometry.

References

1. Kinlough-Rathbone, R. L., Packham, M. A., and Mustard, J. F. (1983). In *Measurements of platelet function* (ed. L. A. Harker and T. S. Zimmerman), pp. 64–91. Churchill Livingstone, New York.
2. Kaplan, K. L. and Owen, J. (1983). In *Measurements of platelet function* (ed. L. A. Harker and T. S. Zimmerman), pp. 115–25. Churchill Livingstone, Edinburgh.
3. Levine, S. P. (1986). In *Biochemistry of platelets* (ed. D. R. Phillips and M. A. Shuman), pp. 378–415. Academic Press, Orlando.
4. George, J. N. and Shattil, S. J. (1991). *N. Engl. J. Med.*, **324**, 27.
5. Shattil, S. J., Cunningham, M., and Hoxie, J. A. (1987). *Blood*, **70**, 307.
6. Abrams, C. and Shattil, S. J. (1991). *Thromb. Haemost.*, **65**, 467.
7. Ejim, O. S., Powling, M. J., Dandona, P., Kernoff, P. B., and Goodall, A. H. (1990). *Thromb. Res.*, **58**, 519.
8. Wehmeier, A., Tschope, D., Esser, J., Menzel, C., Nieuwenhuis, H. K., and Schneider, W. (1991). *Thromb. Res.*, **61**, 271.
9. Santos, M. T., Valles, J., Marcus, A. J., Safier, L. B., Broekman, M. J., Islam, N., *et al.* (1991). *J. Clin. Invest.*, **87**, 571.
10. LaRosa, C. A., Rohrer, M. J., Rodino, L. J., Benoit, S. E., Barnard, M. R., and Michelson, A. D. (1994). *J. Vasc. Surg.*, **19**, 306.
11. Michelson, A. D., Ellis, P. A., Barnard, M. R., Matic, G. B., Viles, A. F., and Kestin, A. S. (1991). *Blood*, **77**, 770.
12. Kestin, A. S., Ellis, P. A., Barnard, M. R., Errichetti, A., Rosner, B. A., and Michelson, A. D. (1993). *Circulation*, **88**, 1502.
13. Rajasekhar, D., Kestin, A. S., Bednarek, F. J., Ellis, P. A., Barnard, M. R. and Michelson, A. D. (1994). *Thromb. Haemost.*, **72**, 957.
14. Hansen, S. R. and Harker, L. A. (1988). *Proc. Natl. Acad. Sci. USA*, **85**, 3184.
15. Eidt, J. F., Allison, P., Nobel, S., Ashton, J., Golino, P., McNatt, J., *et al.* (1989). *J. Clin. Invest.*, **84**, 18.

16. Kelly, A. B., Marzec, U. M., Krupski, W., Bass, A., Cadroy, Y., Hanson, S. R., *et al.* (1991). *Blood*, **77**, 1006.
17. Michelson, A. D. (1994). *Blood Coagul. Fibrinolysis*, **5**, 121.
18. Laudano, A. P. and Doolittle, R. F. (1978). *Proc. Natl. Acad. Sci. USA*, **75**, 3085.
19. Plow, E. F. and Marguerie, G. (1982). *Proc. Natl. Acad. Sci. USA*, **79**, 3711.
20. Adelman, B., Gennings, C., Strony, J., and Hanners, E. (1990). *Circ. Res.*, **67**, 941.
21. Vu, T.-K. H., Hung, D. T., Wheaton, V. I., and Coughlin, S. R. (1991). *Cell*, **64**, 1057.
22. Yamamoto, N., Greco, N. J., Barnard, M. R., Tanoue, K., Yamazaki, H., Jamieson, G. A., *et al.* (1991). *Blood*, **77**, 1740.
23. McEver, R. P. (1990). *Blood Cells*, **16**, 73.
24. Phillips, D. R., Charo, I. F., Parise, L. V., and Fitzgerald, L. A. (1988). *Blood*, **71**, 831.
25. Shattil, S. J., Hoxie, J. A., Cunningham, M., and Brass, L. F. (1985). *J. Biol. Chem.*, **260**, 11107.
26. Abrams, C., Deng, J., Steiner, J., O'Toole, T., and Shattil, S. (1994). *J. Biol. Chem.*, **269**, 18781.
27. Michelson, A. D. and Barnard, M. R. (1987). *Blood*, **70**, 1673.
28. Michelson, A. D. (1992). *Semin. Thromb. Hemost.*, **18**, 18.
29. Hourdille, P., Heilmann, E., Combrie, R., Winckler, J., Clemetson, K. J., and Nurden, A. T. (1990). *Blood*, **76**, 1503.
30. Ruggeri, Z. M. (1991). *Prog. Hemost. Thromb.*, **10**, 35.
31. Rinderknecht, H. (1962). *Nature*, **193**, 167.
32. Shattil, S. J., Budzynski, A., and Scrutton, M. C. (1989). *Blood*, **73**, 150.
33. Johnston, G. I., Pickett, E. B., McEver, R. P., and George, J. N. (1987). *Blood*, **69**, 1401.
34. Kestin, A. S., Valeri, C. R., Khuri, S. F., Loscalzo, J., Ellis, P. A., MacGregor, H., *et al.* (1993). *Blood*, **82**, 107.
35. Coller, B. S., Peerschke, E. I., Scudder, L. E., and Sullivan, C. A. (1983). *Blood*, **61**, 99.
36. Montgomery, R. R., Kunicki, T. J., Taves, C., Pidard, D., and Corcoran, M. (1983). *J. Clin. Invest.*, **71**, 385.
37. Michelson, A. D. and Barnard, M. R. (1993). *Blood*, **81**, 1408.
38. Abrams, C. S., Ellison, N., Budzynski, A. Z., and Shattil, S. J. (1990). *Blood*, **75**, 128.
39. Michelson, A. D. (1987). *J. Lab. Clin. Med.*, **110**, 346.
40. Ginsberg, M. H., Frelinger, A. L., Lam, S. C., Forsyth, J., McMillan, R., Plow, E. F., *et al.* (1990). *Blood*, **76**, 2017.
41. Lages, B., Shattil, S. J., Bainton, D. F., and Weiss, H. J. (1991). *J. Clin. Invest.*, **87**, 919.
42. Sims, P. J., Wiedmer, T., Esmon, C. T., Weiss, H. J., and Shattil, S. J. (1989). *J. Biol. Chem.*, **264**, 17049.
43. Sims, P. J., Faioni, E. M., Wiedmer, T., and Shattil, S. J. (1988). *J. Biol. Chem.*, **263**, 18205.
44. Bevers, E. M., Comfurius, P., and Zwaal, R. F. (1991). *Blood Rev.*, **5**, 146.
45. Schroit, A. J. and Zwaal, R. F. (1991). *Biochim. Biophys. Acta*, **1071**, 313.
46. Gilbert, G. E., Sims, P. J., Wiedmer, T., Furie, B., Furie, B. C., and Shattil, S. J. (1991). *J. Biol. Chem.*, **266**, 17261.
47. Wiedmer, T., Shattil, S. J., Cunningham, M., and Sims, P. J. (1990). *Biochemistry*, **29**, 623.

48. Fox, J. E., Austin, C. D., Reynolds, C. C., and Steffen, P. K. (1991). *J. Biol. Chem.*, **266**, 13289.
49. Dachary-Prigent, J., Freyssinet, J. M., Pasquet, J. M., Carron, J. C., and Nurden, A. T. (1993). *Blood*, **81**, 2554.
50. Mann, K. G., Nesheim, M. E., Church, W. R., Haley, P., and Krishnaswamy, S. (1990). *Blood*, **76**, 1.
51. Jy, W., Horstman, L. L., Arce, M., and Ahn, Y. S. (1992). *J. Lab. Clin. Med.*, **119**, 334.
52. Wiedmer, T., Hall, S. E., Ortel, T. L., Kane, W. H., Rosse, W. F., and Sims, P. J. (1993). *Blood*, **82**, 1192.
53. Rajasekhar, D., Barnard, M. R., Bednarek, F. J., Benoit, S. E., and Michelson, A. D. (1993). *Blood*, **82**, 163a.
54. Thiagarajan, P. and Tait, J. F. (1991). *J. Biol. Chem.*, **266**, 24302.
55. Thiagarajan, P. and Tait, J. F. (1990). *J. Biol. Chem.*, **265**, 17420.
56. Chang, C. P., Zhao, J., Wiedmer, T., and Sims, P. J. (1993). *J. Biol. Chem.*, **268**, 7171.
57. Davies, T. A., Drotts, D., Weil, G. J., and Simons, E. R. (1988). *Cytometry*, **9**, 138.
58. Jennings, L. K., Dockter, M. E., Wall, C. D., Fox, C. F., and Kennedy, D. M. (1989). *Blood*, **74**, 2674.
59. Cattaneo, M., Kinlough-Rathbone, R. L., Lecchi, A., Bevilacqua, C., Packham, M. A., and Mustard, J. F. (1993). *Blood*, **70**, 221.
60. Shattil, S. J., Haimovich, B., Cunningham, M., Lipfert, L., Parsons, J. T., Ginsberg, M. H., *et al.* (1994). *J. Biol. Chem.*, **269**, 14738.
61. LaRosa, C. A., Rohrer, M. J., Benoit, S. E., Barnard, M. R., and Michelson, A. D. (1994). *Blood*, **84**, 158.
62. Shattil, S. J., Cunningham, M., Wiedmer, T., Zhao, J., Sims, P. J., and Brass, L. F. (1992). *J. Biol. Chem.*, **267**, 18424.
63. Zamarron, C., Ginsberg, M. H., and Plow, E. F. (1990). *Thromb. Haemost.*, **64**, 41.
64. Frelinger, A. L., Lam, S. C., Plow, E. F., Smith, M. A., Loftus, J. C., and Ginsberg, M. H. (1988). *J. Biol. Chem.*, **263**, 12397.
65. Frelinger, A. L., Cohen, I., Plow, E. F., Smith, M. A., Roberts, J., Lam, S. C., *et al.* (1990). *J. Biol. Chem.*, **265**, 6346.
66. Stenberg, P. E., McEver, R. P., Shuman, M. A., Jacques, Y. V., and Bainton, D. F. (1985). *J. Cell Biol.*, **101**, 880.
67. Larsen, E., Celi, A., Gilbert, G. E., Furie, B. C., Erban, J. K., Bonfanti, R., *et al.* (1989). *Cell*, **59**, 305.
68. Nieuwenhuis, H. K., van Oosterhout, J. J., Rozemuller, E., van Iwaarden, F., and Sixma, J. J. (1987). *Blood*, **70**, 838.
69. Febbraio, M. and Silverstein, R. L. (1990). *J. Biol. Chem.*, **265**, 18531.
70. Boukerche, H. and McGregor, J. L. (1988). *Eur. J. Biochem.*, **171**, 383.
71. Aiken, M. L., Ginsberg, M. H., and Plow, E. F. (1987). *Semin. Thromb. Hemost.*, **13**, 307.

Identification, isolation, and characterization of platelet glycoproteins mediating platelet adhesion

JOHN L. McGREGOR, ODILE GAYET, NATHALIE MERCIER, LILIAN McGREGOR, and ELZA CHIGNIER

1. Introduction

Platelets play a vital role in haemostasis by the formation of a plug or thrombus at a site of vessel wall injury. The function of these anucleated cells is largely dependent on the presence of a number of glycoproteins. Moreover, adhesion and aggregation of platelets to disrupted atheroma plaque, leading in some cases to vessel occlusion, is also mediated by glycoproteins. The importance of glycoproteins in platelet functions has led to extensive work, using various techniques, to identify structural/functional sites on these glycoproteins implicated in interacting with various ligands. The aim of this chapter is to describe a number of techniques used in studying glycoproteins involved in platelet adhesion to extracellular matrix proteins or to leucocytes.

Work over this past decade has shown that over 40 glycoproteins are present on the platelet surface. Some of these glycoproteins (GPIIb–IIIa/$\alpha_{IIb}\beta_3$, GPVn–IIIa/$\alpha_v\beta_3$, GPIb–IX, GPV, GPIa–IIa/$\alpha_2\beta_1$, GPIc–IIa/$\alpha_5\beta_1$, GPIc*–IIa/$\alpha_6\beta_1$, GMP140/P-selectin/CD62, PECAM-1/CD31) have been extensively characterized and shown to be members of the integrin, selectin, and superimmunoglobulin families. It is of interest to note that a majority of these platelet glycoproteins are also present on resting or activated endothelial cells. Absence of some of these glycoproteins, such as GPIIb–IIIa, GPIb–IX, GPIa–IIa, on platelets from patients with congenital disorders leads to a lack of platelet adhesion or aggregation. Moreover, monoclonal antibodies directed against these glycoproteins effectively block platelet functions (1).

2. Adhesion of platelets to collagen and other extracellular matrix proteins

For adhesion experiments, platelets are washed according to a modification of the method by Mustard (2). Washed platelets are then ^{51}Cr-labelled and added to plastic wells coated with extracellular matrix proteins such as collagen, laminin, or fibronectin (3). Adhesion of platelets is performed in the presence or absence of monoclonal antibodies, peptides, or small organic molecules that may block such adhesion.

Protocol 1. Platelet adhesion

Equipment and reagents

- Hood for labelling and handling radioactive substances
- γ-Counter
- Bench centrifuge
- Prostaglandin E$_1$ (PGE$_1$) (20 ng/ml) (Sigma)
- D-Phenylalanine-L-proline-L-arginine chloromethyl ketone (PPACK) (Calbiochem) 10^{-6} M
- Apyrase, grade III (1.3 mg/ml) (Sigma)
- ^{51}Cr (in NaOH solution) (1 mCi/ml) (Amersham)
- Bovine serum albumin, fraction V (Boehringer Diagnostics)
- Immulon-1 removal strips, bearing 12 flat-bottom wells (Dynatech Laboratories Inc.)

- ACD anticoagulant: 1.4% (w/v) citric acid, 2.5% (w/v) sodium citrate, 2% (w/v) glucose pH 4.3–4.5
- Tyrode's buffer: 140 mM NaCl, 3 mM KCl, 12 mM NaHCO$_3$, 0.4 mM NaH$_2$PO$_4$.H$_2$O, 1 mM MgCl$_2$.6H$_2$O, 2 mM CaCl$_2$.2H$_2$O, 0.35% (w/v) BSA, 0.1% (w/v) glucose, pH 7.33 with Hepes
- Calcium-free Tyrode's buffer: 140 mM NaCl, 3 mM KCl, 12 mM NaHCO$_3$, 0.4 mM NaH$_2$PO$_4$.H$_2$O, 2 mM MgCl$_2$.6H$_2$O, 0.35% (w/v) BSA, 0.1% (w/v) glucose, pH 7.33 with Hepes
- Fibronectin, laminin, collagen type I and III (Sigma)

A. Washing and labelling platelets

1. Draw blood from healthy consenting donors, discarding the first 1 ml, into ACD in a ratio of 1 ml of ACD to 6 ml of blood.

2. Centrifuge at 150 *g* for 25 min at 37 °C to obtain platelet-rich plasma (PRP).

3. Carefully remove PRP, recentrifuging if necessary to remove red blood cell contaminants, and incubate for 10 min at 37 °C following addition of 20 ng/ml of PGE$_1$. Addition of PGE$_1$ greatly helps to prevent platelet activation.

4. Centrifuge the PRP for 15 min at 1100 *g* and 37 °C, and resuspend the pellet in 10 ml calcium-free Tyrode's buffer containing PGE$_1$ (20 ng/ml), PPACK (10^{-6} M), and apyrase (130 µg/ml).

5. Add ^{51}Cr (5 µCi/ml of washed platelets) and leave for 30 min at 37 °C.

6. Centrifuge ^{51}Cr-labelled platelets at 1100 *g* for 10 min at 37 °C, resuspend the pellet in calcium-free Tyrode's buffer containing PGE$_1$ (20 ng/ml) and apyrase (130 µg/ml), and leave for 10 min at 37 °C. Take an aliquot for counting the number of platelets.

---

7. Recentrifuge at 1100 g for 10 min at 37°C, resuspend the pellet in calcium-free Tyrode's buffer containing 1% BSA, PGE$_1$ (20 ng/ml), and apyrase (26 µg/ml), and incubate at 37°C until required.

B. Labelled platelet adhesion to collagen, laminin, or fibronectin

1. Coat Immulon-1 removal strips, bearing 12 flat-bottom wells, with 10 µg/ml laminin, collagen, or fibronectin (100 µl/well). Laminin and fibronectin are left incubating overnight at 4°C. Collagen is left for 3 h at 37°C.

2. Block wells with calcium-free Tyrode's buffer containing PGE$_1$ (20 ng/ml) and 1% BSA for 90 min at room temperature. Monoclonal antibodies, peptides, or small organic molecules that are to be tested are incubated at different concentrations in phosphate-buffered saline (50 µl/well) on the collagen coated wells (or other extracellular matrix proteins) for 60 min at room temperature prior to the addition of ^{51}Cr-labelled platelets.

3. Add ^{51}Cr-labelled platelets to the wells (50 µl, 2.5×10^7 platelets/well) and incubate for 30 min at room temperature. Wash three times with calcium-free Tyrode's buffer containing 1% BSA. Strips of wells are then cut off and radioactivity counted in a γ-counter.

3. Surface labelling techniques combined with one- or two-dimensional SDS–PAGE

As previously indicated a large number of glycoproteins are present on the platelet surface. Resting or activated washed human platelets are radioactively labelled at the surface by techniques specific for proteins or glycoproteins. These labelled platelets samples are then analysed by either one-dimensional discontinuous sodium dodecyl sulfate (SDS) polyacrylamide gel electrophoresis or by a high resolution two-dimensional separation system involving isoeletric focusing in the first dimension and SDS–polyacrylamide gel electrophoresis in the second. Radioactive labelling techniques, if used for the first time, should be performed with great care and under the guidance of a safety officer.

Protocol 2. Labelling platelet membrane glycoproteins

Equipment and reagents

- Hood used for handling radioactive substances
- Bench centrifuge
- Water-bath
- Freezer (–70°C)
- Phosphate-buffered saline (PBS) pH 7.4
- *Vibrio cholerae* neuraminidase (Behringwerke, Marburg-Lahn, Germany)

Protocol 2. *Continued*

- Galactose oxidase (4 U/ml) (Kabi, Stockholm, Sweden)
- Sodium metaperiodate (0.0002 M)
- Glycerol solution
- Lactoperoxidase (Sigma)
- ^{125}I
- ACD anticoagulant (see *Protocol 1*)
- $[^3H]NaB_3H_4$ (5–20 Ci/mmole) (Amersham)
- CGS: 0.012 M sodium citrate, 0.03 M glucose, 0.12 M NaCl pH 6.5
- TENA: 0.01 M Tris, 0.005 M EDTA, 0.154 M NaCl pH 7.4

A. Washing platelets

1. Draw blood into ACD (1 vol. of ACD to 6 vol. of blood). Centrifuge at 150 *g* for 10 min to obtain PRP. Remove residual contaminating red and white blood cells by a further centrifugation at 150 *g* for 10 min.

2. Centrifuge PRP at 1100 *g* for 15 min and wash the platelet pellet according to the method of Massini and Lüscher (4) modified by the addition of EDTA.

3. Gently resuspend the platelet pellet in CGS containing 0.005 M EDTA and wash twice in that solution. Further wash the platelet pellet in TENA, count, and resuspend in PBS at a concentration of 10^9/ml.

B. Neuraminidase, galactose oxidase, and $[^3H]NaB_3H_4$ labelling (5)

1. Resuspend washed platelets in PBS and incubate with 10 U/ml of *Vibrio cholerae* neuraminidase for 15 min at 37 °C.

2. Wash once in TENA and resuspend in PBS. Add galactose oxidase to platelets (10^9/ml) and incubate for 5 min at 37 °C.

3. Increase the volume of the platelet suspension to 10 ml by addition of TENA buffer and centrifuge. Resuspend in PBS and incubate with $[^3H]NaB_3H_4$ (0.5 mCi) for 15 min at room temperature under a hood.[a]

4. Wash labelled platelets twice in 10 ml of TENA and solubilize for polyacrylamide gel electrophoresis.

C. Sodium metaperiodate and $[^3H]NaB_3H_4$ labelling (3)

1. Incubate 1 ml of platelets (10^9/ml) at melting ice temperature (0 °C) and in complete darkness with 0.002 M sodium metaperiodate for 10 min.

2. Terminate reaction by addition of 0.2 ml of 0.2 M glycerol solution, wash the platelet pellet twice with 10 ml TENA, and resuspend in PBS.

3. Incubate with $[^3H]NaB_3H_4$ is as described in part B.

D. Lactoperoxidase + $Na^{125}I$ labelling (3)

1. Add carrier-free $Na^{125}I$ (0.25 mCi) to 1 ml of platelets (10^9/ml).[b]

2. Add lactoperoxidase (2.5 nmole) followed by addition of five 10 µl aliquots of 0.003 M H_2O_2 at 10 sec intervals. The platelet suspension is gently shaken during the addition of H_2O_2.

3. Wash platelets two times with 10 ml of TENA and solubilize for gel electrophoresis.

[a] Aliquots of NaB_3H_4 (0.5 mCi) are prepared from a stock solution in an appropriate hood made to handle a volatile radioactive substance, snap frozen, and stored at –70°C.
[b] An alternative labelling method is to use carrier Iodo-Beads from Pierce (Rockford, IL, USA), coated with chloramine-T which when rehydrated in a solution containing $Na^{125}I$ will subsequently label platelet proteins.

Protocol 3. Polyacrylamide gel electrophoresis

Equipment and reagents

- Heating block
- Eppendorf microcentrifuge
- Sodium dodecyl sulfate (SDS) (2%)
- 0.5 M Tris pH 6.8
- Platelet pellets
- N-ethylmaleimide (Sigma)
- Dithiothreitol (Sigma)
- 10% sucrose or 10% glycerol
- Protein assay procedure
- Bromophenol blue (0.03%, w/v)

- Gel apparatus
- Acrylamide: N,N′-methylene bisacrylamide (bis) (30 : 0.8, w/w)
- 1.5 M Tris–HCl pH 8.8
- 20% SDS (w/v)
- H_2O
- TEMED
- 10% ammonium persulfate
- 10% sodium persulfate

A. Preparation of sample

1. Resuspend labelled platelet pellets in 100 μl of 0.05 M Tris pH 6.8 and 2% SDS.

2. Heat samples immediately to 100°C for 10 min.

3. Remove an aliquot for protein determination, e.g. by the Lowry *et al.* (6) or a rapid Coomassie brillant blue assay (7).

4. For non-reduced samples, add N-ethylmaleimide (2 mM) before SDS solubilization; for reduced samples, add dithiothreitol (0.04 M) and heat at 100°C for 5 min.

5. Increase density of cooled sample by addition of sucrose (10%) or glycerol (10%) and add a drop of bromophenol blue (0.03%) as a tracking dye. Microcentrifuge samples before SDS–PAGE according to the method of Laemmli (8).

B. One-dimensional SDS–polyacrylamide gel electrophoresis (3)

1. Set-up gel apparatus using 1.5, 1, or 0.75 mm spacers.

2. Prepare a 10% SDS–polyacrylamide separating gel by addition of the following:
   - acrylamide : bis (30 : 0.8)[a]   10 ml
   - 1.5 M Tris–HCl pH 8.8 (0.375 M)   7.5 ml
   - 20% SDS (w/v)   150 μl

Protocol 3. *Continued*

- TEMED   30 µl
- H_2O 12.0 ml
- 10% sodium persulfate   300 µl

Allow to set.

3. Prepare a 3% stacking gel by addition of the following:
   - acrylamide : bis (30 : 0.8)   2 ml
   - 1.5 M Tris–HCl pH 8.8 (0.375 M)   5 ml
   - 20% SDS (w/v)   100 µl
   - TEMED   20 µl
   - H_2O 12.8 ml
   - 10% ammonium persulfate   200 µl

   Allow to set.

4. Add samples (40 or 80 µg of protein)[b] in 10 µl volumes and electrophorese at 80–100 V until the bromophenol blue marker reaches
   the bottom of the gel slab.

[a] Polyacrylamide is a neurotoxic substance and should be handled with adequate precautions.
Alternatively, solutions can be purchased.
[b] For PAS (periodic acid–Schiff's) stained gels the electrophoresed sample should contain
aproximately 200 to 300 µg protein.

3.1 Two-dimensional O'Farrell polyacrylamide gel separation system

Characterization of human blood platelet membrane glycoproteins by their
isoelectric point (pI) and apparent molecular weight (M_r) is performed
according to the technique of O'Farrell (9) as previously described (10,11).
For platelet glycoproteins we have obtained a good pI separation using Pharmalytes 5–7 and 3.5–10. The O'Farrell polyacrylamide gel separation technique is described in Chapter 9. Additional details that may be useful in this
method are given below.

(a) Isoelectric focusing (IEF). IEF lysis buffer may contain either *N*-ethyl-
   maleimide (NEM) (0.001 M), for samples that need to be electrophoresed in the first dimension under non-reducing conditions, or
   dithiothreitol for samples that need to be electrophoresed under reducing conditions. We have obtained good separations using Pharmalytes
   (5–7) (1.6%), Pharmalytes (3.5–10) (0.4%). The established pH gradient
   can be determined by using Pharmacia isoelectric focusing calibration
   kits containing proteins, stained by Coomassie blue after IEF, that have
   specific pI. Platelet samples prepared in lysis buffer, run under non-
   reducing or reducing conditions, containing 80 µg of protein are loaded
   on IEF gels.

(b) Staining of gels. Polyacrylamide gels at the end of the electrophoretic run are fixed and washed in a methanol (40%)/glacial acetic acid (7%) solution to remove SDS. Proteins on gels are visualized by Coomassie (12) or silver staining (13,14). For staining glycoproteins the periodic acid–Schiff's (PAS) silver staining procedure can be used (15). Densitometry scanning is performed on wet slab gels.

(c) Fluorography and indirect autoradiography (3). Gels are prepared for fluorography by immersing them in a special solution available for this purpose from Amersham or New England Nuclear. Alternatively, the solutions can be prepared as indicated by Bonner and Laskey (16). Treated gels are then dried on to Whatman filter paper number 3MM and exposed at –70°C to a pre-flashed RP Royal X-OMAT, new film, Amersham, or an Agfa Curix II. To obtain the maximum amount of information it may be necessary to expose films for several days. Films are processed according to the manufacturer's instructions. For indirect autoradiography fixed polyacrylamide gels are sandwiched between pre-flashed Royal X-OMAT film and two Cronex lightning plus scintillation screens (Dupont) and left at –70°C for a few hours or overnight.

4. The combined use of FPLC and gas phase sequencing techniques to isolate and characterize platelet glycoproteins

Glycoproteins present on the platelet surface can be separated by fast protein liquid chromatography techniques (FPLC). A number of these glycoproteins can be isolated to a high degree of purity, in a native state, by the use of two-dimensional gel chromatographic techniques. These samples are then analysed by discontinuous SDS–polyacrylamide gel electrophoresis, Western blotted, or characterized by N terminal gas phase sequencing.

Protocol 4. Triton X-114 platelet membrane extraction followed by tandem anion exchange and size exclusion FPLC (17)

Equipment and reagents

- Ultracentrifuge
- Bench centrifuge
- Sonicator
- Water-bath
- FPLC system
- Pharmacia K16/40 glass column (400 x 16 mm)
- Q-Sepharose fast flow gel column
- Superloop

- Mono-Q HR10/10 prepacked column (100 x 10 mm)
- Superose 12HR 10/30 column (300 x 10 mm)
- Western blotting apparatus
- Gas phase sequencer
- Berol 185
- Triton X-114
- Washed platelets (5 x 10^9/ml)

Protocol 4. *Continued*

- Solubilization buffer: 1% Triton X-114 (v/v), 10 mM Tris–HCl pH 7.4, 0.1 mM leupeptin, 5 mM EDTA
- Triton X-114 sucrose beds: 3 ml of 6% sucrose prepared in 10 mM Tris–HCl pH 7.4, 154 mM NaCl, 1 mM EDTA, and 0.06% Triton X-114
- Starting buffer: 0.5% Berol 185 in 20 mM Tris–HCl pH 7.4
- Final buffer: 0.5% Berol 185 in 20 mM Tris–HCl pH 7.4 containing 1 M NaCl
- Mobile phase for gel filtration: 0.5% Berol 185, 1 mM EDTA in 0.1 M Tris–HCl pH 7.4

Method

1. Resuspend washed platelets (5×10^9/ml) in 10 mM Tris–HCl pH 7.4, 0.1 mM leupeptin, 5 mM EDTA, and sonicate at 4 °C.

2. Centrifuge platelet sample at 4 °C for 20 min at 9000 *g*.

3. Remove supernatant and centrifuge at 4 °C for 60 min at 100 000 *g*.

4. Solubilize platelet pellet membrane with 1% Triton X-114 (v/v), 10 mM Tris–HCl pH 7.4, 0.1 mM leupeptin, 5 mM EDTA for 30 min, and then centrifuge at 100 000 *g*, 4 °C for 30 min.

5. Layer 2 ml of the supernatant on 3 ml of 6% sucrose prepared in 10 mM Tris–HCl pH 7.4, 154 mM NaCl, 1 mM EDTA, and 0.06% Triton X-114.

6. Incubate tubes containing the extracted supernatant and the sucrose bed at 37 °C for 5 min and centrifuge at 25 °C for 10 min at 1100 *g*.

7. Collect the detergent phase, present as a yellow pellet in each tube, and add to a Q-Sepharose fast flow gel column (packed into a Pharmacia K16/40 glass column, 400 × 16 mm) connected to a FPLC system.

8. Equilibrate the Q-Sepharose column in 20 mM Tris–HCl pH 7.4 (starting buffer). The detergent phase of the Triton X-114 platelet membrane is diluted in the starting buffer, to reduce its viscosity, and loaded on the Q-Sepharose column using a superloop. Wash the column with the starting buffer until the optical density returns to baseline.

9. A non-ionic detergent gradient, 0–0.5% Berol 185, is generated over 90 min at a flow rate of 4 ml/min to further remove Triton X-114 contaminants and to equilibrate the column with that detergent.

10. Elute proteins from the Q-Sepharose column using a 0–1.0 M NaCl gradient generated over 90 min at a flow rate of 4 ml/min. The starting buffer is 0.5% Berol 185 in 20 mM Tris–HCl pH 7.4, and the final buffer is 0.5% Berol 185 in 20 mM Tris–HCl pH 7.4 containing 1 M NaCl.

11. Dilute the peaks eluted from the Q-Sepharose column with the starting buffer to reduce their NaCl concentration and inject via a superloop into a Mono-Q HR10/10 prepacked column (100 × 10 mm) connected to the FPLC system.

12. Elute proteins from the Mono-Q column using a 0–1.0 M NaCl gradient generated over 70 min at a flow rate of 4 ml/min. Starting and final buffers are the same as those used for the Q-Sepharose column.

13. Concentrate peaks eluted from the Mono-Q column in an Amicon ultrafiltration cell (model M-3) to a volume of 400 µl. Inject samples into a Superose 12HR 10/30 column (300 × 10 mm), via a superloop, connected to the FPLC system. The mobile phase contains 0.5% Berol 185, 1 mM EDTA in 0.1 M Tris–HCl pH 7.4, at a flow rate of 0.4 ml/min. The total separation time is 75 min.

14. Separate eluted peaks from the different phases of FPLC chromatography on an SDS–PAGE Laemmli system.

15. Electrophoresed samples can be Western blotted and protein bands identified either by the use of staining monoclonal antibodies and/or N terminal gas phase sequencing (see *Protocol 5*).[a]

[a] Alternatively, separated protein bands can be characterized by two-dimensional tryptic peptide map analysis (18).

Protocol 5. Tandem lectin affinity and Mono-Q anion exchange FPLC chromatography (19,20)

Equipment and reagents

- Ultracentrifuge
- Bench centrifuge
- Sonicator
- Water-bath
- FPLC system
- Pharmacia HR10/10 (100 mm x10 mm)
- Superloop
- Mono-Q HR10/10 prepacked column (100 × 10 mm)
- Western blot
- Gas phase sequencer (Applied Biosystems)
- WGA–Sepharose 6MB

- Polyvinylidene difluoride membrane (Immobilion PVDF) (Millipore)
- Sodium deoxycholate (1%) (Merck, Darmstadt, Germany)
- Solubilization buffer: 1% (w/w) sodium deoxycholate in 10 mM Tris–HCl pH 8.2, 5 mM EDTA, 0.5 mg/ml leupeptin
- Loading buffer: 10 mM Tris–HCl pH 8.2, 0.5% DOC, 5 mM EDTA
- Eluting buffer: 2.5% (w/v) *N*-acetylglucosamine (Sigma)
- Ponceau S

Method

1. Treat platelet membranes for 30 min at 4°C with solubilization buffer.

2. Centrifuge the solubilized membrane suspension at 4°C for 30 min at 100 000 *g* and load the supernatant on to a lectin affinity column.

3. Pack the WGA–Sepharose 6MB into a glass column (HR10/10, 100 mm x10 mm), connect to a FPLC, and equilibrate in the loading buffer.

4. Load the supernatant of the platelet membranes on to the flow column (flow rate 0.5 ml/min) and then extensively wash with the loading buffer.

Protocol 5. *Continued*

5. Elute glycoproteins bound to the WGA–Sepharose 6MB with 2.5% (w/v) *N*-acetylglucosamine.

6. Dialyse eluted glycoproteins overnight against 10 mM Tris–HCl pH 7.4, 0.1% Lubrol PX and then run on a Mono-Q anion exchange column (HR5/5, 50 mm × 5 mm) as indicated in *Protocol 4*.

7. Characterize glycoproteins eluted from the Mono-Q column by monoclonal antibody affinity chromatography, immunoprecipitation, and Western blotting.[a]

[a] Glycoproteins separated by SDS–PAGE, using either the modification of Hunkapillar and Hood (21) or that introduced by Moos *et al.* (22), are transferred to a polyvinylidene difluoride membrane by the method of Matsudaira (23). Proteins immobilized on PVDF membrane are Ponceau S stained, excised, and sequenced using an automatic gas phase sequencer.

5. Generation and use of monoclonal antibodies to isolate and characterize glycoproteins involved in platelet adhesion (24–27)

Monoclonal antibodies can be produced against platelet glycoproteins either by immunizing mice with intact resting or activated platelets, isolated platelet membranes, a mixture of isolated glycoproteins obtained by affinity chromatography, or via the use vectors inducing expression of the protein of interest in mice. Handling animals for the production of hybridoma should follow the rules established by the French National Institute of Health (INSERM) or its equivalent in other countries.

5.1 Immunization schedule using intact platelets

(a) Day 1: Washed platelets resuspended in a Tyrode buffer, in the absence of bovine serum albumin, are diluted in 1 : 1 ratio with complete Freund's adjuvant. Six mice are injected with this mixture (50 μg of platelet proteins/animal) into the peritoneum.

(b) Day 14: The immunization is repeated but in incomplete Freund's adjuvant.

(c) Day 35: Injection of day 14 is repeated.

(d) Day 45: Blood is carefully collected from each animal by a tail bleed. Tubes bearing the collected blood is left overnight at room temperature and then microcentrifuged for 30 min. Isolated serum is tested at different dilutions against platelets in an ELISA or dot blot system for reactivity.

(e) Day 56: The mouse having the serum that gives the best response against platelet glycoproteins is selected for splenectomy. The selected animal is boosted by intravenous injection, in the tail, of 50 µg platelets. The other five animals are given a further injection, via the peritoneum, of 50 µg platelets in the presence of incomplete Freund's adjuvant.

(f) Day 59: Splenoctomy of the best responder is performed and the isolated spleen is used in the fusion.

Protocol 6. Generation of monoclonal antibodies

Equipment and reagents

- sp2/O-Ag14 (mouse myeloma cell line)
- RPMI 1640 containing sodium pyruvate, 2 mM glutamine, penicillin–streptomycin (200 U/ml), 10% fetal calf serum
- Polyethyleneglycol (PEG 4000) (Boehringer)
- Hypoxanthine aminopterin thymidine
- 96-well microtitreplates
- Petri dish
- Fetal calf serum
- Bovine serum albumin, fraction V (Boehringer Diagnostics)
- Isotyping kit (Amersham)
- Pristane (2,6,10,14-tetramethyl-pentadecane)

- Phosphate-buffered saline (sterile)
- Phosphate buffer pH 8.2: 0.14 M $Na_2HPO_4.2H_2O$ adjusted to pH 8.2 with NaH_2PO_4
- Phosphate buffer pH 6: 0.14 M $NaH_2PO_4.2H_2O$ adjusted to pH 6 with Na_2HPO_4
- 1 M Tris pH 9
- 1 M Tris pH 9 dialysed against PBS and concentrated
- Protein A–Sepharose column
- Citrate buffer pH 4.5: 0.1 M sodium citrate adjusted to pH 4.5 with citric acid
- Citrate buffer pH3: 0.1 M sodium citrate adjusted to pH 3 with sodium acetate

A. Myeloma cell culture

1. Thaw a tube of sp2/O-Ag14 (mouse myeloma cell line) ten days prior to the fusion and amplify cells in complete medium (RPMI 1640 containing sodium pyruvate, 2 mM glutamine, and 10% fetal calf serum) in order to have 60×10^6 cells at the day of the fusion.

2. Wash cells three times in RPMI 1640 medium without fetal calf serum. Count an aliquot of cells before the third centrifugation by diluting 1 : 1 in Trypan blue. Resuspend the pellet in 2 ml of RPMI without serum and keep in cell incubator at 37 °C.

B. Excision of the spleen

1. Sacrifice the best responding mouse following the guide-lines of the relevant health authorities.

2. Fix the mouse on to a dissection plate, spray with 70% ethanol, and cut open using sterile dissection tools.

3. Place the excised spleen in a Petri dish containing RPMI 1640 medium.

C. Preparation of lymphocytes

1. Transfer the spleen into a Petri dish containing 12 ml of RPMI 1640 medium and perfuse several times with 1 ml of medium to eliminate red blood cells.

Protocol 6. *Continued*

2. Remove about 1 mm of the two extremities of the spleen and transfer into another Petri dish containing 14 ml of medium.

3. Manually extrude spleen cells by the use of 1 ml syringes and 21 G needles, transfer to a tube, and leave decanting for 12 min at room temperature.

4. Take a sample of the supernatant, count the cells, and centrifuge for 10 min at 500 *g* at room temperature.

5. Wash cells once in RPMI 1640, resuspend in 5 ml of the same medium, and keep at 37 °C.

6. The ratio used for the fusion of lymphocytes (isolated from the spleen) to myeloma cells (sp2/O cells) is 5 : 1 but it can also be 10 : 1. The number of sp2/O cells necessary to achieve a 5 : 1 ratio is added to the 5 ml of medium containing the isolated lymphocytes (see step 5).

7. Increase the volume of the suspension to 20 ml with RPMI medium and add 100 ml of PEG 4000.

8. Incubate cells for 1 h at 37 °C.

D. Fusion

1. Centrifuge cell suspension for 15 min at 37 °C.

2. Add 1 ml of PEG to the pellet over a period of 1 min by gentle shaking. Leave 30 sec before gently adding 10 ml of RPMI over 5 min, followed by 10 ml over 2 min, and finally 10 ml.

3. Centrifuge suspension for 15 min at 25 °C.

4. Resuspend cell pellet at 2×10^5 cells/ml in RPMI 1640 containing sodium pyruvate, 2 mM glutamine, penicillin–streptomycin (200 U/ml), 10% fetal calf serum, and hypoxanthine aminopterine thymidine (50 x), and add to a 96-well microtitreplate.

5. Grow hybridomas for ten days with two changes of medium.

6. Test hybridomas by ELISA. Positive wells are passed in 24-well or 6-well plates in complete medium/hypoxanthine thymidine (50 x), and hybridomas amplified, cloned, and frozen in fetal calf serum/DMSO (10%).

E. Cloning and subcloning of hybridomas

1. Cloning and subcloning are carried out by limit dilutions. Add one drop of cells to 20 ml of complete medium and deliver 200 µl of suspension to half of the wells in a 96-well microtitreplate.

2. Add 10 ml of medium to the remaining suspension and deliver to the

second half of the plate. Continue until you have five plates with a ratio in the last one of one cell/well.

3. Grow clones for ten days without changing medium.

4. Test wells by ELISA, positive wells are amplified, subcloned (same protocol as for cloning), and frozen.

F. Isotyping of monoclonal antibodies

1. The class of heavy and light chains of monoclonal antibody is determined by using an isotyping kit according to the manufacturer's instructions (Amersham).

G. Production of ascites

1. Inject mice intraperitoneally with 200 μl of Pristane 10 to 21 days before injection of one million hybridoma cells in sterile PBS.

2. Wait ten days and anaesthetize the mouse. Collect ascites fluid in heparinized tubes.

3. Centrifuge at 3000 *g* for 10 min at 4°C. Supernatants rich in monoclonal antibody are then stored at –20°C.

H. Purification of monoclonal antibodies[a]

1. Thaw ascites, microcentrifuge, and dilute (1 : 1) in phosphate-buffered saline.

2. Adjust pH to 8.2 with 1 M Tris pH 9, and layer on top of the protein A–Sepharose column (Pharmacia).

3. Allow the sample to penetrate and equilibrate the protein A–Sepharose column (0.5 ml/min) in phosphate buffer pH 8.2.

4. Wash the column until baseline recovers its initial level. Elute IgG_1 with phosphate buffer pH 6, IgG_{2a} with citrate buffer pH 4.5, and IgG_{2b} with citrate buffer pH 3.

5. Neutralize eluted fraction with 1 M Tris pH 9, dialyse against PBS, and concentrate.

6. Determine protein concentration. Purified monoclonal antibody is stored at –20°C in the presence of 1% BSA.

[a] Murine IgG have the property to bind, by their Fc region, to protein A of *Staphylococcus aureus*. Therefore, they can be purified by affinity on a protein A–Sepharose column.

6. Platelet–leucocyte interactions

Activated platelets are known to interact with leucocytes via a number of glycoprotein receptors (e.g. P-selectin, CD36, $\alpha_v\beta_3$). Such an interaction can be characterized by observing the numbers of activated platelets rosetting around leucocytes. In rats, platelets and PMNs are obtained by drawing blood via a heart puncture. Platelet–leucocyte interactions can then be tested in the presence or absence of peptides or monoclonal antibodies directed against glycoproteins that are thought to play a role in such cell–cell interactions. The following method was used to investigate platelet–leucocyte rosetting.

Protocol 7. Human platelet–leucocyte rosetting (26)

Equipment and reagents

- Bench centrifuge
- Water-bath
- Phase-contrast microscope
- Cell incubator
- Laminar flow hood
- Bovine serum albumin, fraction V (Boehringer Diagnostics)
- ACD anticoagulant (see *Protocol 1*)
- Tyrode's buffer (see *Protocol 1*)
- Calcium-free Tyrode's buffer (see *Protocol 1*)

- Washed platelets (1 x 10^8/ml)
- U937 monocytic cells in exponential growth
- RPMI 1640 supplemented with Hepes and 0.5% BSA
- D-Phenylalanine-L-proline-L-arginine chloromethyl ketone (PPACK) (Calbiochem) (10^{-6} M)
- Minisorb tubes (Nunc)
- Neubauer counting chamber

Method

1. Wash U937 cells twice with RPMI 1640 supplemented with Hepes and 0.5% BSA. Resuspend at 3 × 10^6/ml and keep on ice throughout the experiment.

2. Activate platelets with 0.3 U/ml thrombin for 10 min and stop reaction with 10^{-6} M PPACK.

3. Mix platelets (50 μl) with U937 cells (100 μl) in Minisorb tubes and leave for 30 min at 4°C.

4. Count the number of platelets rosetting around U937 cells in a Neubauer counting chamber under a phase-contrast microscope. A rosette consists of at least two platelets around a U937 cell.

Protocol 8. Measurement of rat platelet–leucocyte interactions (28)

Equipment and reagents

- Ultracentrifuge
- Bench centrifuge
- Water-bath
- Phase-contrast microscope
- Sterile ACD anticoagulant for rat blood: 0.8% (w/v) citric acid, 2.2% (w/v) sodium citrate, 2.45% (w/v) glucose, pH 3–4.5
- Tyrode's buffer (see *Protocol 1*)

- Calcium-free Tyrode's buffer (see *Protocol 1*)
- Tris–glycine solution: 250 mM/litre Tris, 500 mM/litre glycine
- Bovine serum albumin, fraction V (Boehringer Mannheim)
- Dulbecco Eagle medium (DEM) (Gibco, 41966-029)
- Sterile 6% dextran solution

- Sterile Ficoll–histopaque, density 1077 (Sigma)
- Sterile 0.9% NaCl solution
- Sterile 0.2% NaCl solution
- Sterile 1.6% NaCl solution
- Sodium pentobarbital (Sanofi, France)
- EDTA (2%)
- Bovine thrombin (Hoffman La Roche, Diagnostica, Basel, Switzerland)
- D-Phenylalanine-L-proline-L-arginine chloromethyl ketone (PPACK) (Calbiochem) (10^{-6} M)
- Paraformaldehyde

A. Isolating and washing rat platelets

Animal handling follows the rules established by French National Institute of Health and Medical Research.

1. Anaesthetize the rat by intraperitoneal injection (0.11 ml/100 g of body weight) of sodium pentobarbital. Blood is obtained by heart punction and collected, after discarding the first millilitre, on ACD in a ratio of 2.5 ml of ACD to 7.5 ml of blood.

2. Centrifuge tubes bearing blood samples at 500 g for 15 min at 37 °C to obtain platelet-rich plasma (PRP). Carefully remove PRP, pool, and leave for 5 min at room temperature. The remaining blood sample is used for isolation of leucocytes (see below).

3. Centrifuge the PRP for 15 min at 1100 g at 37 °C, resuspend the pellet in calcium-free Tyrode's buffer containing 0.2% EDTA, and leave for 5 min at room temperature.

4. Centrifuge the platelet suspension for 15 min at 1100 g at 37 °C, and resuspend in 10 ml of calcium-free Tyrode's buffer. Leave the suspension for 5 min at room temperature. Count the platelets.

5. Centrifuge the platelet suspension for 15 min at 1100 g at 37 °C, and resuspend in calcium-free Tyrode's buffer at 10^8 platelets/ml. Leave the suspension for 5 min at room temperature.

6. Take two tubes of 7 ml of the platelet suspension. One for platelet activation and the other to serve as a control.

7. Activate platelets with 0.15 U/ml bovine thrombin for 10 min without stirring; stop the reaction with 10^{-6} M PPACK.

8. Centrifuge both tubes for 15 min at 1100 g at 37 °C, and resuspend the pellets in 10 ml of calcium-free Tyrode's buffer. Fix the platelet suspensions using paraformaldehyde (8%) by incubation for 1 h at room temperature. Add 1 ml of Tris–glycine solution and incubate for 15 min at room temperature.

9. Wash fixed platelets three times using the calcium-free Tyrode's buffer.

B. Isolating rat PMNs

1. Reconstitute blood samples to their former volume with sterile 0.9% NaCl and rock gently. Add sterile 6% dextran solution (1 : 10, v/v) and

Protocol 8. *Continued*

> mix gently. Leave for 30 min in a slanted position at room tempera-
> ture to allow red blood cells to sediment. Gently move tubes to a
> vertical position and leave for 5 min.

2. Prepare sterile 15 ml Falcon tubes containing 3 ml of Ficoll (1017 density). Carefully layer the plasma overlaying the red blood cells on the
   Ficoll. Centrifuge at 400 *g* for 30 min at 15°C.

3. Discard the supernatant and the ring containing the mononucleated
   cells. Resuspend the pellet containing PMNs in 40 ml of sterile 0.9%
   NaCl.

4. Centrifuge tubes at 300 *g* for 10 min at 15°C, and discard supernatant.
   Lyse red blood cells by adding 0.2% NaCl (10 ml) and then 1.6% NaCl
   (10 ml) agitating throughout.

5. Centrifuge tubes at 300 *g* for 10 min at 15°C. Discard the supernatant. Resuspend the pellet with 40 ml of sterile 0.9% NaCl and wash
   three times. Count the PMNs and resuspend in DMEM at $2–3 \times 10^7$
   cells/ml.

6. Determine platelet–leucocyte interactions by incubating 50 µl of
   washed rat platelet suspension (resting or activated) at 2×10^8
   platelets/ml with 20 µl neutrophil suspension at $2–3 \times 10^7$ cells/ml;
   maintain continuous agitation at 4°C for 30 min as described by Jungi
   et al. (29).

7. Use of PCR to identify glycoproteins involved in platelet adhesion (30)

Evidence that high quality RNA can be isolated from platelets has allowed
molecular biology techniques to be adapted to the study of platelet adhesion
glycoproteins. Polymerase chain reaction (PCR) technology has been extensively used for the molecular characterization of mutations in platelets of
patients with genetic disorders such as Glanzmann thrombasthenia or
Bernard–Soulier syndrome. These studies have provided a substantial
amount of information about platelet function.

The guanidine isothiocyanate/phenol/chloroform technique for the isolation of total RNA originally published by Chomczinski and Sacchi (31) was
adapted for the extraction of total platelet RNA (32,33). RNA is extremely
sensitive to RNases and extreme care must be taken to prevent contamination: we therefore recommend wearing gloves for all manipulations and using
disposable plastic in preference to glassware. All solutions must be treated
with diethylpyrocarbonate (DEPC) and autoclaved.

Protocol 9. Platelet RNA extraction

Equipment and reagents

- Microcentrifuge
- Spectrophotometer (260/280 nm)
- Horizontal agarose gel eletrophoresis system
- Lysis buffer: 4 M guanidinium thiocyanate, 25 mM sodium citrate pH 7.0, 0.5% sarcosyl, 0.1 M 2-mercaptoethanol
- 2 M sodium acetate pH 4
- Water saturated phenol (Sigma)
- Chloroform/isoamyl alcohol (24 : 1, v/v)
- Isopropanol
- 75% ethanol
- DEPC treated water (Sigma)
- Platelet-rich plasma (5×10^9 platelets)
- Eppendorf tubes
- Agarose (Sigma)

Method

1. Add 100 μl lysis buffer per 5×10^9 platelets.[a]

2. Add 100 μl 2 M NaAc, 1 ml water saturated phenol, and 200 μl chloroform/isoamyl alcohol to 1 ml platelet lysate.

3. Vortex and chill on ice for 15 min.

4. Centrifuge at 11000 *g* for 20 min and transfer the upper aqueous phase containing the RNA into a new Eppendorf tube.

5. Add an equal volume of isopropanol and allow the RNA to precipitate for at least 30 min at –20°C.

6. Microcentrifuge at 11000 *g* for 15 min and pour off supernatant.

7. Resuspend the pellet in 100 μl lysis buffer and perform a second isopropanol precipitation under the same conditions as above (steps 5 and 6).

8. Wash the pellet with 75% ethanol, air dry, and resuspend in an appropriate volume of DEPC treated water.[b,c,d]

[a] Since platelet RNA is relatively unstable it is advisable to store samples as lysates (up to six month at –80°C) and perform the extractions just before use.
[b] The concentration of RNA can be determined by measuring the OD_{260} of a sample aliquot: one OD_{260} unit corresponds to an RNA concentration of 40 μg/ml.
[c] Sample purity can be estimated from the ratio OD_{260}/OD_{280} which should range between 1.8 and 2. Protein or phenol contamination would decrease this ratio.
[d] Visualization of ribosomal RNAs after agarose gel electrophoresis and ethidium bromide staining is a good indication of the sample quality. Undegraded RNA should show sharp 28 and 18S rRNA bands, the 28S band staining being twice as intense as for the 18S band.

Protocol 10. Reverse transcription and PCR amplification

Equipment and reagents

- Microcentrifuge
- Spectrophotometer (260/280 nm)
- Thermocycler
- Random hexanucleotides p(dN)₆ (10 μM) (Boehringer Mannheim)
- Water-bath
- Oligo(dT)₁₅₋₁₈ (10 μM) (Boehringer Mannheim)
- MMLV-RT (Moloney murine leukaemia virus reverse transcriptase) (Gibco BRL)

Protocol 10. *Continued*

- RT buffer (10 x) (BRL)
- PCR buffer: 50 mM KCl, 0.04% gelatin (4 ×)
- *Taq* DNA polymerase (Amplitaq, Perkin Elmer)
- RNasin (BRL)
- dNTP set (Pharmacia)
- Mineral oil (Sigma)

A. Reverse transcription

1. Denature 2 µg platelet total RNA at 75 °C for 10 min. Chill on ice.
2. Add the following:
    - 250 µM dATP, dTTP, dGTP, and dCTP
    - 1 µM primer (p(dN)$_6$ or (dT)$_{15-18}$)[a]
    - 40 U RNasin
    - 500 U MMLV-RT
    - 10 × RT buffer (5 µl)
    - DEPC treated H$_2$O to a final volume of 50 µl
3. Incubate the reaction at 42 °C for 45 min.
4. Inactivate the reverse transcriptase at 95 °C for 5 min.

B. PCR amplification

1. To the RT reaction, add the following:
    - 4 × PCR buffer (25 µl)
    - 1 µM sense oligonucleotide
    - 1 µM antisense oligonucleotide

    Adjust the reaction volume to 99.5 µl.
2. Denature the samples at 99 °C for 7 min.
3. Incubate at the annealing temperature for 5 min.
4. Microcentrifuge (11 000 g) briefly to collect condensation.
5. Add 2.5 U *Taq* DNA polymerase and overlay with a drop of mineral oil to prevent evaporation.
6. Incubate again at the annealing temperature for 5 min.
7. Carry out 30 rounds of amplification under the following conditions:
    - denaturation, 60 sec at 94 °C
    - annealing, 90 sec at the annealing temperature[b]
    - elongation, 120 sec at 72 °C
8. Perform a final extention step at 72 °C for 7 min.

[a] First strand cDNA is reverse transcribed using either 'random hexanucleotides p(dN)$_6$', or 'oligo(dT)$_{15-18}$' depending on the position of the fragment to be amplified on the messenger sequence.
[b] The annealing temperature is set to 5 °C below the fusion temperature of the oligonucleotide. The fusion temperature can be estimated from the formula: FT = 2 AT + 4 GC.

The purified PCR fragments are inserted into a pUC (or pUC-derived) plasmid vector containing M13 sequences complementary to universal sequencing primers. The multiple cloning site of these vectors is contained within the β-galactosidase gene. Introducing an insert into the polylinker causes an interruption of the β-galactosidase gene. Thus, in the presence of X-Gal and IPTG, recombinant clones will form white colonies in contrast to the wild-type vector which will develop a blue colour.

Protocol 11. Subcloning

Equipment and reagents

- TAE buffer (50 x): 242 g Tris base, 57.1 ml glacial acetic acid, 37.2 g $Na_2EDTA.2H_2O$, 1 litre
- Gel loading buffer (6 x): 0.25% bromophenol blue, 0.25% xylene cyanol, 15% Ficoll 400
- Horizontal agarose gel electrophoresis system
- Geneclean (Bio 101)
- 10 mM ATP (Pharmacia)
- T4 DNA ligase and 10 x ligase buffer (Biolabs)
- SOC media: 2% bactotryptone, 0.5% bacto yeast extract, 10 mM NaCl, 2.5 mM KCl, 10 mM $MgCl_2$, 10 mM $MgSO_4$, 20 mM glucose

- LB broth/agar: 1% bactotrytone, 0.5% bacto yeast extract, 10 mM NaCl, 1.5% agar
- 100 mg/ml ampicillin (1000 x stock solution) (Sigma)
- 40 mg/ml X-Gal (5-bromo-4-chloro-3-indolyl-β-D-galactopyranoside) in dimethylformamide (Sigma)
- 100 mg/ml isopropyl-β-D-thiogalactopyranoside (IPTG)
- Incubator (37°C)
- Gyratory shaker incubator
- Competent *E. coli* XL1 Blue (Stratagene)
- pUC19 (Stratagene)

A. PCR analysis and fragment recovery

1. Add 1 × gel loading buffer and separate PCR products on an agarose gel.

2. Excise fragments from the gel and purify by gene cleaning or electro-elution.

B. Ligation and transformation of competent E. coli cells

1. Mix together:
   - 50 ng plasmid
   - purified PCR fragment (amount equivalent to a molar ratio insert : vector, 1 : 5)
   - 10 × ligase buffer (1 µl)
   - 500 µM ATP
   - 400 U T4 DNA ligase

   Make up to 10 µl and incubate at 12°C overnight.

2. Transform 100 µl competent[a] *E. coli* cells with 1 µl ligation reaction according to the technique described by Hanahan (34).

3. Incubate on ice for 30 min.

4. Transfer the tube to a 37°C water-bath for 60 sec.

149

Protocol 11. *Continued*

5. Add 400 µl pre-warmed SOC media and incubate at 37 °C for 60 min in a gyratory shaker incubator.

6. Spread transformed bacteria on LB agar plates containing 100 µg/ml ampicillin, 25 µl (40 mg/ml) X-Gal, and 40 µl (100 mg/ml) IPTG. Invert the plate and leave in a 37 °C incubator overnight.

C. Selection of recombinant clones

1. Inoculate 20 µl of the following PCR reaction cocktail with a few cells from white isolated colonies with the following:
   - 1 × *Taq* DNA polymerase buffer
   - 1 µM sense oligonucleotide
   - 1 µM antisense oligonucleotide
   - 0.5 U *Taq* DNA polymerase[b]

2. Perform 25 cycles of PCR amplification under the conditions described in *Protocol 10*.

3. Analyse PCR products on agarose gel.

[a] Competent cells are highly sensitive to mechanical lysis caused by pipetting. All mixing should be done by swirling or tapping the tube gently.
[b] Most thermostable DNA polymerases used in PCR add single adenosines to the 3′ end of polymerization products. Therefore, insertion of PCR products into a plasmid vector requires either:
(a) A polishing step of the PCR fragment to create blunt-ends: different enzymes such as the T7 DNA polymerase or the Klenow fragment can be used.
(b) In the presence of dTTP alone, the *Taq* DNA polymerase will add 3′ T-overhangs to the blunt-ended vector.
(c) Modified vectors with a 3′ T-overhang are commercially available and can be used for direct insertion of the PCR products (TA cloning, Invitrogen).

Double-stranded DNA minipreparations and sequencing reactions are performed according to the protocol described by Kraft *et al.* (35). The sequencing reaction is a modification of the Sequenase protocol.

Protocol 12. Sequencing

Equipment and reagents

- Centrifuge
- Microcentrifuge
- Sequencing gel apparatus
- Sequenase version 2 (USB)
- 5 M potassium acetate pH 4.8
- 1 mg/ml DNase-free RNase A (DNases are inactivated by boiling for 10 min)
- 1 : 1 (v/v) Tris pH 8 saturated phenol / chloroform
- 70% and 100% ethanol
- [³⁵S]dATP (3000 Ci/mmol, Amersham)
- Gel dryer
- X-ray films (Kodak XAR-5)
- Autoradiography cassettes
- Incubation buffer: 50 mM glucose, 10 mM EDTA, 25 mM Tris pH 8
- 0.2 M NaOH, 1% SDS
- Phenol/chloroform (1 : 1, v/v)
- 5 M NaCl

- 13% PEG
- 2 M NaCl, 2 mM EDTA
- 1 M Tris–HCl pH 4.5
- 3 M sodium acetate

A. *Plasmid minipreparation[a]*

1. Spin down saturated overnight cultures.

2. Resuspend cells in 100 µl of an ice-cold solution containing 50 mM glucose, 10 mM EDTA, 25 mM Tris pH 8. Incubate for 5 min at room temperature.

3. Add 200 µl of a freshly prepared solution of 0.2 M NaOH, 1% SDS. Mix samples gently by inversion and incubate on ice for 5 min.

4. Add 150 µl of ice-cold 5 M potassium acetate pH 4.8. Mix briefly by inversion and incubate on ice for 5 min.

5. Centrifuge at 11 000 *g*, 4 °C, for 10 min and transfer the supernatant to a new Eppendorf. Add RNase A (50 µg/ml) and incubate at 37 °C for 30 min.

6. Add an equal volume of phenol/chloroform, vortex, and spin for 2 min.

7. Transfer the aqueous phase into a fresh tube and ethanol precipitate. Wash the pellet with 70% ethanol, air dry, and resuspend in 16.8 µl H_2O.

8. Add 3.2 µl NaCl (5 M) and 20 µl PEG (13%). Mix well and incubate on ice for 30 min.

9. Centrifuge at 11 000 *g* for 10 min. Wash the pellet with 1 ml ice-cold 70% ethanol and resuspend in 20 µl H_2O.

B. *Sequencing reaction*

1. Add 2 µl of a freshly prepared solution of 2 M NaOH, 2 mM EDTA. Mix well and incubate at room temperature for 5 min.

2. On ice, add sequentially 8 µl 1 M Tris–HCl pH 4.5 and 3 µl 3 M sodium acetate. Add 75 µl 100% ethanol and allow DNA to precipitate on dry ice for 10 min.

3. Centrifuge at 11 000 *g*, 4 °C, for 5 min. Wash the pellet with 200 µl ice-cold 70% ethanol, air dry, and resuspend in 7 µl H_2O.

4. Add 1 µl sequencing primer (provided by the kit) and 2 µl 5 × Sequenase buffer (provided by the kit). Mix and incubate at 37 °C for 30 min.

5. Prepare four tubes containing 2.5 µl of one of the four termination mixes (ddGTP, ddATP, ddTTP, ddCTP) (provided by the kit). Pre-warm at 37 °C.

6. To the annealing mix, add 1 µl 0.1 M DTT, 2 µl 1 : 5 diluted labelling mix (provided by the kit), 0.5 µl (4 mCi) [^{35}S]dATP, and 2 µl 1 : 8

Protocol 12. *Continued*

diluted Sequenase enzyme (provided by the kit). Incubate at room temperature for 5 min.

7. Transfer 3.5 µl labelling reaction into each of four termination mix tubes and incubate at 37 °C for 5 min.

8. Add 4 µl stop solution (provided by the kit) containing the dye markers to each tube.

9. Denature samples at 70 °C for 3 min and load on a sequencing gel (6% acrylamide, 8 M urea). Run the gel at 1500 V in 1 × TBE buffer until the blue dye runs off. Dry gel and expose to X-ray film for at least 16 h.

[a] A 3 ml saturated overnight culture from the selected clones provides sufficient amounts of material for a sequencing reaction.

References

1. McGregor, J. L. (1995). In *Immunopharmacology of platelets* (ed. M. Joseph). Academic Press, London.
2. Mustard, J. F., Perry, D. W., Ardlie, N. G., and Packham, M. A. (1972). *Br. J. Haematol.*, **22**, 193.
3. Parmentier, S., Catimel, B., McGregor, L., Leung, L., and McGregor, J. L. (1991). *Blood*, **78**, 2021.
4. Massini, P. and Lûscher, E. F. (1974). *Biochim. Biophys. Acta*, **372**, 109.
5. McGregor, J. L., Clemetson, K. J., James, E., and Dechavanne, M. (1979). *Thromb. Res.*, **16**, 437.
6. Lowry, O. H., Rosenbrough, N. J., Farr, A. L., and Randall, R. J. (1951). *J. Biol. Chem.*, **193**, 265.
7. Read, S. M. and Northcote, D. H. (1981). *Anal. Biochem.*, **116**, 53.
8. Laemmli, E. K. (1970). *Nature*, **227**, 680.
9. O'Farrell, P. H. (1975). *J. Biol. Chem.*, **250**, 4007.
10. McGregor, J. L., Clemetson, K. J., James, E., Lûscher, E. F., and Dechavanne, M. (1980). *Biochim. Biophys. Acta*, **599**, 473.
11. McGregor, J. L., Clemetson, K. J., James, E., Capitanio, A., Greenland, T., Lûscher, E. F., *et al.* (1981). *Eur. J. Biochem.*, **116**, 379.
12. Holbrook, I. B. and Leaver, A. G. (1976). *Anal. Biochem.*, **75**, 634.
13. Merril, C. R., Goldman, D., and Van Keuren, M. L. (1982). *Electrophoresis*, **3**, 17.
14. Morrissey, J. H. (1981). *Anal. Biochem.*, **117**, 307.
15. Kapitany, R. A. and Zebrowski, E. J. (1973). *Anal. Biochem.*, **56**, 361.
16. Bonner, R. A. and Laskey, A. D. (1975). *Eur. J. Biochem.*, **56**, 335.
17. McGregor, J. L., Catimel, B., Parmentier, S., Clezardin, P., Dechavanne, M., and Leung, L. (1989). *J. Biol. Chem.*, **264**, 501.
18. McGregor, J. L., Clemetson, K. J., James, E., Clezardin, P., Dechavanne, M., and Lûscher, E. (1982). *Biochim. Biophys. Acta*, **689**, 513.
19. Catimel, B., Parmentier, S., Leung, L., and McGregor, J. L. (1991). *Biochem. J.*, **279**, 419.

20. Catimel, B., Leung, L., El Ghissassi, H., Mercier, N., and McGregor, J. L. (1992). *Biochem. J.*, **284,** 231.
21. Hunkapillar, M. J. and Hood, L. E. (1983). In *Methods in enzymology* (ed. H. W. Hirsc and S. N. Timasheff), Vol. 91, pp. 486–93. Academic Press, London.
22. Moos, M., Nguyen, N. Y., and Liu, T. Y. (1988). *J. Biol. Chem.*, **263,** 6005.
23. Matsudaira, P. (1987). *J. Biol. Chem.*, **262,** 10035.
24. McGregor, J. L., Brochier, J., Wild, F., Follea, G., Trzeciak, M. C, James, E., *et al.* (1983). *Eur. J. Biochem.*, **131,** 427.
25. McGregor, J. L., McGregor, L., Bauer, A. S., Catimel, B., Brochier, J., Decha-vanne, M., *et al.* (1986). *Eur. J. Biochem.*, **159,** 443.
26. Parmentier, S., McGregor, L., Catimel, B., Leung, L., and McGregor, J. L. (1991). *Blood*, **77,** 1734.
27. Daviet, L., Buckland, R., Puente-Navazo, M. D., and McGregor, J. L. (1995). *Biochem. J.*, **305,** 221.
28. Chignier, E., Sparagano, M. H., McGregor, L., Thillier, A., Pellechia, D., and McGregor, J. L. (1994). *Comp. Biochem. Physiol.*, **109 A,** 881.
29. Jungi, T. W., Spycher, M. O., Nydegger, J. E., and Barandum, S. (1986). *Blood*, **67,** 629.
30. Wyler, B., Daviet, L., Bortkiewicz, H., Bordet, J. C., and McGregor, J. L. (1993). *Thromb. Haemost.*, **70,** 500.
31. Chomczynski, P. and Sacchi, N. (1987). *Anal. Biochem.*, **162,** 156.
32. Newman, P. J., Gorki, J., White II, G. C., Gidwitz, S., Cretney, C. J., and Aster, R. H. (1989). *J. Clin. Invest.*, **82,** 739.
33. Djaffar, I., Vilette, D., Bray, P. F., and Rosa, J. P. (1991). *Thromb. Res.*, **62,** 127.
34. Hanahan, D. (1983). *J. Mol. Biol.*, **166,** 557.
35. Kraft, R., Tardiff, J., Krauter, K. S., and Leinwand, L. A. (1988). *Biotechniques*, **6,** 544.

Monoclonal antibodies to platelet cell surface antigens and their use

J. MICHAEL WILKINSON

1. Introduction

The introduction of the technique of monoclonal antibody (mAb) preparation in 1975 revolutionized the study of cell surface molecules, and this has been as true for platelets as for any other type of cell. mAb have been used both to characterize molecules previously defined by other methods and also to identify new molecules, by immunization of mice with whole platelets or platelet plasma membrane fractions. Like any other cell type, platelets express a wide variety of cell surface proteins whose surface density may vary from tens to tens of thousands of molecules per cell. Many of the major surface glycoproteins are involved in the wide variety of adhesive interactions which platelets are able to undergo (1) and whose activity is tightly controlled during platelet activation. This control may be by conformational changes in existing cell surface molecules, notably in GPIIb–IIIa to reveal its fibrinogen (Fg) binding site, or by modulation of the level of cell surface expression, as for the platelet selectin, GMP 140. Other major surface glycoproteins, such as the CD9 antigen, have, as yet, no known or well defined function. There are in addition many minor surface proteins, which include receptors of various types and many other molecules of unknown function. mAb may thus be used for the definition of those proteins which are present on the surface of either resting or activated platelets, both in qualitative or quantitative terms. They may also be used for affinity purification, as described in Chapter 7, for further structural and functional characterization. In addition, the exquisite specificity of mAb for a single epitope on a particular protein means that they can be used as probes for particular structures or functions. A variety of mAb has been described, some of which are able to inhibit aggregation and activation while others are able to promote these functions. Hence they are ideal reagents for the characterization of the activities which are responsible for the transformation of resting discoid platelets into multicellular aggregates.

It is impossible within the compass of a short chapter to provide a comprehensive list of the very large number of mAb which have been shown to recognize structures on the platelet surface, and no attempt has been made to do so. Most of the commercial suppliers of immunological reagents carry such mAb in their listings and should provide an appropriate characterization for each one. In most cases it will be necessary to refer to the original literature for more precise details of reactivity. The mAb which are listed here are representative of those which cause platelet aggregation or activation, or which are able to inhibit those activities, and others which can be used to monitor the state of platelet activation.

2. Platelet activation by mAb to cell surface molecules

There are a number of mAb whose addition to a platelet suspension has been shown to cause activation or aggregation. An understanding of the reasons for these activities is important both because such activation may interfere with the use of the mAb for other purposes and also because it may illuminate basic platelet functions. Three such mechanisms have been identified:

- activation through the platelet Fc receptor (FcγRII)
- complement activation
- direct activation of the Fg binding site on GPIIb–IIIa

Each of these will be considered in turn. Stimulation of signalling through FcγRII is probably the most common cause of mAb-induced aggregation and the expression and signalling functions of the FcγRII on platelets will be considered first.

2.1 FcγRII-mediated activation

2.1.1 The platelet Fc receptor

Three types of Fcγ receptors, FcγRI, FcγRII, and FcγRIII, are expressed on haemopoietic cells (2). In comparison with other cell types, Fc receptor expression on platelets is comparatively simple and is restricted to the FcγRII, or CD32, molecule, a 40 kDa glycoprotein. FcγRII is coded for by three closely linked genes, FcγRIIA, B, and C, which can give rise to at least six isoforms by alternative splicing. In platelets only the FcγRIIA form is expressed, as a single transmembrane isoform, which has two polymorphic variants. Individuals can be divided into high responders (HR) or low responders (LR) either on the basis of a CD3-dependent T cell proliferation assay or by using anti-FcγRII mAb. There are population differences in the expression of these two forms, with 70% of Caucasian individuals being HR and 30% LR, while in Asian populations the percentages are 15% HR and 85% LR. The basis of the polymorphism is a single amino acid substitution at

Table 1. mAb to FcγRII

mAb	Subclass	Alleles	Supplier	Reference
IV.3	IgG$_{2b}$	Both	Medarex	5
41H16	IgG$_{2a}$	R/R131		6
CIKM5	IgG$_1$	Both		7
KU79	IgG	Both		8
KB61	IgG$_1$	Both		9
2E1	IgG$_{2a}$	Both	Immunotech	10

position 131 of an Arg (R131), in HR individuals, for a His (H131) in LR individuals. Most mAb to FcγRII recognize both forms, but 41H16 binds strongly to R131 but only weakly or not at all to H131 (see *Table 1*). Individuals can be classified into three groups on the basis of the 41H16/IV.3 binding ratio as determined by flow cytometry (3). These groups correspond to R/R131 and H/H131 homozygous and R/H131 heterozygous individuals. Reproducible variations in the level of expression of FcγRII on platelets from different individuals are also found. While the levels of expression of FcγRII may vary from 1600 to 4600 molecules per platelet in different individuals, these levels are stable over an extended period. There is no significant difference in levels of expression between the three different groups.

FcγRII is a low affinity receptor which will only bind aggregated IgG. It shows selectivity in binding to the various subclasses of both human and mouse IgG. For human this is $3 > 1 = 2 > 4$, while for mouse the order is $1 > 2b > 2a = 3$. The cytoplasmic region of FcγRII contains an activation motif which is thought to bind to a src-family tyrosine kinase. Cross-linking of receptors by binding of aggregated IgG leads to kinase activation, with consequent triggering of intracellular signalling pathways leading to cell activation (4). This sequence of events appears to hold true for all cells expressing FcγRIIA and its consequences for platelet activation are discussed below.

2.1.2 Activation through the FcγRII

Platelet activation via the FcγRII has been investigated using the anti-FcγRII mAb, IV.3 (see *Table 1*). Washed platelets were incubated with IV.3 and then cross-linked with F(ab')$_2$ goat anti-mouse IgG (GAM). No aggregation occurred after binding of IV.3 but subsequent cross-linking of FcγRII with GAM in a stirred platelet suspension gave a strong aggregation response. This type of aggregation was also observed when another anti-FcγRII mAb, KU79, was used, showing that this is a general phenomenon associated with the cross-linking of platelet FcγRII (11).

The first characteristic of the aggregation response to be noted is that it is preceded by a lag phase which is inversely related to the concentration of

GAM used. This lag phase is interpreted as being due to the need to reach a sufficient degree of cross-linking before activation is triggered. Activation is accompanied both by an increase in inositol phosphate turnover and by the mobilization of intracellular Ca^{2+}.

Treatment of platelets with the IgG_1 anti-FcγRII mAb, CIKM5, causes aggregation without the need for GAM cross-linking. This mAb, and other IgG_1 anti-FcγRII mAb, can clearly bind to the FcγRII both through their antigen binding site and their Fc, whereas IgG_{2a} and IgG_{2b} mAb only bind via the antigen binding site and require further cross-linking to cause activation. Anti-FcγRII mAb cause aggregation of LR (H/H131) platelets, either directly or after GAM cross-linking, to much the same extent as they do HR (R/R131) platelets (12). This confirms that the difference between the molecules is in their ability to bind IgG rather than their capacity to initiate intracellular signalling events.

2.1.3 mAb Fc interaction with FcγRII

mAb to a number of different platelet surface antigens have been shown to cause platelet aggregation and activation in a manner which is very similar to that described above for cross-linking of FcγRII. Where full investigations have been carried out, it is clear that activation is stimulated via the FcγRII. *Table 2* lists some of the well characterized mAb which show this effect, together with others which illustrate the range of antigens involved. This list is in no way exhaustive and many other mAb show similar effects; it is also probable that activating mAb to other antigens will be identified in the future. The characteristics of all these mAb is that, with the exception of 50H.19, which is discussed below, they are all of the IgG_1 subclass. Aggregation in all cases occurs following a concentration-dependent lag phase and is inhibitable by the anti-FcγRII mAb, IV.3. In most cases Fab or F(ab')$_2$ are not effective in causing aggregation and inhibit activation by whole antibody. Aggregation is accompanied by dense granule secretion, as measured by 5-HT release, and by the mobilization of intracellular Ca^{2+}. In a number of cases variations in the aggregation response between platelets from different donors have been noted and this correlates with FcγRII allele expression. *Table 2* illustrates the range of surface proteins to which activating mAb are directed. It appears that most IgG_1 mAb to the CD9 and CD36 antigens will act as activators, whereas only a limited number of those to GPIIb–IIIa act in this way. A number of mAb to minor surface components, including CD69 and β$_2$-microglobulin, will also cause aggregation. It is likely that antigen clustering is required for activation and that proteins must be free to diffuse in the plasma membrane. No mAb to the major cell surface protein, GPIb–IX, which is anchored to the membrane skeleton (see Chapter 11), have been shown to cause aggregation. Activation could take place as a result of cross-linking of antigen and FcγRII either on the same or on adjacent platelets. While both are possible, the consensus view is that mAb binding causes

Table 2. mAb which cause platelet activation

mAb	Subclass	CD antigen	Antigen	M_r (kDa)	Surface expression (molecules/cell)	Conc. of mAb (µl/ml)	Inhibition by: Fab	IV.3	Reference
ALB6	IgG$_1$	CD9	–	25	35–65 000	2	Fab	+	13,14
SYB1	IgG$_1$	CD9	–	25	35–65 000	2	F(ab')$_2$	+	15
50H.19	IgG$_{2a}$	CD9	–	25	35–65 000	10	†	+	16
6C9	IgG$_1$	CD41/CD61	GPIIb–IIIa	140/105	40–65 000	0.4	‡	ND	17
P256	IgG$_1$	CD41/CD61	GPIIb–IIIa	140/105	40–65 000	3	‡	+	18
PM6/248	IgG$_1$	CD41/CD61	GPIIb–IIIa	140/105	40–65 000	2	F(ab')$_2$	+	19
OKM5	IgG$_1$	CD36	GPIV	88	25 000	2	F(ab')$_2$	ND	20
8A6	IgG$_1$	CD36	GPIV	88	25 000	5	ND	+	3
Leu23	IgG$_1$	CD69	–	34/28	ND	12	Fab	ND	21
B2.62.2	IgG$_1$	–	β$_2$m	13	ND	10	F(ab')$_2$	+	22
LeoA1	IgG$_1$	–	–	67	1200	1.5	ND	+	23
JS1	IgG$_1$	–	–	155	ND	20	F(ab')$_2$	+	24

ND: not determined; †: immobilized F(ab')$_2$ causes activation; ‡: F(ab')$_2$ causes partial aggregation.

clustering of antigen on one platelet which then presents an immune complex to the FcγRII of an adjacent platelet, thus triggering activation.

The response obtained is similar, regardless of the surface density of the antigen involved, although it is related to the nature and density of surface expression of FcγRII on the platelets of any individual (3). The optimal activating concentration of any mAb is in the range of 1–10 µg/ml, which again is not related to the surface density of the antigen.

2.2 Complement-mediated activation

A number of antiplatelet mAb which are of the IgG_{2a} and IgG_{2b} subclass cause platelet aggregation and activation, which is not inhibitable by mAb IV.3. Further investigation shows that this is due to platelet lysis, mediated by C1q fixation. The complement dependence of this phenomenon can be demonstrated by resuspending washed or gel filtered platelets, before stimulation, in serum which has been heat treated (57 °C, 30 min) or absorbed with an antiserum to C1q. Both treatments inhibit activation. Complement-mediated aggregation has been demonstrated for mAb to both CD9 and GPIIb–IIIa. As with FcγRII-mediated activation, it is probable that, for complement fixation to occur, there is a requirement for mAb-induced clustering of antigen on the cell surface.

Platelets express a C1q receptor (C1qR), a 67 kDa transmembrane protein, and can be activated either by immobilized C1q or by soluble C1q complexes. This aggregation is accompanied by the release of granule contents and the activation of Fg binding by GPIIb–IIIa. It can be inhibited by an IgM mAb to the C1qR, II1/D1 (25). It is likely that mAb-stimulated, complement-mediated aggregation occurs through this mechanism.

Although the subclass dependence of FcγRII- or complement-mediated activation is, on the whole, clear cut, two IgG_{2a} anti-CD9 mAb, BU16 and 50H.19, have been reported to give activation, in the presence of heat inactivated serum, which is inhibitable by mAb IV.3. These mAb are clearly capable of activating platelets by either mechanism, depending on the conditions.

2.3 Direct activation of Fg binding to GPIIb–IIIa

Activation of integrins switches them from a resting state to an activated state which is able to bind ligand; this conformational transition is accompanied by the exposure of 'ligand-induced binding sites' (LIBS). mAb which recognize such binding sites on GPIIb–IIIa may be able to stabilize the conformation of the Fg binding site or cause its exposure and hence induce aggregation in the presence of Fg. Details of two well characterized mAb which possess this property are shown in *Table 3*. Characteristically, these mAb are able to cause aggregation of platelets by stimulation of Fg binding, but this is not accompanied by secretion or other activation reactions. Aggregation in both cases can be stimulated by Fab fragments, ruling out both the

Table 3. mAb causing GPIIb–IIIa activation

mAb	Subclass	Antigen	Binding sites/platelet	Reference
D33C	IgG$_1$	GPIIb	44 000	26
D3GP3	IgG$_1$	GPIIIa	5000	27,28

involvement of FcγRII and agglutination by cross-linking. It has been postu-lated that activating mAb such as these may alter the equilibrium in favour of the Fg binding form, however the fact that the anti-GPIIIa mAb, D3GP3, can only bind to a minority of the GPIIb–IIIa molecules on the platelet surface suggests that this may not always be the case.

As noted in *Table 2*, the F(ab')$_2$ fragments of two of the anti-GPIIb–IIIa mAb which are able to cause FcγRII-mediated activation, 6C9 and P256, cause aggregation, but without any accompanying activation. Unlike D33C and D3GP3, Fab fragments of these mAb are not effective in this respect, and it is not clear why divalent fragments are required. It is probable, there-fore, that P256 and 6C9 are able to cause platelet aggregation by two different mechanisms.

2.4 Characteristics of mAb-induced platelet aggregation

From the foregoing it is clear that each of the three types of mAb-induced aggregation has its own characteristics and that they can be distinguished by a number of preliminary experimental manipulations. These need to address the following questions:

(a) Is aggregation accompanied by a full activation response, including gran-ule secretion, as measured by 5-HT release, and by Ca^{2+} mobilization?

(b) Is aggregation inhibited by prior incubation with anti-FcγRII mAb, par-ticularly mAb IV.3?

(c) Is aggregation still observed when F(ab')$_2$ or Fab fragments are used. Is there a difference between the response to F(ab')$_2$ and Fab?

(d) Is aggregation still observed when gel filtered platelets, with or without added Fg, are used or when platelet-rich plasma is reconstituted with heat treated plasma or serum?

(e) Are there differences in response between individual donors. Can these be related to the FcγRII phenotype?

With experiments designed to test these various possibilities, it should be possible to distinguish between mAb which cause direct aggregation and those which are dependent on the FcγRII or the C1qR. As indicated previously, it should not be forgotten that a single mAb may operate through more than one mechanism.

3. mAb which recognize platelet activation antigens

Platelet activation by physiological agonists gives rise to degranulation and the incorporation of both granule and lysosomal membranes into the cell surface membrane. Integral proteins of granule and lysosomal membranes thus become exposed at the cell surface and may be used as markers of activation. mAb to these proteins may be used to monitor the activation process. Below are given brief descriptions of the most important of such antigens, and *Table 4* gives details of some of the mAb which recognize them.

3.1 CD62

The CD62 antigen, otherwise known as P-selectin, GMP 140, or PADGEM, is an integral membrane protein of 140 kDa found in the α granules of resting platelets and in the Weibel–Palade bodies of endothelial cells (35). It is a member of the selectin family of adhesion molecules and recognizes carbohydrate ligands related to sialyl Le^x. Activation of platelets with either strong agonists, such as thrombin, or weak ones, such as ADP, causes a rapid translocation of CD62 to the cell surface where it mediates adhesion, principally to neutrophils. Anti-CD62 mAb have been used to monitor platelet activation and some, but not all, are able to inhibit platelet adhesion to neutrophils (see *Table 4*).

3.2 CD63

The CD63 antigen is a 30–60 kDa integral membrane protein of lysosomal membranes whose function is unknown. It was originally described in platelets but has since been shown to be of wide distribution. It belongs to the newly recognized tetraspan protein family, which also includes the CD9, CD37, and CD53 molecules (36). Thrombin stimulation causes the antigen to

---

Table 4. mAb to activation antigens

Molecule	mAb	Subclass	Activity	Reference
CD62	S12	IgG$_1$	Weak inhibition	29
CD62	AC1.2	IgG$_1$	No inhibition	30
CD62	CLB-thromb/6	IgG$_1$	Strong inhibition	31
CD63	RUU SP2.28	IgG$_{2b}$		32
CD63	H5C6	IgG$_1$		33
Granulophysin	D503	IgG$_1$		29
Granulophysin	D519	IgG$_{2a}$		29
Granulophysin	D545	IgG$_1$		29
LAMP-1	H5G11	IgG$_1$		34
LAMP-2	H4B4	IgG$_1$		34

---

be expressed on the platelet surface where it becomes a major protein constituent. Its level of expression increases from 650 molecules per unstimulated platelet to 12 600 after stimulation (32). The platelet dense granule protein, granulophysin, is also present in lysosomal membranes, with a similar distribution to CD63. Current evidence strongly suggests that CD63 and granulophysin are the same molecule (37).

3.3 LAMP-1 and LAMP-2

These lysosome-associated membrane proteins (LAMP) are, like CD63, integral proteins of the lysosomal membrane. In the platelet both have been shown to be heavily glycosylated molecules of around 110 kDa (38). Surface expression of these proteins requires activation by a strong agonist such as thrombin, ADP being ineffective. After activation, levels of expression are an order of magnitude less than those of CD63, there being less than 2000 molecules of each per platelet. LAMP-1 and LAMP-2 have recently been given the Leucocyte Workshop designations of CD107a and CD107b, respectively.

4. mAb which inhibit platelet aggregation

The final topic to be considered is those mAb which are able to inhibit the major platelet function of Fg binding, and hence aggregation. A considerable number of inhibitory mAb have been described, some of which recognize the GPIIb–IIIa complex and some either GPIIb or GPIIIa. A limited number are described briefly in this section and are shown in *Table 5*.

The first, and possibly most interesting, is the IgM mAb, PAC1, which has been shown to recognize a neo-epitope on GPIIb–IIIa, revealed when platelets are activated. The uniqueness of PAC1 lies in the fact that the site recognized is the Fg binding site itself and the sequence of part of the mAb binding site has been shown to mimic that of Fg. PAC1 is thus not only an inhibitor of aggregation but also an activation marker. PAC1 Fab has recently been produced in a baculovirus expression system. The specificity of the Fab is the same as that of the whole IgM, but the binding affinity is lower. This system allows mutations to be introduced into the antigen binding site in order to explore the basis of the specificity. It may also prove to be a useful way of producing Fab fragments which are difficult to prepare by other means (39).

Three other mAb which inhibit aggregation are shown in *Table 5*. They inhibit Fg binding by interacting with different sites near to, but separate from, the Fg binding site. 7E3 and its F(ab′)$_2$ fragment have been extensively used, both *in vitro* and *in vivo*, to inhibit aggregation.

Table 5. mAb which inhibit fibrinogen binding

mAb	Subclass	Antigen	Reference
PAC1	IgM	GPIIb–IIIa	40
10E5	IgG$_{2a}$	GPIIb–IIIa	41
7E3	IgG$_1$	GPIIb–IIIa	42
M148	IgG$_1$	GPIIb–IIIa	43

5. Immunodetection of cell surface proteins

A variety of methods using mAb to study platelet surface proteins are available. The major fluorescence methods are described in Chapters 6 and 14, while those for surface labelling and immunoprecipitation are given in Chapter 7. Methods described here are for ELISA assays and for immunoblotting. The ELISA methods given (*Protocol 1*) use both whole, formaldehyde fixed platelets, and purified or partially purified protein fractions as target antigens, to be detected by the direct binding of mAb. The ELISA technique is capable of very great variation and assays can be designed which involve sandwich techniques in which the antibody rather than the antigen is immobilized. A full discussion of such methods is beyond the scope of this book. Western blotting methods are a useful alternative to immunoprecipitation. Proteins either from whole platelets, solubilized by boiling in SDS buffer, or from purified membrane fractions may be separated by SDS–PAGE, transferred electorphoretically to nitrocellulose membrane, and analysed by probing with appropriate mAb. It should, however, be borne in mind that only a minority of mAb, particularly of those to membrane glycoproteins, give positive results in Western blotting. Thus the mAb to be used must be chosen with care and proteins must be run on SDS–PAGE both before and after reduction of disulfide bonds.

Protocol 1. ELISA techniques

Equipment and reagents

- Phosphate-buffered saline (PBS) (10 ×): 80 g NaCl, 2 g KCl, 11.5 g NaHPO$_4$, 2 g KH$_2$PO$_4$ per litre (dilute as required)
- To flick-wash plates: fill wells with wash solution, flick out into sink, and blot inverted plate on to paper towel to remove excess liquid
- Dissolve *o*-phenylene diamine (OPD) (Sigma, P9029) in MeOH at 10 mg/ml—store 1 ml aliquots in microcentrifuge tubes at –20°C
- 96-well Nunc Immunoplates
- Phosphate–citrate buffer pH 5.0: make stock solutions of 0.05 M citric acid and 0.1 M Na$_2$HPO$_4$—add 48.6 ml citric acid to 51.4 ml Na$_2$HPO$_4$
- ELISA substrate solution: make up 1 ml OPD solution (1 mg) to 25 ml with phosphate–citrate buffer, add 10 µl 30% H$_2$O$_2$ (make up *immediately* before use and keep

A. Preparation of fixed platelet plates

1. Add 50 µl of poly-L-lysine solution (Sigma, P1024) (1 mg/100 ml in PBS) to each well. Leave for 30 min at room temperature and flick out.

---

2. Suspend formaldehyde fixed platelets at 40×10^6/ml in PBS. Add 50 µl per well. Centrifuge in microtitre plate holders at 2000 r.p.m. for 5 min.

3. Add 50 µl 0.05% glutaraldehyde in PBS per well. Leave for 15 min at room temperature.

4. Flick wash plates two or three times with PBS.

5. Add 150 µl gelatin in PBS (20 mg/100 ml) and leave for 1 h at room temperature.

6. Plates may be stored at –20 °C until required.

B. Preparation of protein-coated plates

1. Dissolve protein, at 10 µg/ml, in 0.05 M Na_2CO_3 pH 9.6 (1.59 g Na_2CO_3, 2.93 g $NaHCO_3$, 0.2 g NaN_3 per litre). Add 100 µl per well.

2. Incubate overnight at 4 °C.

C. Assay procedure

1. Wash plates three times in PBST (0.05% Tween 20 in PBS).

2. Add 50 µl of mAb solution to each well, with duplicates for all tests, and appropriate positive and negative controls. Leave for 30 min at room temperature.

3. Wash three times with PBST.

4. Add 100 µl peroxidase-conjugated goat anti-mouse Ig H+L (Bio-Rad, 170–6516), diluted in PBST. The optimal dilution must be determined by titration. Leave for 1 h at room temperature.

5. Wash five times with PBST.

6. Add 150 µl OPD solution per well. Leave for 30 min at room temperature in the dark.

7. Add 50 µl 2 M H_2SO_4 to stabilize colour.

8. Read absorbance at 495 nm in a microtitre plate reader.

Protocol 2. Western blotting

Equipment and reagents

- SDS–PAGE separations should be carried out as described in Chapter 7—the following procedure is described for use with Bio-Rad or Hoeffer mini-gels
- Gels should be stained with Coomassie blue and destained with 7% acetic acid/25% MeOH—they may be stored before blotting in destain solution for an indefinite period
- Cathode buffer: 25 mM Tris, 40 mM amino caproic acid, 20% MeOH
- Anode buffer 1: 25 mM Tris, 20% MeOH
- Anode buffer 2: 300 mM Tris, 20% MeOH
- Semi-dry electroblotter (Sartorius or similar)
- Nitrocellulose membrane, cut to size of gel

Protocol 2. *Continued*

- Whatman 3MM filter paper, cut to be 1 cm larger all round than gel
- Wash buffer: PBS containing 0.3% Tween 20
- Peroxidase substrate: dissolve 50 mg diaminobenzidine (DAB) (Sigma, D8001) in 100 ml PBS and add 100 μl 30% H_2O_2

A. Discontinuous blotting

1. Equilibrate stained gel in SDS–PAGE running buffer (0.25 M Tris, 1.92 M glycine pH 8.3), containing 1% SDS, for 30 min.

2. Soak three sheets of filter paper in cathode buffer and place on cathode plate.

3. Place gel on paper.

4. Rinse nitrocellulose in distilled water and place on gel, making sure that there are no bubbles between them by rolling with a glass rod.

5. Cover with two sheets of filter paper soaked in anode buffer 1 and complete the sandwich with one sheet of filter paper soaked in anode buffer 2.

6. Cover with cathode plate and run at 40 mA/gel for about 2 h. During this time the Coomassie blue stain will dissociate from the proteins and will be transferred to the membrane, it provides an image of the original gel but does not interfere with immunostaining. The efficiency of protein transfer may be checked by restaining the gel. It is probable that some high M_r proteins will only give partial transfer.

7. Block the nitrocellulose membrane by storing in 1.5% gelatin in PBS at 4 °C, overnight, or longer, if need be.

B. Immunostaining

1. Dissolve gelatin by warming and wash blot in several changes of wash buffer. Cut membrane into appropriate tracks with a scalpel blade. A slotted block of appropriate size is convenient for subsequent incubations, together with a rocking table. Square plastic Petri dishes (Bibby-Sterilin) are suitable for incubating larger blots.

2. Incubate strips with mAb for 1 h at room temperature. For tissue culture supernatant this may be undiluted. For ascites or purified Ig, a dilution should be made in wash buffer. Determine the optimal dilution by titration.

3. Wash with at least three changes of wash buffer.

4. Incubate with peroxidase-conjugated anti-mouse Ig, diluted in wash buffer. Again, determine the optimal dilution by titration.

5. Wash with at least three changes of wash buffer.

6. Add substrate. Allow brown bands to form and wash in distilled water before background develops. Transfer strips to glass plate to dry, keeping out of the light.

6. mAb preparations

In the past mAb have been prepared in the laboratory either as tissue culture supernatant or as ascites fluid, however, both ethical considerations and legislative constraints on animal usage suggest that tissue culture methods should now be the method of choice. Culture supernatant is suitable for many applications but for some studies, particularly where quantitative data is required, purified IgG must be used. This is obviously the case for the preparation of F(ab')$_2$ and Fab fragments. Yields of purified IgG of between 1–2 μg/ml may be expected.

Purification of IgG can be accomplished simply, by chromatography on protein A–Sepharose, with a minimum of equipment. This is described in *Protocol 3*. Preparation of F(ab')$_2$ and Fab fragments depends on the subclass of the IgG involved. The methods given in *Protocols 4* and *5* are for IgG$_1$. For a discussion of the conditions appropriate for other mouse IgG subclasses, reference should be made to Parham (44). Digestion times and enzyme:substrate ratios must be determined by pilot experiments for each mAb. The final product should be assessed by SDS–PAGE under both non-reducing and reducing conditions. In non-reducing gels IgG will have an M_r of 150 kDa, F(ab')$_2$ of 100 kDa, and Fab of 50 kDa. Under reducing conditions IgG heavy (H) and light (L) chains will have M_r of 50 kDa and 25 kDa, respectively, while both F(ab')$_2$ and Fab will give a doublet at 25 kDa of L chain and Fd fragment.

Protocol 3. Purification of IgG

Equipment and reagents

- Protein A–Sepharose (Pharmacia)
- Small chromatography column, approx. 10 cm × 1 cm (e.g. Bio-Rad Econo-column)
- Peristaltic pump
- Binding buffer: 1.5 M glycine, 3 M NaCl, adjusted to pH 8.9 with 5 M NaOH
- Elution buffers: 100 mM citric acid, adjusted to pH 6.0, 5.0, and 4.0 with 5 M NaOH
- Wash buffer: 100 mM citric acid, adjusted to pH 3.0 with 5 M NaOH
- Spectrophotometer for OD$_{280}$ measurement

Method

1. Suspend protein A–Sepharose in H$_2$O and pack into column (about 4 cm).

2. Wash column with five volumes of wash buffer and equilibrate with binding buffer. All steps should be carried out at room temperature.

3. Clarify culture supernatant by centrifugation and, if necessary, filtration through glass fibre filter paper (Whatman GF/C) to prevent column blockage.

4. Add solid glycine and NaCl to culture supernatant to make it 1.5 M in glycine and 3 M in NaCl, and adjust pH to 8.9 with 5 M NaOH.

Protocol 3. *Continued*

5. Pass supernatant through column at a rate of about 1 ml/min, using peristaltic pump.

6. Wash column with binding buffer until OD_{280} falls to baseline.

7. Elute IgG with Na citrate buffers of pH 6.0, 5.0, and 4.0 in descending order. Collect 1 ml fractions (fractions may conveniently be collected by hand) and monitor protein elution by measuring OD_{280}. IgG_1 will be eluted at pH 6.0, IgG_{2a} at pH 5.0, and IgG_{2b} and 3 at pH 4.0.

8. Pool eluted fractions, adjust pH to 7.0 with 2 M Tris, and dialyse against PBS.

9. Estimate yield by measuring OD_{280} and using an extinction coefficient of 1.4 per mg/ml.

10. Wash column with wash buffer and re-equilibrate with binding buffer.

Protocol 4. Preparation of $F(ab')_2$ fragments

Equipment and reagents

- See *Protocol 3*
- Pepsin (Sigma, P6887)

- $2 \times$ SDS–PAGE sample buffer: 4% SDS, 0.2 mM dithiothreitol, 120 mM Tris–HCl pH 6.8, 0.02% bromphenol blue

Method

1. Dialyse IgG into 0.1 M Na citrate pH 4.0, and adjust to 5 mg/ml.

2. Add 3% (w/w) of pepsin to IgG and incubate at 37 °C.

3. Follow time course of reaction by digestion of a small amount of IgG, remove samples at approx. 1 h intervals over 24 h, and boil with an equal volume of $2 \times$ SDS–PAGE sample buffer for 1 min (8–12 h digestion may be optimal).

4. Monitor cleavage by SDS–PAGE under reducing conditions to determine optimal cleavage time.

5. Use same conditions for bulk digestion.

6. Stop reaction by adjusting pH to 7.0.

7. Pass digest through protein A–Sepharose column to remove uncleaved IgG and Fc fragment, using conditions for IgG purification (*Protocol 3*). $F(ab')_2$ fragments will pass through the column unretarded and may be monitored by collecting fractions and measuring OD_{280}. Little dilution should be encountered during this process.

Protocol 5. Preparation of Fab fragments

Equipment and reagents

- See *Protocol 4*
- Papain (Sigma, P4762)
- 100 mM cysteine (freshly prepared)
- 10 mM NaEDTA
- 1 M iodoacetamide

Method

1. Dialyse IgG into 0.1 M Na acetate pH 5.5, and adjust to 5 mg/ml. Make 10 mM in cysteine and 1 mM in EDTA.

2. Add 1% (w/w) papain and follow time course of reaction as in *Protocol 4*. The concentration of papain may need to be varied to obtain optimal cleavage.

3. Stop reaction by addition of 1 M iodoacetamide to give final concentration of 0.1 M.

4. Remove uncleaved IgG and Fc by passing through protein A–Sepharose as described in *Protocol 4*.

References

1. Kieffer, N. and Phillips, D. R. (1990). *Annu. Rev. Cell Biol.*, **6**, 329.
2. van de Winkel, J. G. J. and Anderson, C. L. (1991). *J. Leuk. Biol.*, **49**, 511.
3. Tomiyama, Y., Kunicki, T. J., Zipf, T. F., Ford, S. B., and Aster, R. H. (1992). *Blood*, **80**, 2261.
4. Ravetch, J. V. (1994). *Cell*, **78**, 553.
5. Looney, R. J., Abraham, G. N., and Anderson, C. L. (1986). *J. Immunol.*, **136**, 1641.
6. Zipf, T. F., Lauzon, G. J., and Longenecker, B. M. (1983). *J. Immunol.*, **131**, 3064.
7. Pilkington, G. R., Lee, G. T. H., Michael, P. M., Garson, O. M., Kraft, N., Atkins, R. C., *et al.* (1986). In *Leucocyte typing II* (ed. E. L. Reinherz, B. F. Haynes, L. M. Nadler, and I. D. Bernstein), p. 353. Springer-Verlag, New York.
8. Willis, H. E., Bowder, B., Feister, A. J., Mohankumar, T., and Ruddy, S. (1988). *J. Immunol.*, **140**, 234.
9. Pulford, K., Ralfkiaer, E., Macdonald, S. M., Erber, W. N., Falini, B., Gatter, K. C., *et al.* (1986). *Immunology*, **57**, 71.
10. Farace, F., Mitjavila, M.-T., Betaieb, A., Dokhelar, M. C., Wiels, J., Finale, Y., *et al.* (1988). *Cancer Res.*, **48**, 5759.
11. Anderson, G. P. and Anderson, C. L. (1990). *Blood*, **76**, 1165.
12. Osborne, J. M., Brandt, J. T., Chacko, G. W., and Anderson, C. L. (1995). In *Leukocyte typing V: white cell differentiation antigens* (ed. S. Schlossman, L. Boumsell, W. Gilks, J. Harlan, C. Kishimoto, J. Morimoto, *et al.*), p. 1251. Oxford University Press, Oxford.

13. Boucheix, C., Soria, C., Mirshahi, M., Soria, J., Perrot, J.-Y., Fournier, N., *et al.* (1983). *FEBS Lett.*, **161,** 289.
14. Worthington, R. E., Carroll, R. C., and Boucheix, C. (1990). *Br. J. Haematol.*, **74,** 216.
15. Carroll, R. C., Worthington, R. E., and Boucheix, C. (1990). *Biochem. J.*, **266,** 527.
16. Griffith, L., Slupsky, J., Seehafer, J., Boshkov, L., and Shaw, A. R. E. (1991). *Blood*, **78,** 1753.
17. Modderman, P. W., Huisman, H. G., Van Mourik, J. A., and Von dem Borne, A. E. G. Kr. (1988). *Thromb. Haemost.*, **60,** 68.
18. Bachelot, C., Rendu, F., Boucheix, C., Hogg, N., and Levy-Toledano, S. (1990). *Eur. J. Biochem.*, **190,** 177.
19. Hornby, E. J., Brown, S., Wilkinson, J. M., Mattock, C., and Authi, K. S. (1991). *Br. J. Haematol.*, **79,** 277.
20. Ockenhouse, C. F., Magowan, C., and Chulay, J. D. (1989). *J. Clin. Invest.*, **84,** 468.
21. Testi, R., Pulcinelli, F., Frati, L., Gazzaniga, P. P., and Santoni, A. (1990). *J. Exp. Med.*, **172,** 701.
22. Rubinstein, E., Boucheix, C., Urso, I., and Carroll, R. C. (1991). *J. Immunol.*, **147,** 3040.
23. Scott, J. L., Dunn, S. M., Jin, B., Hillam, A. J., Walton, S., Berndt, M. C., *et al.* (1989). *J. Biol. Chem.*, **264,** 13475.
24. Horsewood, P., Hayward, C. P. M., Warkentin, T. E., and Kelton, J. G. (1991). *Blood*, **78,** 1019.
25. Peerschke, E. I. B., Reid, K. B. M., and Ghebrehiwet, B. (1993). *J. Exp. Med.*, **178,** 579.
26. Gulino, D., Ryckewaert, J.-J., Andrieux, A., Rabiet, M.-J., and Marguerie, G. (1990). *J. Biol. Chem.*, **265,** 9575.
27. Kouns, W. C., Wall, C. D., White, M. M., Fox, C. F., and Jennings, L. K. (1990). *J. Biol. Chem.*, **265,** 20594.
28. Kouns, W. C. and Jennings, L. K. (1991). *Thromb. Res.*, **63,** 343.
29. McEver, R. P. and Martin, M. N. (1984). *J. Biol. Chem.*, **259,** 9799.
30. Larsen, E., Celi, A., Gilbert, G. E., Furie, B. C., Erban, J. K., Bonfanti, R., *et al.* (1989). *Cell*, **59,** 305.
31. Admiraal, L. G., Daams, G. M., Bos, M. J. E., and Von dem Borne, A. E. G. Kr. (1989). In *Leucocyte typing IV: white cell differentiation antigens* (ed. W. Knapp, B. Dörken, W. R. Gilks, E. P. Rieber, R. E. Schmidt, H. Stein, *et al.*), p. 1041. Oxford University Press, Oxford.
32. Nieuwenhuis, H. K., van Oosterhout, J. G., Rozemuller, E., van Iwaarden, F., and Sixma, J. J. (1987). *Blood*, **70,** 838.
33. Hildreth, J. E. K., Derr, D., and Azorsa, D. O. (1991). *Blood*, **77,** 121.
34. Mane, S. M., Marzella, L., Bainton, D. F., Holt, V. K., Cha, Y., Hildreth, J. E. K., *et al.* (1989). *Arch. Biochem. Biophys.*, **268,** 360.
35. McEver, R. P. (1991). *Thromb. Haemost.*, **66,** 80.
36. Horejsí, V. and Vlcek, C. (1991). *FEBS Lett.*, **288,** 1.
37. Nishibori, M., Cham, B., McNicol, A., Shalev, A., Jain, N., and Gerrard, J. M. (1993). *J. Clin. Invest.*, **91,** 1775.
38. Febbraio, M. and Silverstein, R. L. (1992). *Blood*, **80,** 1470.
39. Abrams, C., Deng, Y.-J., Steiner, B., O'Toole, T., and Shattil, S. J. (1994). *J. Biol. Chem.*, **269,** 18781.

40. Shattil, S. J., Hoxie, J. A., Cunningham, M., and Brass, L. F. (1985). *J. Biol. Chem.*, **260,** 11107.
41. Coller, B. S., Peerschke, E. I., and Scudder, L. E. (1983). *J. Clin. Invest.*, **72,** 325.
42. Coller, B. S. (1985). *J. Clin. Invest.*, **76,** 101.
43. Jones, D., Fritchy, J., Garson, J., Nokes, T. J. C., Kemshead, J. T., and Hardisty, R. M. (1984). *Br. J. Haematol.*, **57,** 621.
44. Parham, P. (1983). *J. Immunol.*, **131,** 2895.

Measurement of protein phosphorylation, kinase activity, and G protein function in intact platelets and membrane preparations

ISOBEL A. WADMAN, KANWAR VIRDEE,
DENISE S. FERNANDEZ, CHRISTINE L. WASUNNA,
and RICHARD W. FARNDALE

1. Introduction

We have collated in this chapter methods for locating or determining the activity of platelet signalling proteins. SDS–PAGE provides a means of separating the proteins, their labelling is achieved either by covalent or affinity methods, and they are usually detected on film, either by autoradiography or Western blotting. The preparation of platelets and platelet membranes from Blood Transfusion Service concentrates, together with basic electrophoretic methods, are described in Section 1. Methods for protein phosphorylation and the determination of kinase activity are described in Section 2, and for GTP binding proteins in Section 3. We expect that the reader will modify the precise conditions of the methods to suit their particular need; the protocols below will provide a starting point from which these and other assays may be developed.

A detailed review is beyond the scope of this chapter and although leading references are included, these are not intended to be comprehensive, rather to provide examples of the techniques discussed.

1.1 Platelet and membrane preparation from blood bank concentrates

We regularly use platelet concentrates supplied within 24 hours of collection by the Regional Blood Transfusion Service. In our experience, stored at room temperature over several days on a Stovall BellyDancer rocking table (setting 2; Scotlab), signalling pathways in these platelets are as active as in platelets freshly obtained from whole blood, but we recommend that this should be verified especially where platelet responses which may decline quickly after collection of human blood, such as to ADP, are to be measured. The procedure is essentially similar to that used to prepare platelets from whole blood (see Chapter 1). Although it is seldom absolutely necessary, you may include inhibitors (apyrase 20–100 µg/ml, or aspirin 100 µM, or indomethacin 10 µM) to facilitate resuspension after the second and subsequent centrifugation steps. Usually $2–5 \times 10^{10}$ platelets can be obtained from a single pack of concentrate.

Protocol 1. Preparation of platelets from concentrates

Equipment and reagents

- A platelet concentrate, containing platelets from one unit of blood in 50 ml
- Bench centrifuge (MSE Centaur is used below, of $r_{max} = 15$ cm)
- Clear polystyrene centrifuge tubes (10–15 ml)
- Buffer P: 145 mM NaCl, 5 mM KCl, 1 mM MgSO$_4$, 10 mM glucose, 25 mM Hepes, 0.5 mM EGTA pH 7.3

Method

1. Centrifuge up to 10 ml platelet concentrate at 180 *g* (1200 r.p.m.) for 15 min, to pellet contaminating red cells.

2. Remove the supernatant platelet suspension together with any platelet pellet, carefully avoiding the small underlying pellet of red cells. Add inhibitors to the platelets as appropriate.

3. Centrifuge the platelet suspension at 800 *g* (2000 r.p.m.) for 15 min. Discard the supernatant.

4. Resuspend the pellet in about one-quarter its original volume of buffer P.

5. Count platelet suspension, using a haemocytometer or electronic cell counter, and dilute to 10^9 platelets/ml.

Several of the methods described below can only be used with permeabilized platelet preparations (see Chapter 5). *Protocol 2* can be used to prepare a suitable crude membrane fraction from bloodbank platelet concentrates. The preparation is stable for several weeks and each concentrate yields 1.5 ml of membrane fraction with a protein content of 10–20 mg/ml.

Protocol 2. Preparation of platelet membrane fraction

Equipment and reagents

- Polypropylene centrifuge tubes (50 ml)
- Teflon-on-glass homogenizers of 10 ml and 50 ml volume
- Ultracentrifuge capable of 70 000 *g*
- Liquid nitrogen
- Buffer A: 120 mM NaCl, 12.9 mM Na$_3$ citrate, 30 mM glucose
- Buffer B: 5 mM EDTA, 5 mM Tris pH 7.4
- 1 mM KHCO$_3$

Method

1. Make each platelet concentrate up to 5 ml in buffer A, and centrifuge at 180 *g* for 15 min. Save the supernatant platelet suspensions, carefully remove platelet pellets from contaminating red cells beneath them, and add them to the platelet suspensions.

2. Centrifuge the platelets at 1000 *g* for 15 min, then discard the supernatant. Resuspend the pellet in hypotonic buffer B (5 ml/platelet concentrate pack).

3. Dispense into 1.5 ml polypropylene tubes, and freeze in liquid nitrogen.

4. Allow the platelets to thaw at room temperature, pool them, and disrupt further with ten strokes of the large homogenizer. Repeat steps 3 and 4.

5. Centrifuge at 70 000 *g* for 30 min. Remove the supernatant.[a]

6. Resuspend and homogenize the pellet in 10 ml buffer B, and centrifuge at 70 000 *g* for 30 min.

7. Resuspend in 1 mM $KHCO_3$ (1.5 ml per platelet concentrate), homogenize (ten strokes), and dispense in 100 μl portions into uncapped polypropylene tubes.

8. Store under liquid nitrogen or at −70 °C until required.

[a] Retain a portion of the supernatant, cytosol fraction for ADP-ribosylations using cholera toxin; store at −80 °C. See *Protocol 10*.

1.2 General procedures used in protein separation and detection

The following procedures are common to several of the techniques described below.

(a) Electrophoresis. A mini-gel format, such as the Hoefer Mighty Small apparatus, with 10% or 11% acrylamide gels, 1.5 mm thick, accommodates a sample volume of 50 μl, and allows proteins to be separated quickly. The loss of molecular weight resolution occasioned by using mini-gels is substantially offset by the decreased bandwidth compared with larger format gels. 2 × Laemmli's buffer (20 g/litre SDS, 0.5 g/litre bromophenol blue, 125 mM Tris pH 6.8, 20% glycerol (v/v), to which 10% β-mercaptoethanol (v/v) is added immediately before use) is used throughout, except with the MAP kinase assay (*Protocol 9*).

(b) Electroblotting. Non-radioactive samples can be transferred to PVDF membranes (Immobilon P, Millipore) using a semi-dry blotting apparatus, e.g. the Hoefer TE77. A current of 0.8 mA/cm² (about 40 mA per gel) for 2 h gives good protein transfer with, as electrolyte, 150 mM glycine, 25 mM Tris pH 8.3, containing 20% (v/v) methanol. As an alternative, especially with radiolabelled samples, a wet blotting system (e.g. Hoefer TE52 Transphor) running at a current of 1 A for 3 h, or 0.5 A overnight, can be used with the same electrolyte. This is especially useful as a means of electroeluting unbound, contaminating radiolabel from blots.

(c) Hybridization methods. Several protocols require equilibration with radio-labelled materials, e.g. $[\alpha\text{-}^{32}\text{P}]\text{GTP}$ or $[\gamma\text{-}^{32}\text{P}]\text{ATP}$, which is usually performed in a rolling hybridization oven (e.g. Hybaid Micro-4). This will accommodate several intact blots (or gels in *Protocol 9*) in a glass hybridization tube, with as little as 5 ml of medium, or a single blot can be processed in 50 ml polypropylene tubes. If one or two lanes only are to be processed, with correspondingly smaller fluid volumes, these will fit adequately into polystyrene universal vials (Sterilin). Where overnight denaturation or renaturation steps are included, or to wash radiolabel from blots, square polystyrene culture dishes (10×10 cm) (Sterilin) are ideal, using a minimum fluid volume of 12 ml. The reciprocal motion provided by the Hoefer Red Rocker is efficient for this application.

(d) Detection methods. Routinely, radiolabelled proteins are detected on pre-flashed Fuji RX film by autoradiography at $-70\,^{\circ}\text{C}$, using a single intensifying screen. In the MAP kinase assay, slightly higher sensitivity may be obtained using Kodak X-OMAT film, or by using the Molecular Dynamics PhosphorImager. In Western blots of G protein subunits, the enhanced chemiluminescence method (ECL, Amersham) is used, exposing to Hyperfilm-ECL for up to 60 min.

1.3 Isoelectric focusing (IEF) methods for platelet proteins

The separation of platelet proteins may call for isoelectric focusing methods. Such methods are time-consuming, and it may be difficult to ensure that proteins enter the isoelectric focusing gel uniformly. The following section describes a method which may prove to have general utility. It is relatively rapid and requires an inexpensive accessory kit to be used with the Hoefer Mighty Small mini-gel apparatus.

Signalling proteins, especially G proteins, may exist as multiple isoforms which can be separated on the basis of their differing isoelectric points. Heterogeneity in pI may arise either through expression of different transcripts, or mutants, or by post-translational covalent modification: phosphorylation of both G_i and G_s has been suggested to modulate their function (1), and attachment of neutral species, such as myristate, palmitate, or arachidonate, to charged amino acid residues might alter their ability to dissociate (2). Fatty acylation renders the G protein hydrophobic, contributing to the difficulty, when analysing G proteins by IEF, of ensuring uniform and high levels of entry into the tube gel. Secondly, correspondingly higher levels of protein need to be used with 2D methods, since the protein of interest is distributed between several spots rather than concentrated in a single band as in conventional SDS–PAGE. A procedure which we have found useful to study both platelet phosphoproteins and G protein subunits by IEF is described below. An alternative approach to IEF of G proteins has been detailed elsewhere (3).

Protocol 3. Sample preparation for IEF

Equipment and reagents

- Carbonic anhydrase pI markers (2.5 mg/ml each) (Sigma, C3666, C6403, and C6653), which have nominal pI of 5.4, 5.9, and 6.6, respectively (in our hands these ran at somewhat different pI than their stated value)
- K_2CO_3 (5 mM and 500 mM)
- Ultrapure urea (solid and 9.5 M)
- DTT (25 and 100 mg/ml)
- Nonidet P-40
- Stirrer and microcentrifuge
- Either a platelet membrane preparation containing, after experimental manipulation, 1 mg protein in 100 µl of suspension in 25 mM Tris pH 7.5, or intact platelets at 10^9/ml in buffer P (see *Protocol 1*)

A. Platelet membranes

1. To 100 µl membranes, add 2 µl K_2CO_3 (500 mM) and 114 mg ultrapure urea.

2. Stir vigorously using a small magnetic stirrer until urea has dissolved (about 10 min).

3. Add 10 µl DTT (100 mg/ml), 4 µl Nonidet P-40, and 4 µl of each pI marker.

4. Stir vigorously for 10 min, remove stirrer bar, and centrifuge at 10 000 *g* for 15 min.

B. Intact platelets

1. To 50 µl platelet suspension, activated as desired, add 1 ml ice-cold buffer P.

2. Centrifuge at 10 000 *g* for 1 min and discard the supernatant.

3. Add 40 µl of 9.5 M urea containing 5 mM K_2CO_3.

4. Disrupt platelets by freezing in liquid nitrogen, then thawing at 30°C for 10 min with vortexing.

5. Add 10 µl of 9.5 M urea, containing 25 mg/ml DTT and 10% (v/v) Nonidet P-40, and mix well.

6. Centrifuge at 10 000 *g* for 15 min.

The supernatants from *Protocols 3A* and *3B* are suitable for loading into IEF gels. The conditions described in *Protocol 4A* are adequate to establish the necessary pH gradient (5.8–8.5) and to resolve the platelet proteins according to their pI. After the first dimension run, the IEF tubes may either be stored at –20°C until ready for the second dimension separation, or processed immediately. Molecular weight (M_r) is resolved using a conventional 1.5 mm thick, mini-gel format with an 11% gel to improve the discrimination of proteins from ampholytes (which stain with Coomassie blue).

Protocol 4. Isoelectric focusing

Equipment and reagents

- Hoefer SE 220 tube gel adapters (each holds six IEF tubes). To prevent the gels extruding from their tubes during electrofocusing, a slight constriction is introduced by rotating one end of each IEF tube in a hot gas burner flame. This also serves to identify the lower end of the tube for manipulation after running.
- Hoefer glass IEF tubes, cleaned by soaking in 1 M NaOH for 1 h, rinsing thoroughly, soaking in chromic acid overnight, rinsing exhaustively in distilled water, and drying in an oven immediately prior to use. (After use, and NaOH cleaning, it is convenient to store the IEF tubes in chromic acid.)
- Equilibration buffer: 125 mM Tris pH 6.8, 2.5% SDS, 10% glycerol, 0.025% bromophenol blue, 5 mM DTT
- 4 ml of the IEF gel mix, sufficient for 12 tubes, containing: 2.2 g ultrapure urea, 532 µl of 28.4% acrylamide/1.6% bisacrylamide, 800 µl Nonidet P-40 (10%, v/v), 200 µl Pharmalytes pH 5–8, and 50 µl Pharmalytes pH 4.5–5.4 (Sigma), 740 µl water, and 6 µl ammonium persulfate (10%, w/v)—this provides a 4.3% total acrylamides, 5.4% cross-linked, gel containing 9.2 M urea and 2% total Pharmalytes

- 1 ml disposable syringes fitted with silicone rubber tubing to adapt them to the IEF tube, and a rack from which these can be suspended (see *Figure 1a*)
- Nitrogen cylinder
- 1000 V power supply
- Glass microscope slides
- 2.5 ml polystyrene test-tubes, e.g. Luckham LP3
- A small diameter pH electrode, e.g. Corning, 476540
- 11% gels for molecular weight resolution (M_r calibration is accommodated by inserting a small piece of 1.5 mm thick Teflon at one end into the stacking gel to form a single well for M_r markers)
- TEMED
- 20 mM NaOH
- 10 mM H_3PO_4
- 125 mM Tris pH 6.8
- Agarose (10 mg/ml) in stacking gel buffer: 125 mM Tris pH 6.8, containing 0.1% SDS
- M_r markers, e.g. Rainbow markers (Amersham)
- Ponceau S (1 g/litre) (Sigma) in acetic acid (5%, v/v)

A. First dimension

1. The mix should be stirred until the urea has dissolved, then degassed by bubbling N_2 through it from a fine capillary tube for 10 min, and finally 4 µl TEMED added. With each IEF tube attached to its syringe, draw up gel mix to about 5 mm from the top of the tube. Suspend the tube by the syringe (*Figure 1a*) until the gel has polymerized (1–2 h), then remove the tubes from their syringes.

2. Lubricate the IEF tubes slightly and insert them into the tube gel adapter. Grease the adapter with silicone grease and clamp it to the gel apparatus.

3. Fill the upper reservoir, and flush the tops of the tubes with degassed 20 mM NaOH.

4. Fill the lower reservoir, and flush the lower end of each tube (using a syringe and bent needle), with degassed 10 mM H_3PO_4.

---

5. Load 20–25 µl sample containing 80–100 µg protein into the top of the tube. Load blank sample buffer into at least one tube for pH gradient determination.
6. Run for 3.5 h at 1000 V.

B. *Processing and second dimension*

1. Using the Hoefer tube gel extractor with a syringe filled with 125 mM Tris pH 6.8, gently extrude the gel from the IEF tube, making sure its orientation is preserved throughout.
2. Carefully manoeuvre the gel into a 2.5 ml polystyrene test-tube and add 0.5 ml equilibration buffer. Keep the tubes horizontal for 10–15 min, agitating occasionally, or leave on a rocking table.
3. Hold the tube gel on a clean microscope slide adjacent to the M_r resolving gels, and slide it into the gap between the plates above the stacking gel (see *Figure 1b*). Expel bubbles from beneath the tube gel by gentle pressure with a spacer, and seal the tube in place using about 100 µl of agarose in stacking gel buffer, melted by heating to about 50 °C.
4. M_r standards are loaded into their well, and gels are run at 20 mA/gel until the dye front has just emerged (about 2 h).
5. To measure the pH gradient in the blank IEF tube gels, extrude them on to a clean glass plate, using water in the tube gel extraction syringe, and rinse in water briefly. Cut them into 5 mm lengths, equilibrating each of these in 0.5 ml water for 2 h, with occasional vortexing, and measure the pH.
6. The separated proteins may be stained conventionally. If proteins are to be immunodetected, however, gels are immediately transferred to blotting buffer (see Section 1.2b) and after 10–15 min equilibration, electroblotting is performed. After this, proteins can be stained using Ponceau S.

Figure 2 shows the IEF method applied to phosphoproteins in intact platelets, treated with collagen, where multiple species at 29 and 47 kDa are resolved (*Figure 2c*) or with prostaglandin E_1, where phosphorylation of 47 and 20 kDa proteins is suppressed, and new labelled proteins at about 40 and 22 kDa (*Rap1b*) (see Section 2.2) can be observed (*Figure 2b*).

2. Methods for the detection of protein phosphorylation

2.1 General objectives

Many signalling pathways culminate in the activation of specific protein kinases, and the platelet provides an excellent model in which such events

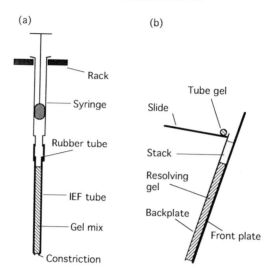

Figure 1. Preparing and handling IEF tube gels. (a) The arrangement used to load gel mix into the IEF tube. (b) Transferring the tube gel to the second dimension resolving gel.

may be studied. It was long considered that protein kinase C occupied a central role in platelet function, and its activation can be used as an important and convenient index of early stages of platelet stimulation (4). More recently it has become clear that tyrosine kinases are not only unusually abundant in platelets but also may regulate various platelet signalling pathways including the cytoskeletal reorganization necessary for secretion and aggregation. An understanding of the interplay of the Ca^{2+}/PKC system with tyrosine kinases (for which methods are described in Chapter 10) is essential if the process of platelet activation is to be fully understood. Cyclic nucleotide-dependent protein kinases are recognized as opposing the activatory process in platelets, and this aspect of platelet function is described in Chapter 13.

The following sections provide methods for studying the location and regulation of protein kinases in platelet preparations, using the covalent incorporation of [^{32}P]orthophosphate into platelet proteins, which is achieved either by the use of $^{32}P_i$ to label the metabolic ATP pool of intact platelets, or using [γ-^{32}P]ATP with platelet membrane preparations. Radiolabelled proteins are generally separated by SDS–PAGE. To preserve the phosphorylation state of platelet proteins prior to denaturation, for example if proteins are to be separated later by IEF, it may be necessary to inhibit protein phosphatase activity using EDTA and/or okadaic acid.

2.2 Protein phosphorylation in intact platelets

Most previous studies, for example of the activation of protein kinase C, have used $^{32}P_i$ levels of between 1 and 5 mCi/ml. When labelling in phosphate-free

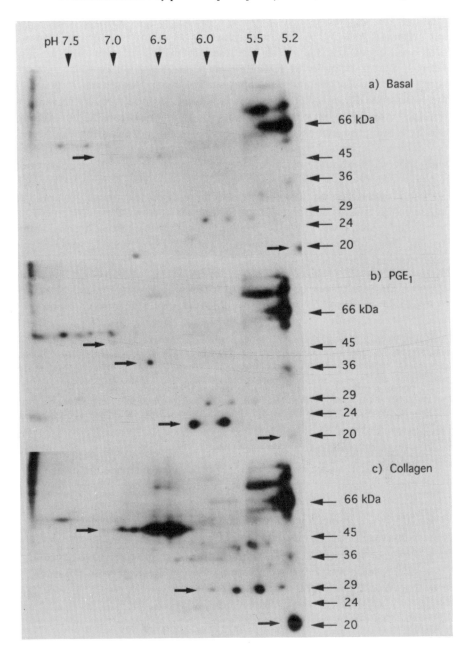

Figure 2. Platelet proteins were radiolabelled and treated with ligand using *Protocols 5* and *6*. Phosphoproteins, discussed in Section 1.3, were separated by IEF using *Protocols 3* and *4*. (a) Basal samples. (b) Treated with 1 μM PGE$_1$. (c) Treated with collagen fibres, 100 μg/ml. M_r markers are shown, together with the measured pH.

medium, this is unnecessarily high, as autoradiographs are over-exposed if left overnight. 100–200 µCi/ml is adequate, or 50 µCi/ml is sufficient for more prolonged exposures. The use of the less penetrative ^{33}P might also be considered, see for example ref. 5. Radiological safety is maintained by manipulating the radiolabel behind a Perspex screen, by shielding emissions above the horizontal during labelling by placing a lead container over the incubation tube (the water-bath effectively absorbs emissions below the horizontal), and by closing the incubation tube in a screw-cap bucket during centrifugation. The MSE Centaur is ideal for this purpose; those microcentrifuges fitted with open rotors should not be considered because tube breakage constitutes a serious potential hazard. *Protocol 5* can be used to label the metabolic ATP pool and *Protocol 6* describes the measurement of protein phosphorylation in intact platelets. This combination of techniques allows an experiment to be completed within a working day, including incubation, electrophoresis, staining and destaining with Coomassie blue (at 60°C in a shaking water-bath), drying the gel, and placing it in a cassette.

Protocol 5. Labelling the metabolic ATP pool of intact platelets

Equipment and reagents
- ^{32}P$_i$ (carrier-free orthophosphate) 10 mCi/ml in dilute HCl (e.g. Amersham, PBS11)
- A bench centrifuge with closed buckets (e.g. MSE Centaur; see *Protocol 1*)
- Screw-top 1.5 ml polypropylene tubes which can stand being boiled without leakage
- A 30°C water-bath
- Buffer P (see *Protocol 1*)

Method

1. Calculate the total volume of platelets, suspended at 10^9/ml (see *Protocol 1*) that is required, allowing 15 or 20 µl of suspension per determination, with a small excess. Pipette this total volume into a screw-top 1.5 ml tube.

2. Add ^{32}P$_i$ to a final level of between 50 and 250 µCi/ml. Up to 10% by volume of radiolabel (Amersham, PBS11) will not cause platelet lysis.

3. Incubate at 30°C for 60 min, then centrifuge at 800 *g* for 10 min. Carefully discard the supernatant, containing ^{32}P$_i$. Resuspend in the original volume of buffer P.

Protocol 6 , which is illustrated using 25 µl samples, the minimum readily handled volume, can be used to activate specific kinases and radiolabel their substrates. These may be separated by electrophoresis. In the simplest case, there may be sufficient resolution of substrates of interest using one-dimensional SDS–PAGE. For example, P47 or pleckstrin (6), serves as an index of protein kinase C activity, and myosin light chain (MLC; P22) is phosphorylated by MLC kinase (*Figure 3a*). Distinct phosphorylated bands, e.g. P24 (GP1Bβ) and P26 (*Figure 3b*), and P22 (*Rap*1b) and P28 (*Figure 4*), reflect cyclic AMP-dependent protein kinase activity. These various proteins may be used as indices of the activity of their respective kinases. It may often be necessary to resolve less prominent substrates, and whilst two-dimensional electrophoresis may be satisfactory (see Section 1.3), immunoprecipitation (see Chapter 5) or other strategies are widely used to separate and concentrate particular radiolabelled proteins. For example, phosphorylated forms of endoplasmic reticulum Ca^{2+} pumps (7) and cytoplasmic phospholipase A_2 (5) have been separated in this way. The small GTP binding protein *Rap*1b was purified chromatographically prior to *in vitro* phosphorylation using exogenous protein kinase (8). Platelet protein phosphorylation is reviewed elsewhere (9).

Protocol 6. Activation of protein kinases in intact platelets

Equipment and reagents
- Platelet suspension (10^9/ml in buffer P), radiolabelled as in *Protocol 5*
- 30°C water-bath and boiling water-bath
- 2 x Laemmli's buffer (see Section 1.2a)
- Buffer P (see *Protocol 1*)

Method

1. Into screw-top 1.5 ml tubes in the 30°C water-bath, dispense kinase activators (hormones or other effectors) in a volume of 5 μl each of buffer P. Two such additions can be accommodated.

2. Start the incubation by adding labelled platelets, to give a total volume of 25 μl.

3. After suitable times, stop the incubation by adding 25 μl Laemmli's buffer. Cap the tube, mix well, and transfer it to the boiling water-bath for 5 min.

4. Proteins are separated by SDS–PAGE.

In *Figure 3a*, the effect of tetradecanoylphorbol acetate (TPA) or collagen on the activation of protein kinase C is shown by the increase in incorporation of radiolabel into P47, or pleckstrin. P22, MLC, is also prominent; the activation of MLC kinase is Ca^{2+}-dependent, although PKC effects a non-activatory phosphorylation event. Hence collagen, which mobilizes platelet calcium, generates a larger P22 signal than TPA, although the reverse is true for pleckstrin phosphorylation.

In *Figure 3b*, forskolin and prostaglandin E_1 were used to activate cyclic AMP-dependent phosphorylation notably of P26, but P24, GPIb is also visible. In addition, these effectors stimulate the phosphorylation of P48 (VASP) and

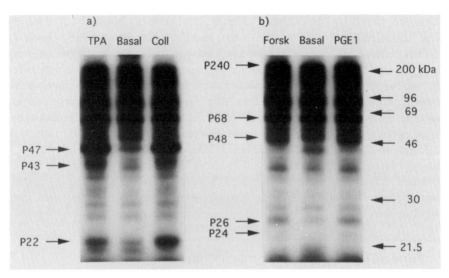

Figure 3. Phosphorylation of intact platelets labelled using *Protocol 5* stimulated by incubation for 2 min, as in *Protocol 6*, with various ligands. The positions of specific substrates mentioned in the text and of M_r markers are indicated. An 11% gel was used. (a) 160 nM TPA (lane 1) and collagen (100 µg/ml, lane 3) are compared with basal activity (lane 2). (b) 10 µM forskolin (lane 1) and 1 µM PGE₁ (lane 3) are compared with basal (lane 2).

there is an increased incorporation into bands of M_r 68 and 240 kDa. *Rap*1b, of M_r 22 kDa, not clearly resolved in *Figure 3b*, is also phosphorylated in cyclic AMP-dependent manner. Cyclic nucleotide-dependent platelet protein phosphorylation is discussed in detail elsewhere (10,11). Note that in *Figure 3b*, basal pleckstrin (*c.* 45 kDa) and MLC (*c.* 21.5 kDa) phosphorylation are reduced by agents which activate cyclic AMP-dependent protein kinase.

Residual [³²P]ATP moves just ahead of the dye front. It is preferable to allow this to emerge into the running buffer, to minimize inadvertent contamination of the resolving portion of the gel from this very hot region during subsequent handling operations.

As an alternative to radiolabelling, we considered the use of Western blotting with antiphosphoserine and antiphosphothreonine monoclonal antibodies (Sigma) to detect P47 phosphorylation in intact platelets. Although these antibodies detected discrete subsets of phosphoproteins, including the P47 region, the phosphorylation pattern did not change on stimulation with TPA or collagen, showing that any increase in net phosphorylation in the P47 region is below the resolution of the method.

2.3 Measurement of protein phosphorylation in platelet membranes

To perform equivalent experiments on membrane preparations, it is necessary to compose an incubation from appropriate effectors and an assay mix including Mg^{2+}, 10–100 µM ATP, and $[\gamma\text{-}^{32}P]$ATP. This offers the advantages that the specific activity of the ATP can be defined and lower levels of radioactivity can be used than in *Protocol 6*. ATP is rapidly depleted by endogenous ATPase activity in membranes. Incubations should therefore be as short as possible, and inclusion of phosphatase inhibitors is recommended, since the rate of dephosphorylation will otherwise soon exceed incorporation of radiolabel. For *Protocol 7*, several days exposure of autoradiographs will be needed.

Protocol 7. Activation of protein kinases in platelet membrane preparations

Equipment and reagents

- Screw-top tubes, water-baths, and Laemmli's buffer as in *Protocol 6*
- Assay mix, including 10 mM Mg^{2+}, 10 µM ATP, and 5 µCi/ml $[\gamma\text{-}^{32}P]$ATP
- Platelet membranes suspended to a concentration of 1–2 mg/ml in 25 mM Tris pH 7.5, containing 1 mM DTT

Method

1. Dispense effectors and assay mix into screw-top tubes to a volume of 25 µl. Equilibrate the tubes in the 30°C water-bath.

2. Start the reaction by adding membranes (25 µl) and mixing.

3. Stop the reaction at suitable times by adding Laemmli's buffer, capping the tube, vortexing, and transferring to the boiling water-bath as in *Protocol 6*.

Figure 4 demonstrates the response of platelet membranes to different effectors, and it is important to note that platelet membranes may give qualitatively different results from intact platelets. For example, it can be seen that phosphatidylserine activated P47 phosphorylation in platelet membranes, whereas even a supramaximal level of TPA was without effect on P47 phosphorylation. We consider that this may reflect either differential distribution (12) of PKC isoforms (or other phosphatidylserine activated kinases) between platelet membrane and cytosolic fractions or their sensitivity to different activators, since the various P47 isoforms demonstrated by IEF in platelet membranes co-migrated with P47 phosphorylated in intact platelets (13). Protein phosphorylation in platelet membranes was also stimulated by Ca^{2+} and by cyclic AMP.

The methods described above allow functional effects of agents of interest to be investigated. They do not examine directly the protein kinases responsible. The use of activators, such as phosphatidylserine or cyclic AMP, as shown in *Figure 4*, may indicate the role of particular kinases in phosphorylation events. More specific tools such as non-hydrolysable analogues of cyclic

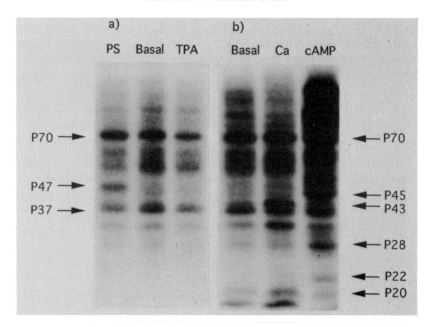

Figure 4. (a) Phosphorylation of P47 in platelet membranes, measured using *Protocol 7*, was stimulated by 2 min incubation with 83 µg/ml phosphatidylserine (PS) but not by 160 nM TPA compared with basal activity. (b) The addition of calcium (Ca) or cyclic AMP (cAMP) provoked the phosphorylation of specific protein bands.

nucleotides have been used to characterize the substrates phosphorylated in response to cyclic AMP-dependent protein kinase (11). Similarly, inhibitors such as Ro31–8220, a specific inhibitor of protein kinase C (14), or peptides derived from the pseudosubstrate regulatory domains of well-characterized protein kinases (15), might allow the role of particular kinases to be deduced.

2.4 Renatured kinase assays

In recent years, the above procedures have been complemented by methods which rely upon the autophosphorylation events which, in some cases, are a prerequisite for the activation of certain protein kinases (15–17). In essence, proteins from intact platelets or membranes, treated with suitable effectors, are separated by SDS–PAGE, and kinase activity is renatured either in the gel or after electroblotting on to suitable membranes. The renatured kinases are then incubated with [γ-^{32}P]ATP. Radiolabel becomes incorporated into the kinase, often in its regulatory domain, and possibly into substrates which co-migrate with it. Alternatively, exogenous substrate can be incorporated into the gel.

2.4.1 Autophosphorylation of renatured proteins on blots

In this way several novel protein kinases have been discovered, and their activation by different effectors has been investigated (18,19). *Protocol 8* provides a method for measuring renatured protein kinase activity on blots. It has been reported that the denaturation step enhanced the detected kinase activity somewhat, as did the use of BSA after renaturation, suggesting that BSA might serve as a substrate for the renatured kinases. Renaturation was absolutely essential, and the KOH wash reduced background radioactivity of the autoradiograph. We use less radioactivity than in the original report, compensating for this by increased reaction time and elevated temperature.

Protocol 8. Autophosphorylation assay for protein kinases

Equipment and reagents

- Platelet proteins, separated by SDS–PAGE and blotted on to PVDF membranes
- Rinse: 50 mM Tris pH 7.5, 100 mM NaCl
- Denaturing buffer: 50 mM Tris pH 8.3, 7 M guanidine–HCl, 50 mM DTT, 2 mM EDTA
- Renaturing buffer: 50 mM Tris pH 7.5, 100 mM NaCl, 2 mM DTT, 2 mM EDTA, 1 g/litre Nonidet P-40, 10 g/litre BSA
- Phosphorylation mix: [γ-^{32}P]ATP (10 μCi/ml), 10 mM MgCl$_2$, 2 mM MnCl$_2$ in 50 mM Tris pH 7.5

- 50 mM Tris pH 7.5
- 50 mM Tris pH 7.5, containing 5% BSA
- 50 mM Tris pH 7.5, containing 0.5 g/litre Nonidet P-40
- 1 M KOH
- 10% acetic acid (v/v)
- 10 cm square polystyrene culture dishes
- 50 ml polypropylene tubes
- Hybridization oven

Method

1. Incubate platelets (10^9/ml) with suitable effectors, then add Laemmli's buffer and boil as *Protocol 6*. Separate proteins by SDS–PAGE (see Section 1.2a).

2. Transfer proteins to PVDF membranes (see Section 1.2b). Rinse briefly, twice.

3. Incubate the blot in denaturing buffer (25 ml) on a rocking table for 1 h at room temperature, then rinse briefly, twice.

4. Replace the rinse with two changes of renaturing buffer and then incubate the blot in renaturing buffer (25 ml) overnight at 4°C on a rocking table.

5. Incubate the blot for 1 h in 50 mM Tris pH 7.5, containing 5% BSA.

6. Place the blot in a 50 ml polypropylene tube together with 2 ml phosphorylation mix. Incubate with rolling at 30°C for 1 h in a hybridization oven.

7. Stop the reaction by carefully discarding the mix. Add 20 ml of 50 mM Tris pH 7.5, and roll for 2 min.

8. Transfer the blot to a square culture dish and wash with four changes (12 ml) of 50 mM Tris for 10 min on a rocking table at room temperature, the third wash containing 0.5 g/litre Nonidet P-40.

Protocol 8. *Continued*

9. Wash for 10 min with 1 M KOH, and rinse (3 × 10 min) with 10% (v/v) acetic acid.

10. Rinse with 50 mM Tris pH 7.5, dry the blot, and prepare an auto-radiograph.

Figure 5 shows the enhanced activity of renatured kinases in intact platelets treated with TPA. There was a significant increase in kinase activity at about 60 and 50 kDa, and a reduction in kinase activity in a band of about 180 kDa.

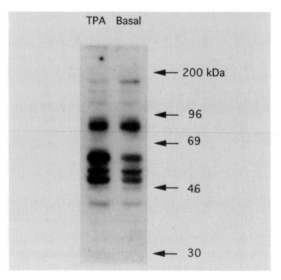

Figure 5. Renatured kinase activity in blotted proteins from intact platelets treated with TPA (160 nM). *Protocol 8* was used to measure kinase activity, and TPA caused a significant increase in the activity of renatured kinases at about 60 and 50 kDa, and a reduction in kinase activity in a band of about 180 kDa.

2.4.2 Assay of MAP kinase by incorporation of MBP into the gel

An elaboration of this approach allows specific substrates to be incorporated into the polyacrylamide gel in which the platelet protein kinases are separated, so that upon renaturation (20), activated kinases find their preferred substrate to hand, and can phosphorylate it. One such technique has enabled the activation of MAP kinases to be examined in platelets, using myelin basic protein incorporated into the gel (21,22), but other kinases may also be specifically detected in this way (20). The method is adapted below for platelet preparations as a phosphorylation assay for MAP kinases. The method may be complemented by measuring the shift in M_r which occurs upon activating the MAP kinases (23), demonstrated in Western blots, or by immunoprecipitation procedures (24).

Protocol 9. The MAP kinase assay

Equipment and reagents

- 5 × 10^7 platelets per sample, incubated with effectors (see *Protocol 4*), and pelleted by centrifugation
- Lysis buffer: 10 mM Tris pH 7.5, 5 mM EDTA, 50 mM NaCl, 30 mM Na$_4$P$_2$O$_7$, 50 mM NaF, 1 mM Na$_3$VO$_4$, 10 mM benzamidine, 1 mM PMSF, 1% Triton X-100, and 10 µg/ml each of leupeptin, aprotonin, and soybean trypsin inhibitor
- 4 × Laemmli's buffer: 200 mM Tris pH 6.8, 400 mM DTT, 8% SDS, 0.5 g/litre bromophenol blue, 40% glycerol
- Buffer M containing 6 M guanidine–HCl

- Gel rinse: 50 mM Tris pH 8, containing 20% (v/v) isopropanol
- Buffer M: 50 mM Tris pH 8, containing 5 mM β-mercaptoethanol
- Buffer M containing Tween 40 (0.04%)
- Reaction mix: 50 mM Tris pH 8, containing 5 mM DTT, 5 mM MgCl$_2$, 1 mM EGTA, 50 µM ATP, and 20 µCi/ml of [γ-^{32}P]ATP
- Myelin basic protein (MBP) (Sigma, M1891) and guanidine–HCl (Sigma, G4630)
- X-ray film, e.g. Kodak X-OMAT

Method

1. Solubilize the platelet pellet by adding 50 µl lysis buffer and holding on ice for 30 min. If necessary, ultrasonicate briefly to disperse aggregated platelets.

2. Clarify lysates by microcentrifuging at 10 000 *g* for 15 min at 4°C. Store the supernatant at –70°C pending assay.

3. Mix 45 µl of the platelet lysate with 15 µl 4 × Laemmli's buffer. Boil the samples for 10 min, and prepare gels using 30 µl of each sample using a 10% gel into which 500 µg/ml MBP was co-polymerized. To conserve MBP, a 0.75 mm thick gel is used. Use the other half of each sample to prepare a Western blot, probed with anti-MAP kinase.

4. Wash the gel twice (30 min) in gel rinse and then twice (30 min) in buffer M.

5. Denature the proteins in the gel by equilibrating it at room temperature with two changes (30 min) of buffer M containing 6 M guanidine–HCl.

6. Allow the proteins to renature by washing the gel in at least five changes of buffer M containing 0.04% (v/v) Tween 40 at 4°C during 40–48 h.

7. Rinse the gel twice in 50 mM Tris pH 8, then incubate for 30–60 min at 37°C with 5 ml reaction mix in a hybridization tube.

8. Remove unincorporated radioactivity by extensive washing of the gel in 5% (w/v) trichloroacetic acid containing 1% (w/v) Na$_4$P$_2$O$_7$ over about two days.

9. MAP kinase activity is detected by drying the gel and either preparing autoradiographs using Kodak X-OMAT film for 24–48 h or using a PhosphorImager.

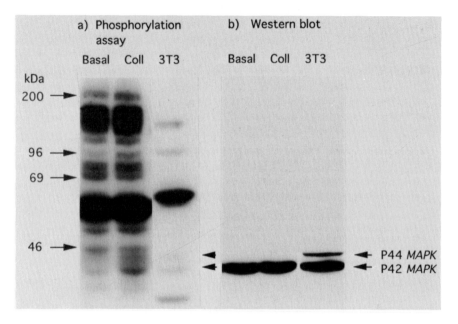

Figure 6. (a) P42 MAP kinase activity stimulated by collagen (100 µg/ml) in intact platelets, was measured as described in *Protocol 9*. 3T3 denotes proteins extracted from 3T3 cells stimulated with TPA, handled similarly, and shows the positions of P44 and P42 MAP kinases. (b) Half of each sample was used to prepare a Western blot, probed with anti-ERK1 (clone MK12, Affiniti, Nottingham) as primary antibody, detected using ECL.

The MAP kinase activity stimulated by collagen, shown in *Figure 6*, is detected in platelets at 42 kDa; this band co-migrates with immunodetected material. Note that the 44 kDa form of MAP kinase, readily demonstrated in Western blots of other tissues, appears to be substantially absent from platelets. Other renaturable kinases provide prominent signals in other protein bands, of similar size distribution but different relative intensity to those shown in *Figure 5*. The detection of stimulated MAP kinase activity is dependent upon MBP being present in the gel, but since the renatured kinase activity of the various bands shown in *Figure 6* is enhanced by the inclusion of MBP in the gel, it is important that the method be complemented by measuring M_r shifts of MAP kinases upon activation (23).

3. Methods for the study of guanine nucleotide binding proteins

The importance of the heterotrimeric G proteins in signalling pathways cannot be overstated. The low molecular weight GTP binding proteins are also becoming recognized in this context, as the regulation and role of *ras* and related gene products in signalling cascades initiated in other cell lineages by growth factors and other stimuli becomes established. Much remains to be revealed, especially regarding the likely function of the small GTP binding proteins in cytoskeletal reorganization and secretion. Not surprisingly, given the importance of such events in platelet activation, the platelet is rich in small GTP binding proteins. In this section, it is intended to provide methods for examining these together with the heterotrimeric G proteins. Protocols are provided for ADP-ribosylation reactions, and for GTP binding methods.

It should be noted that, in permeabilized platelet preparations, these may be complemented by GTPase assays, which have been described elsewhere (3). The latter provide a useful measure of the activation of G proteins stimulated in platelets by treatment with ligands such as thrombin. Furthermore, platelets provide one of the few membrane preparations in which GTPase stimulation by ligands which activate G_s can be demonstrated (3).

3.1 ADP-ribosylation

Bacterial toxins provide a means of covalent insertion of radiolabel ($[\alpha\text{-}^{32}P]$ADP-ribose, from $[\alpha\text{-}^{32}P]$NAD$^+$) into those proteins which possess suitable amino acid sequences in accessible sites. Pertussis toxin, for example, modifies a cysteine residue, the fourth amino acid from the C terminus of the G_i-like G proteins, when these are in their inactive state (25). Platelets possess relatively high levels of G_i2 and G_i3 together with detectable levels of G_i1 (26). Cholera toxin modifies an arginine residue located mid-sequence, close to the GTP binding domain of G_s, and platelets possess modest levels of the lower molecular weight form of G_s. Many other G proteins also possess such an arginine residue, and under some circumstances, cholera toxin can be persuaded to modify G proteins other than G_s. When the guanine nucleotide binding site of G_s is occupied by GTP (or a stimulatory analogue) the protein becomes activated and can accept cholera toxin-mediated ADP-ribosylation; it appears that the guanine nucleotide binding site should be empty for cholera toxin to ADP-ribosylate the equivalent arginine residue of G_i-like G proteins (27). The same consideration may apply to other, non-G_s-like G proteins. It should be noted that cholera and pertussis toxins can be used both to radiolabel G proteins (to detect them or to monitor their activation state) and to saturate them with unlabelled ADP-ribose and hence modify their function quantitatively. Minor adaptations of these protocols will achieve these various ends. Whilst both toxins are taken up readily by many cell types, and are activated intracellularly by reduction, platelets lack the ganglioside necessary for pertussis toxin binding and subsequent internalization; pertussis toxin can therefore only be used on permeable platelet preparations such as membranes. The rate of ADP-ribosylation by pertussis toxin is rather slow. In practise, therefore, quantitative ADP-ribosylation cannot be achieved in semi-permeabilized platelets. Cholera toxin, in contrast, is internalized by platelets and so can be used to ADP-ribosylate G_s in both intact platelets and membranes. However, the latter are deficient in the 21 kDa ADP-ribosylating factor (ARF) needed for catalytic activity, and so membranes must be supplemented with platelet cytosol, which contains ARF.

Recently, an ADP-ribosylation reaction has been elucidated for the small GTP binding protein, *rho*, catalysed by the botulinum C3 transferase (e.g. from UBI, Lake Placid, NY) (28). Asparagine[41] is the target amino acid. This reaction inhibits both cytoskeletal function and the activation of phosphatidylinositol 3-kinase in thrombin treated platelets (29).

The following protocols provide a catch-all method for ADP-ribosylating and radiolabelling platelet membranes with cholera or pertussis toxins, using conditions which will support the activity of either toxin. (Although untested in this laboratory, very similar protocols have been used to ADP-ribosylate *rho* in soluble platelet preparations.) The user will be able to optimize the procedures further to improve labelling for their own needs. The composition of the ADP-ribosylation mix has been thoroughly discussed elsewhere (3,30) but it is worth noting that substituting GDP for GTP may enhance pertussis toxin-mediated labelling, and that, with platelets, there is no need to include thymidine which is often used to inhibit poly-ADP-ribosylation of nuclear material in other cell preparations. Rather high levels of $[\alpha\text{-}^{32}P]NAD$ are needed as the source of ADP-ribose. It is important, therefore, that sample volumes are minimized to reduce radiological hazards, as in *Protocol 5*. Hence, high concentrations of stock materials are used so that correspondingly small volumes are required. The composition of the reaction mix is tabulated within the protocol.

Protocol 10. ADP-ribosylation reactions

Equipment and reagents

- Platelet membranes (10 mg/ml) in 25 mM Tris pH 7.5
- Pertussis toxin (1 mg/ml) (Porton Products)
- Cholera toxin (2 mg/ml) (Sigma, C3012)
- 40 and 62.5 mM DTT
- Water-baths and Laemmli's buffer as in *Protocol 6*
- Wet blotting apparatus (see Section 1.2)

- A reaction mix, formulated from stock materials which may be stored frozen. The volumes used are as follows:

Component	[Stock]	Volume (μl)	[Mix]	[Assay]
ATP	100 mM	6	6 mM	1 mM
MgCl$_2$	100 mM	6	6 mM	1 mM
GTP	1 mM	6	60 μM	10 μM
Nicotinamide	200 mM	33	60 mM	10 mM
Tris pH 7.5	1 M	3	30 mM	5 mM
Either NAD	50 mM	12	6 mM	1 mM
or NAD	1 mM	6	60 μM	10 μM
and $[\alpha\text{-}^{32}P]NAD$			6×10^8 d.p.m./ml	10^8 d.p.m./ml
Water		to 100 μl		

A. Activation of pertussis toxin

1. Mix 1 vol. toxin with 4 vol. 62.5 mM DTT and leave at room temperature for 1 h.

B. *Activation of cholera toxin*

1. Mix 1 vol. toxin with 1 vol. 40 mM DTT, and incubate at 30°C for 20 min.

2. Add 1 vol. water, then keep at room temperature for immediate use.

C. *Reaction*

1. Dispense 4 µl portions of reaction mix, formulated as above, into screw-cap tubes.

2. Add 4 µl activated toxin.[a] Warm the tubes to 30°C in the water-bath.

3. Start the reaction by adding 16 µl platelet membranes in 25 mM Tris pH 7.5.

4. Mix well, incubate for 30 min, stop the reaction by adding 24 µl Laemmli's buffer.

5. Boil the tubes and separate proteins by SDS–PAGE.

6. Transfer the proteins to PVDF membranes using the wet blotting apparatus (see Section 1.2). This elutes the non-specific background (together with unused [α-^{32}P]NAD) which is often found extending from about the 50 kDa proteins to the dye front and which might otherwise obscure bands of interest.

[a] For cholera toxin catalysed reactions, add 4 µl platelet cytosol fraction, and reduce the volume of membranes to be added accordingly.

The reciprocal inhibition observed between the activation of G_i-like G proteins and pertussis toxin catalysed ADP-ribosylation makes the latter a particularly useful tool. The role of G_i-like G proteins in a signalling pathway stimulated by a particular ligand can be inferred if treatment of platelet membranes with the ligand inhibits subsequent ADP-ribosylation, as shown in *Figure 7*, where treatment of platelet membranes with adrenaline, thrombin, or collagen, ligands which activates G proteins which are pertussis toxin substrates, reduced the subsequent incorporation of radiolabel stimulated by pertussis toxin. Conversely, pertussis toxin treatment blocked the downstream effects of these ligands (31). A note of caution should be introduced, however; some effects of pertussis toxin may be mediated by its binding rather than catalytic subunits. It is important in principle, therefore, that the effects of the toxin are shown to depend upon ADP-ribosylation, by omitting NAD from controls, or by testing the binding subunits of the toxin alone.

3.2 Binding of [α-^{32}P]GTP

GTP binding proteins of both classes may be detected by suitable binding assays. In their simplest form, these procedures rely on sufficient renaturation of GTP binding activity occurring during Western blotting that the proteins bind, with high affinity, [α-^{32}P]GTP. (The α-labelled nucleotide is used so

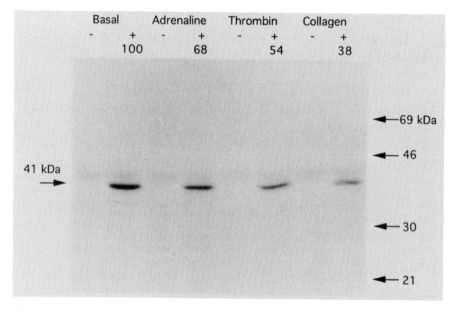

Figure 7. Platelet membranes (35 μg protein) were treated with adrenaline (10 μM), thrombin (1 U/ml), or collagen (100 μg/ml) during an ADP-ribosylation reaction (30 min) stimulated by pertussis toxin (+) as detailed in *Protocol 10*. Blank lanes (−) are controls run without toxin, and basal lanes without ligand are also shown. Densitometry, using a Leica Q500 image analyser, revealed that the ligands suppressed ADP-ribosylation: integrated optical density of the 41 kDa band as a percentage of basal are given beneath the labels.

that labelling persists in the event that GTPase activity is also restored.) Specificity of binding is established by competition with GTP or suitable analogues. This approach is restricted in platelets to the small GTP binding proteins: studies to date have failed to detect significant GTP binding activity in the heterotrimeric G proteins (32–34). It is useful to separate platelet proteins with a higher percentage gel than usual, to assist in resolving the 20–30 kDa region.

Protocol 11. GTP binding in renatured blots

Equipment and reagents

- Platelet proteins, separated by SDS–PAGE and blotted on to PVDF membranes (proteins may be stained with Ponceau S) (Sigma)
- PBS pH 7.5: 6 mM KH_2PO_4, 16 mM Na_2HPO_4, 140 mM NaCl
- Renaturation buffer: 5 mM DTT, 0.5 mM $MgCl_2$, 0.1% (w/v) Triton X-100, 1% BSA in PBS
- Binding buffer: 20 mM Tris pH 7.4, 10 mM $MgCl_2$, 2 mM DTT, 0.1% Triton X-100, 0.3% BSA
- Wash buffer: 5 mM $MgCl_2$, 0.05% Triton X-100 made up in PBS to which 25 mM 2-[*N*-morpholino]ethanesulfonic acid is added, and the pH adjusted to 6.5

Method

1. Rehydrate the blot, then incubate it in a square culture dish with 25 ml renaturation buffer overnight at room temperature on a rocking table.

2. Rinse the blot twice (5 min each) with 20 ml wash buffer.

3. Transfer the blot to a 50 ml polypropylene tube, and add 2.5 ml binding buffer containing 10 µCi [α-^{32}P]GTP. Incubate with rolling for 1 h at room temperature.

4. Carefully discard the radiolabel. Wash the blot in the tube with 20 ml wash buffer.

5. Transfer to a square culture dish and rinse with several changes of cold wash buffer.

6. Dry the blot and prepare an autoradiograph: two days exposure should be sufficient.

7. Parallel incubations should include a GTP binding mix containing 100 µM GTP which will eliminate specific GTP binding bands from the blots.

Figure 8a shows a lane of platelet proteins, prepared as detailed in *Protocol 11*, in which small GTP binding proteins are detected by binding of [α-^{32}P]GTP. Bands of about 18 and 22 kDa are visible, likely *rho* and *rap*1A (smg21), with a prominent band in the 25–27 kDa region. The latter includes *ral*A proteins (33). A 12.5% gel was used, to resolve lower M_r proteins more readily.

3.3 Photoaffinity detection of G proteins

Photoaffinity procedures may be used to detect G proteins in native platelet membranes. 8-azido GTP and GTP-azidoanilide have both been popular in this context, and detailed procedures for the latter are available elsewhere (3). A surprising finding is that [α-^{32}P]GTP itself will serve as a photoaffinity probe, an approach which has also been adapted to study cyclic GMP binding proteins (35). Such methods have been used to establish the association between particular G proteins and receptors. For example, functional coupling of G_q and the thromboxane A_2 receptor has been demonstrated in this way (36).

Protocol 12. Photoaffinity detection of G proteins using [α-^{32}P]GTP

Equipment and reagents

- Platelet membranes or other permeabilized preparations, water-baths as *Protocol 6*
- GTP mix: 200 mM NaCl, 2 mM EGTA, 10 mM MgCl$_2$, 20 mM Tris pH 7.5, with 20% glycerol (v/v), and 80 µCi [α-^{32}P]GTP/ml
- [α-^{32}P]GTP (3000 Ci/mM) (Amersham)
- High-output UV lamp—we have successfully used a 125 W Hanovia lamp fitted with a lowpass filter, emitting light below 366 nm

Protocol 12. *Continued*

Method

1. Incubate platelet membranes (25 µl containing 100 µg protein) at 30 °C for 2–10 min with 25 µl GTP mix. Shield from extraneous UV light during this period.

2. Transfer tubes to an ice-bath, open and expose their contents to UV lamp (at a distance of 5 cm) for 10 min.

3. Stop the reaction with Laemmli's buffer, and boil. Separate proteins by SDS–PAGE, and transfer to PVDF membranes using the wet blotting method, to reduce background labelling.

4. Parallel incubations should include 100 µM GTP, to leave nonspecifically labelled bands. Autoradiographs may need up to 14 days exposure.

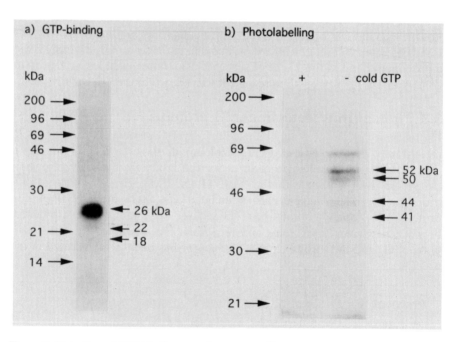

Figure 8. Detection of GTP binding proteins using $[\alpha\text{-}^{32}P]GTP$. (a) Small GTP binding proteins are demonstrated in a blotted platelet particulate fraction, using *Protocol 11*. M_r markers are shown on the *left* and bands of interest on the *right*. A 12.5% gel was used to separate platelet proteins. (b) G proteins are demonstrated in platelet particulate fraction using the photoaffinity procedure described in *Protocol 12*. M_r markers are shown on the *left* and bands of interest on the *right*. A 10% gel was used.

Figure 8b shows the result of an experiment in which platelet membranes, prepared in parallel with those shown in *Figure 8a*, were subjected to UV light in the presence of [α-^{32}P]GTP as detailed in *Protocol 12*. In this case, a 10% gel was used to discriminate better the heterotrimeric G proteins. Bands of about 41 and 44 kDa are clearly visible, which co-migrate with immuno-detected G_i and G_s. Bands of 50–52 kDa which do not correspond to known G proteins are also found, which are attenuated by the inclusion of cold GTP in the reaction mixture. These may correspond to tubulins. A band of about 65 kDa was less sensitive to the presence of GTP in the reaction mix.

Acknowledgements

R. W. F. was supported by CORDA, the heart charity, and the Medical Research Council.

References

1. Sagi-Eisenberg, R. (1989). *Trends Biochem. Sci.*, **14**, 355.
2. Neer, E. J. (1994). *Protein Sci.*, **3**, 3.
3. McKenzie, F. R. (1992). In *Signal transduction: a practical approach* (ed. G. Milligan), pp. 31–56. Oxford University Press, Oxford.
4. Siess, W. (1989). *Physiol. Rev.*, **69**, 58.
5. Kramer, R. M., Roberts, E. F., Manetta, J., Hyslop, P. A., and Jakubowski, J. A. (1993). *J. Biol. Chem.*, **268**, 26796.
6. Tyers, M., Haslam, R. J., Rachubinski, R. A., and Harley, C. B. (1989). *J. Cell. Biochem.*, **40**, 133.
7. Papp, B., Paszty, K., Kovacs, T., Sarkadi, B., Gardos, G., Enouf, J., *et al.* (1993). *Cell Calcium*, **14**, 531.
8. Fischer, T. H., Collins, J. H., Gatling, M. N., and White, G. C. (1991). *FEBS Lett.*, **283**, 173.
9. Gerrard, J. M., Carroll, R. C., Israels, S. J., and Beattie, L. L. (1987). In *Platelets in pathology and biology III* (ed. D. E. McIntyre and J. L. Gordon), pp. 317–51. Elsevier Science Publishers BV, Amsterdam.
10. Waldmann, R., Nieberding, M., and Walter, U. (1987). *Eur. J. Biochem.*, **167**, 441.
11. Eigenthaler, M., Nolte, C., Halbrugge, M., and Walter, U. (1992). *Eur. J. Biochem.*, **205**, 471.
12. Crabos, M., Imber, R., Woodtli, T., Fabbro, D., and Erne, P. (1991). *Biochem. Biophys. Res. Commun.*, **178**, 878.
13. Wadman, I. A. (1992). PhD Thesis, University of Cambridge.
14. Wilkinson, S. E. and Hallam, T. J. (1994). *Trends Pharmacol. Sci.*, **15**, 53.
15. House, C. and Kemp, B. E. (1987). *Science*, **238**, 1726.
16. Smith, J. A., Francis, S. H., and Corbin, J. D. (1993). *Mol. Cell. Biol.*, **128**, 51.
17. Hanks, S. K., Quinn, A. M., and Hunter, T. (1988). *Science*, **241**, 42.
18. Ferrell, J. E. and Martin, G. S. (1989). *J. Biol. Chem.*, **264**, 20723.
19. Kocher, M. and Clemetson, K. J. (1991). *Biochem. J.*, **275**, 301.

20. Kameshita, I. and Fujisawa, H. (1989). *Anal. Biochem.*, **183,** 139.
21. Samiei, M., Sanghera, J. S., and Pelech, S. L. (1993). *Biochim. Biophys. Acta*, **1176,** 287.
22. Papkoff, J., Chen, R.-H., Blenis, J., and Forsman, J. (1994). *Mol. Cell. Biol.*, **14,** 463.
23. Leevers, S. J. and Marshall, C. J. (1992). *EMBO J.*, **11,** 569.
24. Nakashima, S., Chatani, Y., Nakamura, M., Miyoshi, N., Kohno, M., and Nozawa, Y. (1994). *Biochem. Biophys. Res. Commun.*, **198,** 497.
25. Milligan, G. (1988). *Biochem. J.*, **255,** 1.
26. Simonds, W. F., Goldsmith, P. K., Codina, J., Unson, C. G., and Speigel, A. M. (1989). *Proc. Natl. Acad. Sci. USA*, **86,** 7809.
27. Gierschik, P. and Jakobs, K. H. (1987). *FEBS Lett.*, **224,** 219.
28. Aktories, K. and Hall, A. (1989). *Trends Pharmacol. Sci.*, **10,** 415.
29. Zhang, J., King, W. G., Dillon, S., Hall, A., Feig, L., and Rittenhouse, S. E. (1993). *J. Biol. Chem.*, **268,** 22251.
30. Codina, J., Yatani, A., van Dongen, A. M. J., Padrell, E., Carty, D., Mattera, R., *et al.* (1990). In *G proteins* (ed. R. Iyengar and L. Birnbaumer), p. 267. Academic Press, New York.
31. Farndale, R. W., Winkler, A. B., Martin, B. R., and Barnes, M. J. (1992). *Biochem. J.*, **282,** 25.
32. Bhullar, R. P. and Haslam, R. J. (1987). *Biochem. J.*, **245,** 617.
33. Bhullar, R. P., Chardin, P., and Haslam, R. J. (1990). *FEBS Lett.*, **260,** 48.
34. Lapetina, E. G. and Reep, B. R. (1987). *Proc. Natl. Acad. Sci. USA*, **84,** 2261.
35. Tang, K. M., Sherwood, J. L., and Haslam, R. J. (1993). *Biochem. J.*, **294,** 329.
36. Knezevic, I., Borg, C., and LeBreton, G. C. (1993). *J. Biol. Chem.*, **268,** 26011.

10

Tyrosine phosphorylation

EDWIN A. CLARK and JOAN S. BRUGGE

1. Introduction

1.1 A role for tyrosine phosphorylation in signal transduction

One of the central questions in cell biology is how do cells communicate with each other and their environment, and how does an individual cell regulate itself? Characterization of the proteins that regulate extracellular and intracellular signal transduction has lead to an understanding of their role in biochemical pathways involved in cell growth, proliferation, and differentiation. One key regulatory event involves tyrosine phosphorylation of cellular proteins. The enzymes responsible for these phosphorylation events, protein tyrosine kinases (PTKs), fall into two general classes. First, the receptor tyrosine kinases, which have both extracellular (ligand binding) and intracellular (tyrosine kinase) domains that allow them to directly couple external stimuli to intracellular signalling (1). Secondly, the non-receptor tyrosine kinases, which functionally couple with membrane receptors via various protein interaction domains or carry out functions downstream of membrane triggered events. Such coupling allows this class of signal transducers to relay signals from the external environment to the cytoplasm and nucleus (2).

There is ample evidence to suggest that PTKs also play a primary role in platelet signal transduction (reviewed in ref. 3). The binding of numerous platelet agonists to membrane receptors initiates a cascade of events that includes platelet shape change, aggregation, and secretion. Platelet activation by these agonists also triggers polyphosphoinositide turnover, arachidonate metabolism, calcium mobilization and influx, and changes in protein phosphorylation. In particular, agonists such as thrombin, ADP, collagen, thromboxane A_2, and platelet activating factor all induce tyrosine phosphorylation of multiple platelet proteins. Furthermore, numerous signalling molecules associate with PTKs and each other, forming a variety of signalling complexes in resting and agonist-stimulated platelets. The cytoskeleton also appears to be involved in the formation of these complexes and in tyrosine phosphorylation. Finally, tyrosine kinase inhibitors block agonist-induced tyrosine phosphorylation as well as platelet aggregation and secretion. These results suggest that PTKs and tyrosine phosphorylation play a primary role in platelet activation.

1.2 Three waves of agonist-induced tyrosine phosphorylation of platelet proteins

The temporal order of agonist-induced tyrosine phosphorylation can best be described in terms of its regulation by the major platelet integrin receptor, $\alpha_{IIb}\beta_3$. This receptor has been shown to be intimately involved in one of the central events of platelet activation, platelet to platelet aggregation mediated by the binding of fibrinogen. In unstimulated platelets, $\alpha_{IIb}\beta_3$ is not competent to bind fibrinogen. Agonist stimulation induces a conformational change in $\alpha_{IIb}\beta_3$ that allows it to bind fibrinogen which can cross-link these

Table 1. Phosphotyrosine-containing proteins in activated platelets

Protein	M_r	Comments
Src-family kinases		
Src	60 kDa	Activated by integrin-independent mechanism; associated with cytoskeleton, PI3 kinase
Yes	62 kDa	Associated with cytoskeleton, CD36, and GAP
Lyn	54/58 kDa	Associated with cytoskeleton, CD36, and GAP
Fyn	59 kDa	Associated with cytoskeleton, CD36, GAP, and PI3K
Hck	60 kDa	?
Other tyrosine kinases		
Syk	72 kDa	Phosphorylated/activated by integrin-independent and dependent mechanisms
FAK	125 kDa	Phosphorylated/activated by aggregation-dependent mechanism
JAK	130 kDa	?
Signal transducers		
PLCγ	140 kDa	Associated with GAP in unstimulated platelets; associated with rap1B in stimulated platelets
GAP	120 kDa	Associated with Src-family kinases, PLCγ
MAP kinase	42 kDa	Phosphorylated/activated by integrin-independent mechanism
Cortactin	80–85 kDa	Associated with Src in thrombin-stimulated platelets; binds filamentous actin
Other		
FcγRII	40 kDa	Phosphorylated when Fcγ receptor is cross-linked
p110	110 kDa	Phosphorylated by integrin-independent mechanism
p140	140 kDa	Phosphorylation dependent on integrin engagement
p95/97	95/97 kDa	Phosphorylation is aggregation-dependent

receptors on the platelet surface. Finally, if the platelets are stirred, fibrinogen dimers can cross-link $\alpha_{IIb}\beta_3$ on adjacent platelets leading to platelet aggregation (4). Tyrosine phosphorylation in platelets can therefore be divided into four phases: resting platelets; early, integrin-independent; integrin engagement-dependent; and aggregation-dependent (see *Figure 1*). A list of phosphotyrosine-containing proteins in activated platelets is shown in *Table 1*.

First, there are those platelet proteins that are tyrosine phosphorylated in resting platelets (see *Figure 1*, lanes A and E). These proteins include five

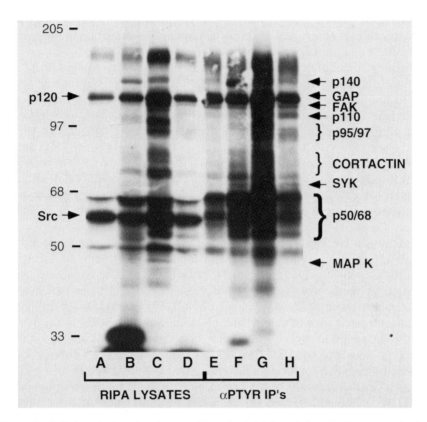

Figure 1. Antiphosphotyrosine immunoblot of platelet proteins. Resting or activated platelets were lysed in RIPA buffer (*Protocol 1C*). The lysates were either solubilized in SDS sample buffer (*Protocol 1D*) or immunoprecipitated with UP28, a rabbit polyclonal antiphosphotyrosine antiserum (*Protocol 2*). The samples were then electrophoresed on an SDS–polyacrylamide gel and immunoblotted for phosphotyrosine-containing proteins (*Protocol 3*). A–D are the RIPA lysates and E–H are the UP28 (antiphosphotyrosine) immunoprecipitates. A, E: resting platelet tyrosine phosphorylation; B, F: integrin engagement-dependent tyrosine phosphorylation (induced by LIBS6); C, G: thrombin-induced, aggregation-dependent tyrosine phosphorylation; D, H: thrombin-induced 'early', integrin-independent tyrosine phosphorylation.

members of the Src-family of non-receptor tyrosine kinases, all of which have molecular weights between 54 and 62 kDa. In resting platelets pp60$^{c\text{-src}}$, the prototypical member of this family, is exclusively phosphorylated at tyrosine 527. Phosphorylation at this site negatively regulates pp60$^{c\text{-src}}$ (5). In addition, an unidentified protein of 120 kDa is also tyrosine phosphorylated in resting platelets. We have found that other platelet proteins may become tyrosine phosphorylated if platelets are prematurely activated during the platelet preparation steps (e.g. during centrifugation and washing of platelets). To avoid this we have found that the inclusion of short-lived platelet activation inhibitors such as prostaglandin E$_1$ (1 µM) and apyrase (1.0 U/ml) in the platelet-rich plasma, and gel filtration of the platelets through Sepharose 2B columns rather than repeated centrifugation and washing, aid in maintaining platelets in an optimally quiescent state (see Chapter 1).

Agonist stimulation of platelets triggers the first wave of agonist-induced tyrosine phosphorylation (see *Figure 1*, lanes D and H). These 'early' events, which are independent of $\alpha_{IIb}\beta_3$, include the tyrosine phosphorylation of GAP (the GTPase activating protein for the small molecular weight G protein p21^{ras}), MAP (mitogen activated protein) kinase, cortactin (a protein that associates with filamentous actin), p72^{syk} (a cytosolic PTK), and an unidentified protein of 110 kDa (6–9). While the specific role(s) of these proteins in platelet physiology remains unknown, their phosphorylation during such an early stage of platelet activation suggests that they may be involved in events that occur rapidly in agonist-stimulated platelets such as platelet shape change, $\alpha_{IIb}\beta_3$ conformational change, and secretion.

Fibrinogen binding to $\alpha_{IIb}\beta_3$ triggers the second wave of agonist-induced tyrosine phosphorylation of p72^{syk} and unidentified proteins of 140 (p140) and 50–68 (p50–68) kDa (see *Figure 1*, lanes B and F). The tyrosine phosphorylation of these proteins is not observed in platelets from patients with Glanzmann thrombasthenia (which do not express $\alpha_{IIb}\beta_3$) or in normal platelets treated with inhibitors that block fibrinogen binding to $\alpha_{IIb}\beta_3$ (such as the tetrapeptide Arg–Gly–Asp–Ser or the monoclonal anti-β_3 antibody 7E3). In addition, specific stimulation of $\alpha_{IIb}\beta_3$ with the antibody LIBS6 (which induces the conformational change in $\alpha_{IIb}\beta_3$ that allows it to bind fibrinogen) in the presence of fibrinogen induces the tyrosine phosphorylation of p72^{syk}, p140, and p50–68 (9,10). The phosphorylation of these proteins probably plays a role in the adhesive and/or cytoskeletal events that follow integrin engagement.

Finally, platelet aggregation induced by fibrinogen cross-linking of $\alpha_{IIb}\beta_3$ on adjacent platelets stimulates the tyrosine phosphorylation of the PTK p125^{FAK} and two unidentified proteins of 95 and 97 kDa (p95/97) (see *Figure 1*, lanes C and G). The tyrosine phosphorylation of these proteins is also dependent on cytoskeletal rearrangements (that are inhibited by cytochalasin D treatment), protein kinase C (PKC), and a rise in intracellular calcium (11,12). Aggregation-dependent events such as activation of the calcium-dependent protease calpain, increases in arachidonate metabolism, cytoskeletal rearrangements, activation of protein tyrosine phosphatases, and secretion may be regulated by these phosphorylation events.

2. Identification of tyrosine phosphorylated proteins in platelets

2.1 Conditions for platelet activation or inhibition of activation

As described above, numerous agonists are capable of inducing platelet activation and tyrosine phosphorylation, and other agents are capable of inducing or inhibiting these events. One variable that makes studies on particular platelet agonists difficult to interpret is that the initial agonist may induce secretion of endogenous agonists that are either stored in platelet granules (e.g. ADP) or synthesized during cellular activation (e.g. thromboxane A_2). Thus, it is important to distinguish the effects of a primary agonist from those induced by a secondary, secreted agonist. This can be done by including cyclo-oxygenase inhibitors such as indomethacin (Sigma, I-7378) (10 μM) which inhibits thromboxane A_2 production, and ADP scavengers such as apyrase (Sigma, A-6535) (10 U/ml).

Numerous other factors can also affect platelet tyrosine phosphorylation. At higher agonist concentrations (e.g. 1.0 U/ml thrombin) it is often difficult to distinguish the three waves of agonist-induced tyrosine phosphorylation, so lower concentrations (0.1 U/ml thrombin) are routinely used. Furthermore, aggregation-dependent tyrosine phosphorylation requires that platelets be stirred (or agitated in some fashion), unless higher platelet concentrations (i.e. 1×10^9/ml) are used. At these platelet concentrations aggregation occurs, even in the absence of stirring, due to the proximity of platelets in the suspension. Finally, if bovine serum albumin (BSA) is present in the platelet suspension buffer, it should be of the highest quality (see *Protocol 3*) since phosphatases present in lower quality preparations of BSA can dephosphorylate proteins present in platelet lysates.

2.2 Preparation of platelet lysates

Many different types of buffers containing detergents such as Triton X-100, NP-40, deoxycholate, and SDS can be used to lyse platelets, depending on the desired result. Lysis with SDS-containing sample buffer is the choice to achieve complete solubilization of platelets; however, the presence of SDS at a concentration higher than 0.1% will preclude the sample being used for immunoprecipitation. Lysis with radioimmunoprecipitation 'RIPA' buffer (see *Protocol 1*C) solubilizes all phosphotyrosine-containing proteins that are detected in an antiphosphotyrosine immunoblot (see *Protocol 3*) and it allows the lysate to be used for immunoprecipitation assays (see *Protocol 2*).

Less stringent buffers containing detergents such as Triton X-100, NP-40, CHAPS, or digitonin help to maintain certain protein–protein interactions in resting or activated platelets (though non-specific interactions must be carefully controlled for using non-immune serum). However, many tyrosine phosphorylated proteins from aggregated platelets are insoluble in such buffers and sediment during lysate clarification (see Chapter 13). A number of different buffer conditions should be tested to determine those that best suit the needs of the experiment performed. We have included three buffers that span a range of stringency conditions, from least (Triton X-100) to most (SDS sample buffer). Also included are directions on how to prepare sodium orthovanadate, a buffer component that is essential for maintaining phosphotyrosine in platelet lysates. It should be noted that divalent cation chelators such as EDTA chelate the sodium orthovanadate and block its ability to inhibit protein tyrosine phosphatases, and should therefore be used at as low a concentration as possible (e.g. 1 mM final concentration in buffer with 1 mM sodium orthovanadate). For more details on the use of orthovanadate as a protein tyrosine phosphatase inhibitor and the analysis of protein phosphorylation, refer to Gordon (13).

Protocol 1. Lysis of platelet suspensions

Equipment and reagents

- Sodium orthovanadate (Fisher Scientific, S454-50)
- 2 × Triton buffer: 2% Triton X-100, 2 mM EGTA, 100 mM Tris pH 7.3 at 4°C
- 2 × RIPA buffer: 2% Triton X-100, 2% sodium deoxycholate, 0.2% SDS, 316 mM NaCl, 2 mM EGTA, 20 mM Tris pH 7.6 at 4°C—the pH of the buffer is critical since the sodium deoxycholate will precipitate out of solution if the pH is too low
- 4 × stock of SDS sample buffer: 280 mM Tris pH 7.2, 40% glycerol, 0.008% bromophenol blue, 8% SDS, 4% β-mercaptoethanol—stir overnight
- Inhibitor stocks: 50 mg/ml leupeptin and 5 M benzamidine in distilled water (stored at −20°C); 100 mM phenyl methyl sulfonyl fluoride (PMSF) in ethanol (stored at 25°C)
- Fisher Vortex Genie 2 (Fisher Scientific)
- Eppendorf Centrifuge 5415 C

A. Preparation of sodium orthovanadate (100 mM)

1. Dissolve 1.84 g sodium orthovanadate in 100 ml distilled water.

2. Heat to boiling while stirring the solution with a magnetic stir bar. Boil for 5 min.

3. Allow the solution to cool to room temperature and add distilled water to return the solution to 100 ml. The stock solution is good for at least one year.

4. If the sodium orthovanadate precipitates out of solution, add an equal volume of distilled water to make a final stock of 50 mM. This stock should remain soluble.

5. To test the sodium orthovanadate solution, lyse thrombin-stimulated/aggregated platelets with an equal volume of 2 × Triton

buffer with or without 2 mM sodium orthovanadate. Analyse the phosphotyrosine-containing proteins by immunoblotting with anti-bodies to phosphotyrosine as described in *Protocol 3* to determine whether the orthovanadate prevented the loss of tyrosine phosphory-lated proteins.

B. Triton X-100 lysis of platelets

1. Add fresh inhibitor stocks (final concentration in 2 × Triton buffer : 1 mg/ml leupeptin, 100 mM benzamidine, 2 mM PMSF, 2 mM sodium orthovanadate) to the 2 × Triton buffer immediately before use.

2. Add an equal volume of 2 × Triton buffer to the platelet suspension (4 × 10^8 platelets/ml) and transfer to an Eppendorf tube. Vortex the sample and place it on ice. To fractionate the sample into Triton solu-ble and insoluble proteins, keep it on ice for 5 min (see Chapter 11). To get optimal solubilization of proteins in this buffer, keep the sample on ice for 30 min.

3. Microcentrifuge for 5 min, 16000 *g* at 4°C. The supernatant can be removed and used as the Triton soluble fraction. Solubilize the pellet in sample buffer (see *Protocol 1D*) or by vortexing for 30 min at 4°C in a starting volume of (RIPA) buffer (see *Protocol 1C*).

4. Microcentrifuge the resolubilized pellet fraction for 5 min, 16000 *g* at 4°C. The supernatant can be removed and used as the Triton insolu-ble, RIPA soluble fraction.

C. RIPA lysis of platelets

1. Add fresh inhibitor stocks (final concentration in 2 × RIPA buffer: 1 mg/ml leupeptin, 100 mM benzamidine, 2 mM PMSF, 2 mM sodium orthovanadate) to the 2 × RIPA buffer immediately before use.

2. Add an equal volume of 2 × RIPA buffer to the platelet suspension and transfer to an Eppendorf tube. Vortex the sample and place it on ice for 5 min.

3. Microcentrifuge for 5 min, 16000 *g* at 4°C. The supernatant can be removed and used as the RIPA soluble fraction.

D. Solubilization of platelet lysates in SDS sample buffer

SDS sample buffer can be used to solubilize platelet proteins in a variety of ways:

1. Add 50 μl of 4 × SDS sample buffer to 150 μl of Triton or RIPA solubil-ized platelet fractions. Vortex and heat to 100°C for 5 min.

2. For the solubilization of the Triton and RIPA insoluble pellets, a volume of 1 × SDS sample buffer (one part 4 × SDS sample buffer plus three parts distilled water) equal to the starting volume of platelets should be

Protocol 1. *Continued*

added. The pellets are extremely insoluble, and should be repeatedly vortexed and heated to 100 °C to insure complete solubilization of the pellet.

3. Optionally, the platelets in suspension can be directly lysed in 100 °C
SDS sample buffer, adding one part 4 × buffer to three parts platelet
suspension. The samples should be thoroughly vortexed and heated
to 100 °C. Platelets should not be pelleted out of suspension by micro-
centrifugation before lysing, as this can lead to inadvertent activation
of the platelets.

2.3 Immunoprecipitation

The choice of immunoabsorbent is more a matter of choice than necessity.
We have found that protein A-containing membranes from formalin fixed *S.
aureus* cells (Pansorbin) are more easily pelleted upon centrifugation and
therefore are used when quantitatively immunoprecipitating, whereas protein A agarose requires less stringent washing and provides a lower background signal. When beginning a protocol, both Pansorbin and protein A
agarose should be tested to determine which suits the needs of the experiment in question.

Protocol 2. Immunoprecipitation of platelet proteins

Equipment and reagents

- Pansorbin: 10% suspension of formalin fixed *S. aureus* cells (Calbiochem-Nov-abiochem Corporation, 507858)
- Protein A agarose (Pierce, 20333)
- RIPA buffer (see *Protocol 1*)
- Triton buffer (see *Protocol 1*)
- Crystallized bovine serum albumin (BSA) (ICN Biomedicals Inc., 809233)
- Triton wash buffer: 1% Triton X-100, 1 mM EGTA, 50 mM Tris pH 7.2, 150 mM NaCl, 1 mM PMSF, 1 mM sodium orthovanadate

- RIPA wash buffer: 1% Triton X-100, 1% sodium deoxycholate, 0.1% SDS, 158 mM NaCl, 1 mM EGTA, 10 mM Tris pH 7.2, 1 mM PMSF, 1 mM sodium orthovanadate
- Rabbit anti-mouse IgG (Organon Teknika Corp., 55480)
- Fisher Vortex Genie 2 (Fisher Scientific)
- Eppendorf Centrifuge 5415 C
- Heat block (VWR Scientific)
- Haematology/chemistry mixer model No. 346 (Fisher Scientific)

A. Preparation of Pansorbin

1. Microcentrifuge the Pansorbin suspension for 1 min in a microcentrifuge at 16 000 *g*. Remove the supernatant and resuspend the
pellet in the starting volume of either Triton or RIPA buffer, depending
on which buffer was used to lyse the platelets (see *Protocol 1*).

2. Incubate 15–30 min at room temperature, microcentrifuge for 1 min at
16 000 *g*, and remove the supernatant. Resuspend the pellet in the
starting volume of either Triton or RIPA buffer containing 1% BSA and
store on ice until needed (good for 24 h).

3. If mouse monoclonal antibodies are being used, incubate 1 μg of rabbit anti-mouse immunoglobulin with each 30 μl of Pansorbin/1% BSA solution for at least 20 min on ice.

B. Immunoprecipitation

1. Pre-clear the platelet lysate (see *Protocol 1*) by adding 30 μl of Pansorbin/1% BSA solution to the lysate and incubating for 30 min at 4°C. The sample should be continuously mixed by placing it on a mixer (see *Equipment* list).

2. Microcentrifuge the sample for 1 min at 16000 *g*, 4°C. The supernatant should be moved to a fresh microcentrifuge tube and 1–5 μg of polyclonal or monoclonal antibody should be added. Vortex and incubate on a mixer for 1–12 h at 4°C. The length of incubation will vary with the antibody used. For best results, the correct incubation time should be experimentally determined.

3. Add 30 μl of Pansorbin/1% BSA solution (or 30 μl of protein A agarose if desired) to the sample. Vortex and incubate on a mixer for 30–60 min at 4°C.

4. Microcentrifuge the sample for 1 min at 16000 *g* to pellet the Pansorbin and wash three times by resuspending the pellet in 700 μl of ice-cold wash buffer and then microcentrifuging. Wash the RIPA lysed samples in RIPA wash and the Triton lysed samples in Triton wash.

5. If the immunoprecipitates are to be electrophoresed and immunoblotted, the pellets should be resuspended in 30–100 μl of SDS sample buffer (see *Protocol 1*) and heated to 100°C for 5 min to elute the immunoprecipitated proteins.[a] Microcentrifuge the sample and load the supernatant on to an SDS–PAGE. If the immunoprecipitates are to be subjected to an *in vitro* kinase reaction, see *Protocol 4*.

[a] Heating the immunoprecipitate to 100°C in the presence of β-mercaptoethanol will reduce the immunoprecipitating antibody disulfide bonds holding the heavy and light chains together. If the detecting antibody used for immunoblotting is the same species as the immunoprecipitating antibody, the heavy chains will be detected. This may interfere in the detection of proteins in the 40–60 kDa range. Since the disulfide bonds holding the heavy and light chains together require boiling to reduce, these chains (one heavy and one light) can be redirected to the 90 kDa range of an SDS–polyacrylamide gel by not boiling the immunoprecipitate.

2.4 Antiphosphotyrosine immunoblotting

The quality of an antiphosphotyrosine immunoblot can vary greatly depending on the care that is taken. Only the highest grade reagents (especially of BSA since impure preparations may contain phosphotyrosine-containing proteins as well as protein tyrosine phosphatases) should be used, and buffers should be filtered before each use to ensure that they are free of particles (living or other). In addition, we have found that the SDS–polyacrylamide gel concentration and time of transfer can greatly affect the detection of phosphotyrosine-containing proteins, as described in *Protocol 3*.

Protocol 3. Antiphosphotyrosine immunoblotting of platelet proteins

Equipment and reagents

- Nitrocellulose: 0.2 μm or 0.45 μm pore size (Schleicher and Schuell)
- Crystallized BSA (ICN Biomedicals Inc., 809233)
- PY20 antiphosphotyrosine antibody (Transduction Laboratories, 11120)
- 4G10 antiphosphotyrosine antibody (Upstate Biotechnology Inc., 05-321)
- Horse-radish peroxidase-conjugate goat anti-mouse immunoglobulin (Bio-Rad Laboratories, 170-6516)
- Nalgene tissue culture filter
- ECL Western blotting kit reagents (Amersham Life Science, RPN2106)
- Transfer apparatus (Hoefer Scientific)
- Orbital shaker (Bellco Biotechnology)
- Rocker platform (Bellco Biotechnology)
- Transfer buffer: 25 mM Tris pH 7.5, 192 mM glycine, 20% methanol, 0.1% SDS
- Western wash buffer: 50 mM Tris pH 7.5, 150 mM NaCl, 0.2% NP-40

Method

1. Fractionate the samples (platelet lysates or immunoprecipitates) on an appropriate SDS–PAGE. Place the gel in transfer buffer and shake on an orbital shaker for 5 min.

2. Cut a piece of nitrocellulose paper to a size that will fit the gel. If the nitrocellulose has been stored at 4°C, it should be hydrated in an immaculately clean dish of hot (but not bubbling hot) distilled water for about 5 min. If the nitrocellulose is stored at room temperature, proceed to the next step.

3. Place the nitrocellulose into the container with the gel and transfer buffer and let them shake together for another 5 min. Lay the nitrocellulose on to the gel between two sheets of filter paper, being careful not to introduce any air bubbles between the gel and nitrocellulose.

4. Transfer the gel. Transferring at 0.5 amps for 75 min is typically best for the 60 kDa region of a 1.5 mM thick, 7.5% polyacrylamide gel, but longer times are often used to achieve a greater degree of transfer of proteins of higher molecular weight.

5. Rinse the nitrocellulose in distilled water in a very clean container for 2 min and then place it in blocking buffer (5% BSA in Western wash buffer) on a rocking platform for 1–12 h. The blocking buffer can be reused by filtering it through a 0.2 μm Nalgene filter and storing at 4°C. In this way the blocking buffer can be used 25 times or more over a six month period.

---

6. Decant the blocking buffer and add antiphosphotyrosine antibodies PY20 and/or 4G10 (each diluted to 1 µg/ml in 3% BSA/Western wash buffer). Incubate with gentle rocking for 90 min at room temperature and then decant the antibody solution. As with the blocking buffer, the primary antibody can be reused by filtering it through a 0.2 µm Nalgene filter and storing at 4°C.

7. Wash the immunoblot with Western wash buffer for 30 min with agitation on an orbital shaker, changing the wash buffer four times.

8. Decant the wash buffer and add horse-radish peroxidase-conjugated goat anti-mouse immunoglobulin (diluted 1 : 10000–20000 in 1% BSA/Western wash buffer). Incubate with gentle rocking for 60 min at room temperature and then decant the antibody solution.

9. Wash with Western wash buffer for 45 min with agitation on an orbital shaker, changing the buffer five times.

10. Prepare the immunoblot for chemiluminescence (ECL) and expose it to film.

3. Analysis of protein tyrosine kinases in platelets

3.1 Immunoprecipitation/kinase assays

To date, five families of protein tyrosine kinases have been identified in platelets. The most abundant tyrosine kinase is Src, which represents as much as 0.4% of total platelet protein (14). Four other members of this family are present in platelets (Fyn, Lyn, Yes, and Hck), though at significantly lower levels (15,16). Thrombin stimulation of platelets induces a two- to fourfold increase in the specific kinase activity of Src, phosphorylation of Src at the site of autophosphorylation (tyrosine 416), and a redistribution to the Triton insoluble (cytoskeletal) fraction upon platelet aggregation (17). While the activation of Src occurs by an integrin-independent mechanism, its redistribution is integrin-dependent. The activation and redistribution of Src suggests that it may be involved in both early, integrin-independent events as well as aggregation-dependent events. Fyn, Lyn, and Yes also redistribute to the cytoskeletal fraction in an integrin-dependent manner (8). In addition, there is evidence suggesting that multiple Src-family members may be activated upon thrombin stimulation:

- Src associates with the actin-filament associated protein cortactin (18)

- Src and Fyn associate with phosphatidylinositol 3-kinase (PI3K) (19)

- Yes, Fyn, and Lyn (but not Src) associate with GAP, the GTPase activating protein for $p21^{ras}$ (6)

In addition, Yes, Fyn, and Lyn (but not Src) associate with glycoprotein IV (GPIV) in unstimulated platelets, suggesting that these kinases may be ideally suited to transduce signals from this cell surface receptor (16).

The focal adhesion kinase (FAK) is a 125 kDa tyrosine kinase that is both tyrosine phosphorylated and activated in platelets in an aggregation-dependent manner (11). This suggests that FAK is not involved in the platelet events that precede platelet aggregation and may play a critical role in those events that occur either concomitant with or following platelet aggregation. In adherent cells, FAK is localized to focal adhesion sites and is phosphorylated upon spreading on extracellular matrices. This suggests a common function for FAK in integrin-mediated events in a variety of cell types.

Syk, a 72 kDa tyrosine kinase, has been identified in platelets (20) and shown to be rapidly activated and tyrosine phosphorylated in thrombin-stimulated platelets by both integrin-independent and integrin engagement-dependent mechanisms (9,21). Syk is also activated by other agonists such as thromboxane A_2, ADP, and collagen as well as the lectin wheat germ agglutinin (9,20,22). In addition, Syk is negatively regulated by calcium (21,22). Thus, Syk may be involved in both early, integrin-independent events as well as those that require integrin engagement.

Two other tyrosine kinase families have been identified in platelets or their precursors (megakaryocytes). JAK 2, a kinase shown to purify with several members of the cytokine receptor family (23), and MATK, a recently cloned tyrosine kinase of megakaryocytic lineage showing closest homology to the Csk tyrosine kinase (24) have yet to be investigated in platelets.

Protocol 4. Immunoprecipitation/kinase assays

Equipment and reagents

- 50 mM acetic acid
- Enolase (Sigma, E-0379)
- Anti-Src antibody (Oncogene Science Inc., OP07L)
- Anti-Syk antibody (Upstate Biotechnology Inc., 06-273)
- Low salt buffer: 100 mM NaCl, 10 mM Tris pH 7.2, 5 mM MnCl$_2$
- Tris–Mn buffer: 10 mM Tris pH 7.4, 5 mM MnCl$_2$
- Syk kinase lysis buffer: 1% Triton X-100, 50 mM Hepes pH 7.5, 75 mM NaCl, 1 mM EGTA

- Kinase reaction buffer: 10 mM Tris pH 7.4, 5 mM MnCl$_2$, 6 µM ATP, 5 µCi [γ-^{32}P]ATP (and 5 µg of activated enolase as an exogenous substrate, if desired)
- Syk kinase mix: 25 mM Hepes pH 7.5, 10 mM MnCl$_2$, 1 µM ATP, 5 µCi [γ-^{32}P]ATP
- Hepes/NaCl buffer: 50 mM Hepes pH 7.5, 150 mM NaCl
- SDS sample buffer (see *Protocol 1*)
- Fisher Vortex Genie 2
- Eppendorf Centrifuge 5415 C
- Heat block (VWR Scientific)

A. Src and FAK in vitro kinase assays

1. Activate enolase at this time if it will be used in the kinase assay as an exogenous substrate. Incubate 1 µl (5 µg) of rabbit muscle enolase with 1 µl of 50 mM acetic acid for each reaction at 37 °C for 15 min. Store on ice until needed.

2. Perform immunoprecipitation assay as described in *Protocol 2*.

3. Pellet the washed immunoprecipitate (see *Protocol 2*) and wash it one additional time in 700 μl of low salt buffer.

4. Add 25 μl of Tris–Mn buffer to the Pansorbin pellet and vortex vigorously to resuspend the pellet.

5. After 5 min at room temperature, add 5 μl of kinase reaction buffer. Vortex, incubate at 30°C for 2 min, and stop the reaction with 30 μl of 2 × SDS sample buffer.[a]

6. Heat the sample for 5 min at 100°C, microcentrifuge for 1 min, and load the sample on to SDS–PAGE. Dry the gel and expose it to film[b] (see *Figure 2A*).

7. For specific activity measurements, duplicate samples should be subjected to SDS–PAGE and immunoblotted to detect kinase protein levels. This then allows a correlation between protein levels and enolase phosphorylation.

B. Syk in vitro kinase assay

1. Syk kinases assays were best performed using Syk kinase lysis buffer for platelet lysis. Wash the immunoprecipitate two times with Syk kinase lysis buffer and one time with Hepes/NaCl buffer.

2. Initiate the kinase assay by adding 20 μl of Syk kinase mix to the immunoprecipitate, vortexing, and incubating the reaction for 4 min at 25°C.

3. Stop the reaction by adding 20 μl of 2 × SDS sample buffer and heating to 100°C for 5 min.

4. Subject the sample to electrophoresis on an SDS–polyacrylamide gel and dry the gel. Expose it to film[b] (see *Figure 2B*).

[a] If the reaction is done in the absence of enolase, the reaction can be stopped by adding 1 ml of low salt buffer and immediately microcentrifuging the sample for 1 min, allowing the unincorporated [γ-^{32}P]ATP to be removed with this wash. Sample buffer can then be added to the pellet and the sample heated, microcentrifuged, and subjected to SDS–PAGE.
[b] Polyacrylamide gels containing ^{32}P-labelled proteins can be rehydrated in 10% methanol, 5% acetic acid and then treated with 1 M KOH for 1 h at 60°C to remove the alkali labile phosphate (phosphoserine and phosphothreonine) (25).

3.2 Platelet proteins associated with protein tyrosine kinases

A number of investigators have used various strategies to identify proteins to which Src-family kinases associate. A strategy has been employed in which various candidate proteins are immunoprecipitated from resting or activated platelets and subjected to an *in vitro* kinase assay. The reaction is then stopped and any complex between the candidate protein and a kinase can be

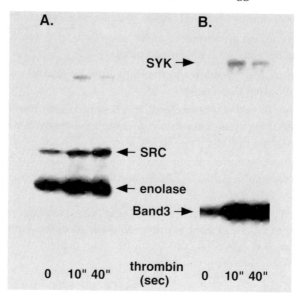

Figure 2. Autoradiograph of Src and Syk immunoprecipitation/kinase assays. (A) pp60[c-src] immunoprecipitated from Triton lysates (see *Protocol 1*) of resting (0) or thrombin treated platelets (for 10 or 40 sec with 0.1 U/ml thrombin) was subjected to an *in vitro* kinase assay using acid denatured rabbit muscle enolase as an exogenous substrate (see *Protocol 4A*). (B) pp72[syk] immunoprecipitated from a modified Triton lysate (see *Protocol 4B*) of resting (0) or thrombin treated platelets (for 10 or 40 sec with 0.1 U/ml thrombin) was subjected to an *in vitro* kinase assay using a glutathione S-transferase fusion protein containing amino acids 1–15 of the erythrocyte protein Band3 as an exogenous substrate as described (*Protocol 4B*). The samples in panel A were subjected to electrophoresis on a 10% polyacrylamide gel and those in panel B on a 12% polyacrylamide gel.

dissociated with SDS. Once the dissociated complex is diluted in buffer (to reduce the SDS concentration to 0.1%), the kinase can be immunoprecipitated with a kinase-specific antibody. In this way, kinases associated with prospective signalling molecules can be identified. Performing similar sorts of experiments, Src-family kinases have been shown to associate with a variety of platelet signalling molecules:

- Fyn, Lyn, and Yes with GPIV in unstimulated platelets (16)
- Fyn, Lyn, and Yes with tyrosine phosphorylated GAP in thrombin-stimulated platelets (6)
- Src with tyrosine phosphorylated cortactin in thrombin-stimulated platelets (18)
- Src with $G_{i\alpha}$ in epinephrine-stimulated (but not thrombin-stimulated) platelets (26)
- Src and Fyn with PI3K in thrombin-stimulated platelets (19)

Such strategies will no doubt aid in identifying protein tyrosine kinases involved in platelet signal transduction.

Protocol 5. Kinase trapping strategy

Equipment and reagents

- Buffer B: 1% Triton X-100, 50 mM NaCl, 1 mM sodium orthovanadate, 1 mM PMSF, 30 mM sodium pyrophosphate, 50 mM NaF, 10 mM Tris pH 7.4
- Buffer A: 1% SDS, 150 mM NaCl, 10 mM Tris pH 7.4
- Heat block (VWR Scientific)

Method

1. Perform immunoprecipitation/kinase assays without exogenous substrates added (see *Protocol 4*). Stop the reaction by adding 100 µl of buffer A and heating the sample to 100°C for 10 min.

2. Dilute the sample in 900 µl of buffer B.

3. Incubate with 30 µl of Pansorbin (see *Protocol 2*) for 30 min to remove immunoglobulin molecules. Microcentrifuge for 1 min at 16000 *g* to pellet the Pansorbin.

4. Move the supernatant to a fresh Eppendorf tube and incubate with 1–5 µg of polyclonal or monoclonal antikinase antibody to immuno-precipitate the autophosphorylated kinase. Adsorb the immunoprecipitated proteins to Pansorbin, wash, and elute as described (*Protocol 2*).

5. Electrophorese the samples on an SDS–polyacrylamide gel, dry the gel, and expose it to film.

3.3 Tyrosine kinase inhibitors and their effects on platelet physiology

To better understand the role of protein tyrosine kinases in platelet signal transduction, a number of kinase inhibitors that show some specificity for protein tyrosine kinases have been employed. Protein tyrosine kinase inhibitors such as tyrphostin, genistein, and erbstatin have been observed to inhibit tyrosine phosphorylation of platelet proteins induced by thrombin, platelet activating factor, thromboxane A_2, and GTPγS (in permeabilized platelets). These inhibitors also affected agonist-induced platelet events such as activation of the integrin $\alpha_{IIb}\beta_3$, platelet aggregation, phosphatidylinositol turnover, calcium mobilization, PKC activation, and serotonin secretion (27–31). These results suggest that protein tyrosine kinases may regulate signalling pathways involved in these platelet events. However, the *in vivo* targets of these kinase inhibitors have not been defined, so it is difficult to rigorously determine the pathways that are affected by these agents.

References

1. Yarden, Y. and Ullrich, A. (1988). *Annu. Rev. Biochem.*, **57,** 443.
2. Cantley, L. C., Auger, K. R., Carpenter, C., Duckworth, B., Graziani, A., Kapeller, R., *et al.* (1991). *Cell*, **64,** 281.
3. Clark, E. A. and Brugge, J. S. (1993). *Trends Cardiovasc. Med.*, **3,** 218.
4. Phillips, D. R., Charo, I. F., and Scarborough, R. M. (1991). *Cell*, **65,** 359.
5. Cooper, J. A., Gould, K. L., Cartwright, C. A., and Hunter, T. (1986). *Science*, **231,** 1431.
6. Cichowski, K., McCormick, F., and Brugge, J. S. (1992). *J. Biol. Chem.*, **267,** 5025.
7. Papkoff, J., Chen, R.-H., Blenis, J., and Forsman, J. (1994). *Mol. Cell. Biol.*, **14,** 463.
8. Fox, J. E. B., Lipfert, L., Clark, E. A., Reynolds, C. C., Austin, C. D., and Brugge, J. S. (1993). *J. Biol. Chem.*, **268,** 25973.
9. Clark, E. A., Shattil, S. J., Ginsberg, M. H., Bolen, J. and Brugge, J. S. (1994). *J. Biol. Chem.*, **269,** 28859.
10. Huang, M.-M., Lipfert, L., Cunningham, M., Brugge, J. S., Ginsbergm, M. H., and Shattil, S. J. (1993). *J. Cell Biol.*, **122,** 473.
11. Lipfert, L., Haimovich, B., Schaller, M. D., Cobb, B. S., Parsons, J. T., and Brugge, J. S. (1992). *J. Cell Biol.*, **119,** 905.
12. Shattil, S. J., Haimovich, B., Cunningham, M., Lipfert, L., Parsons, J. T., Ginsberg, M. H., *et al.* (1994). *J. Biol. Chem.*, **269,** 14738.
13. Gordon, J. A. (1991). In *Methods in enzymology* (ed. T. Hunter and B. Sefton), Vol. 201, pp. 477–82. Academic Press, London.
14. Golden, A., Nemeth, S., and Brugge, J. S. (1986). *Proc. Natl. Acad. Sci. USA*, **83,** 852.
15. Horak, I. D., Corcoran, M. L., Thompson, P. A., Wahl, L. M., and Bolen, J. B. (1990). *Oncogene*, **5,** 697.
16. Huang, M.-M., Bolen, J. B., Barnwell, J. W., Shattil, S. J., and Brugge, J. S. (1991). *Proc. Natl. Acad. Sci. USA*, **88,** 7844.
17. Clark, E. A. and Brugge, J. S. (1993). *Mol. Cell. Biol.*, **13,** 1863.
18. Wong, S., Reynolds, A. B., and Papkoff, J. (1992). *Oncogene*, **7,** 2407.
19. Gutkind, J. S., Lacal, P. M., and Robbins, K. C. (1990). *Mol. Cell. Biol.*, **10,** 3806.
20. Ohta, S., Taniguchi, T., Asahi, M., Kato, Y., Nakagawara, G., and Yamamura, H. (1992). *Biochem. Biophys. Res. Commun.*, **185,** 1128.
21. Taniguchi, T., Kitagawa, H., Yasue, S., Tanagi, S., Sakai, K., Asahi, M., *et al.* (1993). *J. Biol. Chem.*, **268,** 2277.
22. Maeda, H., Taniguchi, T., Inazu, T., Yang, C., Nakagawara, G., and Yamamura, H. (1993). *Biochem. Biophys. Res. Commun.*, **197,** 62.
23. Rodriguez-Linares, B. and Watson, S. P. (1994). *Febs Lett.*, **352,** 335.
24. Bennett, B. D., Cowley, S., Jiang, S., London, R., Deng, B., Grabarek, J., *et al.* (1994). *J. Biol. Chem.*, **269,** 1068.
25. Cooper, J. A. and Hunter, T. (1981). *Mol. Cell. Biol.*, **1,** 165.
26. Torti, M., Crouch, M. F., and Lapetina, E. G. (1992). *Biochem. Biophys. Res. Commun.*, **186,** 440.
27. Dhar, A., Paul, A. K., and Shukla, A. D. (1990). *Mol. Pharmacol.*, **37,** 519.
28. Gaudette, D. C. and Holub, B. J. (1990). *Biochem. Biophys. Res. Commun.*, **170,** 238.

29. Shattil, S. J., Cunningham, M., Wiedmer, T., Zhao, J., Sims, J., and Brass, L. F. (1992). *J. Biol. Chem.*, **267,** 18424.
30. Asahi, M., Yanagi, S., Ohta, S., Inazu, T., Sakai, K., Takeuchi, F., *et al.* (1992). *FEBS Lett.*, **309,** 10.
31. Murphy, C. T., Kellie, S., and Westwick, J. (1993). *Eur. J. Biochem.*, **216,** 639.

11

Study of proteins associated with the platelet cytoskeleton

JOAN E. B. FOX

1. Introduction

1.1 The critical role of the platelet cytoskeleton in regulating platelet function

The platelet cytoskeleton is made up of a network of cross-linked actin filaments that exists throughout the cytoplasm, a microtubule coil that is wound tightly on itself just beneath the membrane, and a membrane skeleton that coats the inner surface of the phospholipid bilayer. There appear to be interconnections between each of these components of the cytoskeleton. Further, the membrane skeleton associates with the cytoplasmic domains of transmembrane receptors. In this way the network of cytoplasmic filaments functions as a scaffold that is linked to the plasma membrane and serves to regulate the contours of the membrane and thus the shape of the cell.

As platelets adhere at a site of injury, they change shape and spread over the damaged area; additional platelets become activated by soluble agonists released at the site of injury; and activation results in changes that enable the platelets to adhere to the original layer of adherent cells, aggregate, change their shape, and extend and retract filopodia in a process in which the cytoskeleton continuously reorganizes and contracts. The result is the formation of a tight platelet plug that continuously pulls in strands of the externally bound fibrin clot. All of these processes involve the platelet cytoskeleton (for a review, see ref. 1). It has been known for many years that the changes in platelet shape are induced as more actin monomers become polymerized into filaments and the network of filaments reorganizes. The retraction of filopodia with their externally bound fibrin clots occurs as the network of filaments binds myosin and tension is generated.

Because of the cytoskeleton's role in regulating the shape and contractile activities of platelets, there has long been considerable interest in identifying the proteins that cross-link the actin filament network, those that induce reorganization of the network, and those that regulate the polymerization of actin filaments in platelets. More recently, it has become apparent that the cytoskeleton does not simply respond to activation by reorganizing, but that it is itself actively involved in regulating the activation process and in regulating the functional activities of signalling molecules.

1.2 The role of the platelet cytoskeleton in transmembrane signalling

Evidence that the cytoskeleton may be involved in regulating platelet activation comes from the observation that signalling enzymes (pp60^{c-src}, pp62^{c-yes}, the p21^{ras} GTPase activating protein, GAP) are recovered with components of the membrane skeleton from detergent lysates of unstimulated platelets (2). Some of the proteins that are rapidly phosphorylated on tyrosine residues when an agonist is added to platelets appear to be associated with the platelet cytoskeleton (2,3), raising the possibility that the cytoskeleton may be involved in regulating early activation-induced events. As platelets adhere to the extracellular matrix or aggregate, adhesive receptors transmit signals that induce cytoskeletal reorganizations and the association of signalling molecules with this structure (1–12). For example, as $\alpha_{IIb}\beta_3$ binds adhesive ligand in a platelet aggregate, it induces signals that cause the cytoskeletal scaffolding to reorganize and several proteins (e.g. phosphatidylinositol 3-kinase (9), calpain (10), pp125^{FAK} (unpublished observations), phospholipase C (11), and pp60^{c-src} (11,12)) to associate with the cytoskeleton. Signalling induced by von Willebrand factor binding to GPIb–IX has also been shown to result in altered association of pp60^{c-src} and phosphatidylinositol 3-kinase with the cytoskeleton (8).

The picture that is emerging is that the cytoskeletal scaffolding in platelets binds signalling molecules, localizing them adjacent to their targets or regulating their activation. It is thought that the reorganization of the cytoskeletal scaffolding in platelets involved in adhesion or aggregation serves to recruit or activate signalling molecules that are required for the motile and contractile events that follow adhesion and aggregation. The finding that cytochalasins, which disrupt the networks of actin within platelets, inhibit adhesive ligand-induced cytoskeletal reorganizations (4), and inhibit adhesive ligand-induced activation of pp125^{FAK} (6) and calpain (10), is consistent with the importance of the cytoskeletal scaffolding in recruiting and activating signalling molecules.

To understand the role of the cytoskeleton in regulating the shape of unstimulated platelets, regulating the activities of signalling enzymes, and inducing contractile events such as migration, shape change, and clot retraction, it will be necessary to have a detailed understanding of the cytoskeletal proteins that make up the cytoskeleton, the interrelationships of these proteins, and the identity of signalling molecules that associate with the cytoskeleton in unstimulated and activated platelets.

2. Cytoskeleton-associated proteins

In order to fully understand the role of cytoskeletal proteins in platelet function, it will be important to determine which proteins are associated with the cytoskeleton in unstimulated platelets, which associate in the very early stages of activation, and which associate as a consequence of occupancy of adhesive receptors. To determine at which stage of activation a protein associates with the cytoskeleton, it is therefore important to precisely define the conditions under which platelet suspensions are activated. Such conditions are defined in Section 2.1.

The method that is most commonly used to determine whether a protein is associated with the cytoskeleton is to lyse the platelets with detergent and to determine whether the protein co-sediments with the detergent insoluble actin filaments. Care must be given to interpreting results obtained by this approach: some proteins may go undetected because they dissociate from the cytoskeleton in detergent lysates, but others may co-sediment with the cytoskeleton because they are themselves inherently insoluble in detergent rather than because they are associated with the insoluble cytoskeleton. Methods are now available that retain cytoskeletons in detergent lysates with much of the organization they have in the intact cell. Methods are also available for assessing whether a protein is insoluble in detergent lysates because it is associated with the cytoskeleton. These methods are discussed in Section 2.2.

Once a protein has been implicated as being associated with the cytoskeleton in detergent lysates, it is desirable to determine whether it is associated with this structure in the intact cell. This criterion for cytoskeletal association has been met for only a few of the proteins that are associated with the platelet cytoskeleton. Methods for investigating the composition of the cytoskeleton in the intact cell are discussed in Section 2.3.

2.1 Methods for obtaining suspensions of platelets

In order to differentiate between proteins that are associated with the cytoskeleton in unstimulated platelets and those that associate as a consequence of platelet activation, it is important to start with platelet suspensions that are isolated in an unstimulated state. Considerable attention has been given to devising means for isolating platelets from plasma under conditions in which inadvertent activation does not take place. Appropriate methods for isolating suspensions of unstimulated platelets are described elsewhere in this book (see Chapter 1).

It is becoming increasingly apparent that in activated platelets some cytoskeletal changes are induced as a consequence of initial agonist-induced signalling, while others are induced as a consequence of the subsequent activation-induced binding of adhesive receptors to their ligands. In order to identify proteins that associate with the cytoskeleton as a consequence of the initial activation of platelets, care must be taken to prevent those changes that occur subsequent to the release of granule contents and binding of adhesive ligand to adhesive receptor. In platelets, transmembrane signalling is induced as a consequence of ligand binding to the fibrinogen receptor ($\alpha_{IIb}\beta_3$) (1–4,6,7,9–12), the collagen receptor ($\alpha_2\beta_1$) (5), and the von Willebrand factor receptor (GPIb–IX) (8). In platelet suspensions, signalling induced by $\alpha_2\beta_1$ can be avoided by using an agonist other than collagen; under these conditions signalling is not induced by GPIb–IX because soluble von Willebrand factor does not normally bind to this receptor. Thus, the major adhesive receptor that induces transmembrane signalling in a suspension of platelets activated with an agonist other than collagen is assumed to be $\alpha_{IIb}\beta_3$, which binds fibrinogen released from activated platelelets. Studies on $\alpha_{IIb}\beta_3$-mediated transmembrane signalling have suggested that binding of ligand to this receptor induces some transmembrane signalling (apparently by inducing dimerization of the receptor) while cross-linking of receptor with antibodies that bind to the ligand binding site induces even more signalling (13–15). In the case of physiological ligand, maximum $\alpha_{IIb}\beta_3$-induced signalling appears to take place if platelet suspensions are stirred. The requirement for stirring may reflect the fact that the increased cell–cell contact induced by stirring accelerates cross-linking of receptor by adhesive ligand. However, it is also possible that a mechanical stress induced by stirring of platelets in which the adhesive receptors on adjacent platelets are cross-linked to each other plays a role in inducing the transmembrane signalling. Whatever the mechanism, it is important to realize that different signals are transmitted and different cytoskeletal reorganizations induced under different conditions, and therefore to take care to activate platelets under defined conditions of adhesive receptor occupancy.

In general, the method that is used to prevent those cytoskeletal reorganizations that are induced as a consequence of $\alpha_{IIb}\beta_3$-induced signalling (and thus, to study those changes that are induced as a consequence of activation *per se*) is to add an agonist to platelet suspensions under conditions in which aggregation is minimized. Because aggregation is the result of cell–cell contact, an effective way of preventing aggregation is to activate the suspensions in the absence of stirring. Even in unstirred suspensions some signalling can be induced (2) perhaps because some cell–cell contact occurs even in unstirred suspensions. One way of minimizing the contact is to be sure that the concentration of platelets in the suspension is not too high. Typically, a concentration of $0.4–1.0 \times 10^9$ platelets/ml is appropriate to minimize cell–cell contact while at the same time providing sufficient platelets for recovery of cytoskeletal fractions. Activation is induced by adding agonist (e.g. 0.1 NIH U/ml of thrombin) to the suspension and inverting the suspensions one or two times; vortexing or stirring must be avoided to prevent cell–cell contact and subsequent platelet aggregation.

Another way to study those events that are induced prior to ligand binding is to utilize conditions under which the binding of adhesive ligand to $\alpha_{IIb}\beta_3$ is prevented. Because fibrinogen binds in a divalent cation-dependent manner, this can be done by including EDTA in the platelet suspension. For example, the Tyrode's buffer described in *Protocol 1* can be used but the magnesium and calcium omitted and 1 mM EDTA included. Another way of preventing adhesive ligand binding to $\alpha_{IIb}\beta_3$ is to include the tetrapeptide, Arg–Gly–Asp–Ser (RGDS), in the platelet suspensions. This tetrapeptide binds to the fibrinogen binding site on the integrin, preventing ligand-induced cross-linking of $\alpha_{IIb}\beta_3$ and transmembrane signalling. RGDS can be obtained from a number of sources (e.g. Peninsula Laboratories); addition of a final concentration of 1 mM RGDS to a platelet suspension 5 min before adding agonist addition is sufficient to inhibit the subsequent agonist-induced aggregation and $\alpha_{IIb}\beta_3$-induced signalling (13,16). Arg–Gly–Glu–Ser, a peptide that does not bind to $\alpha_{IIb}\beta_3$, can be used as a control.

Yet another method that can be used to ensure that a cytoskeletal reorganization is induced by activation *per se* and not as a consequence of $\alpha_{IIb}\beta_3$-induced transmembrane signalling is to perform the studies with platelets from patients with Glanzmann's thrombasthenia, which lack this adhesive receptor. For example, the finding that the tyrosine-phosphorylated protein, cortactin, associates with cytoplasmic actin filaments within seconds of addition of thrombin to platelets from patients with Glanzmann's thrombasthenia (2) indicates that this protein is involved in one of the early cytoskeletal reorganizations that occurs independently of integrin-induced transmembrane signalling. In contrast, pp60$^{c–src}$ is recovered with a cytoskeletal fraction containing cytoplasmic actin from normal platelets but is not recovered with this fraction from thrombasthenic platelets (17). Thus, the association of pp60$^{c–src}$ with this cytoskeletal fraction appears to occur as a consequence of integrin-induced cytoskeletal reorganizations.

Cytoskeletal reorganizations that follow $\alpha_{IIb}\beta_3$-induced transmembrane signalling are typically identified as those that occur only in platelet suspensions that are stirred with thrombin (e.g. 2,17). One problem with detecting changes that occur only in stirred platelet suspensions is that stirred platelets form tight aggregates that can be difficult to solubilize with detergents. Thus, it is important to demonstrate a selective redistribution of proteins to the detergent insoluble fractions in these platelets rather that a general insolubility of platelet proteins in the lysis buffer. Alternatively, the formation of tight aggregates can be prevented by simply flicking the suspensions gently. This method induces aggregation more slowly (the amount of flicking can be controlled to induce the formation of aggregates over a period of 30 minutes, whereas in suspensions stirred in an aggregometer, aggregation is often complete within a minute). Flicking the suspensions is also useful in that it can be used to perform time course experiments that are often not possible in suspensions of stirred platelets. As discussed above, another way of distinguishing cytoskeletal reorganizations that occur as a consequence of $\alpha_{IIb}\beta_3$-induced aggregation from those that occur independently of adhesive receptor-induced signalling is to use conditions in which binding of adhesive ligand to $\alpha_{IIb}\beta_3$ is prevented or to use thrombasthenic platelets. Comparing those changes that occur when normal platelets are stirred with an agonist with those that occur when thrombasthenic platelets are stirred or when inhibitors of fibrinogen binding are included in the incubations allows those changes induced as a consequence of $\alpha_{IIb}\beta_3$-induced transmembrane signalling to be identified.

2.2 Co-sedimentation of proteins with the cytoskeleton in detergent lysates

To get an indication of whether a protein is associated with the cytoskeleton, platelets are normally lysed, detergent insoluble fractions isolated, and the detergent insoluble fractions examined to determine whether the protein of interest is present. This method is based upon the finding that while most proteins are solubilized by detergents, actin filaments are insoluble. Depending on the detergent, other conditions of lysis, and affinity of the interactions, some of the proteins that are associated with actin filaments in the intact cell remain associated in the detergent lysates and can be recovered in association with the actin filaments by centrifugation of detergent extracts.

Actin filaments require high g forces (typically 100 000 g, 2.5 h) to be sedimented. They can be sedimented from detergent lysates at lower g forces only if they are cross-linked into networks or bundles (18). In the past, many of the commonly used lysis buffers allowed the network to disassemble (18). However, lysis buffers are now available that maintain the networks of cytoplasmic actin filaments; the membrane skeleton is retained at the periphery (18). These cytoskeletons can be visualized by electron microscopy. In order to identify proteins present in the cytoskeletons, the detergent lysates are normally centrifuged and proteins identified on SDS–polyacrylamide gels. In the unstimulated platelet, many of the filaments are insufficiently cross-linked to survive the shear forces of centrifugation and require high g forces to be sedimented. However, when platelets are isolated from plasma, they often undergo slight activation such that the networks of pre-existing filaments become more stable; unless steps are taken to prevent or to reverse such activation, the networks are sufficiently stable that they can be sedimented at low g forces (*Figure 1*). Analysis of the low speed, detergent insoluble pellets has identified actin-binding protein and α-actinin (two proteins known to cross-link actin filament networks) and tropomyosin (a protein thought to regulate the association of other proteins with actin filaments in other systems) as components of this network in platelets (*Figure 1A*).

The cytoskeletal changes that allow the actin filament networks to be recovered by low speed centrifugation from detergent lysates appear to occur in platelets in which $\alpha_{IIb}\beta_3$ has not yet become competent to bind ligand (as

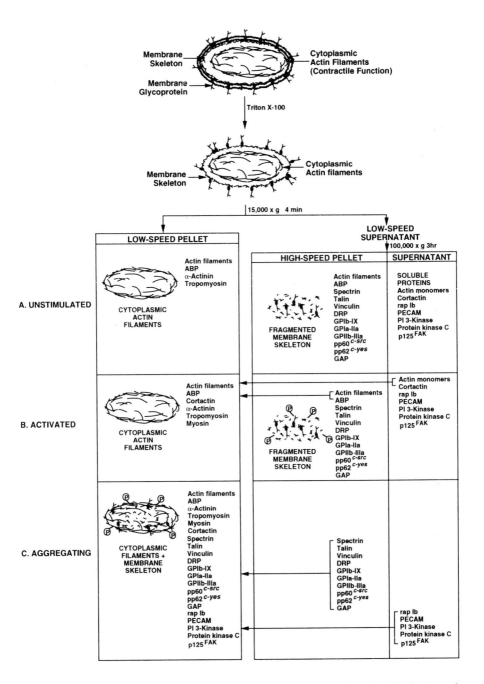

Figure 1. Schematic representation of the platelet cytoskeleton showing distribution of cytoskeletal proteins in Triton X-100 insoluble and soluble fractions from lysates of unstimulated, activated, and aggregated platelets.

detected by the absence of binding of the monoclonal antibody PAC1, a monoclonal antibody that only binds to $\alpha_{IIb}\beta_3$ in its activated state) and increases in the actin filament content that normally occur within seconds of addition of an agonist have not occurred. Thus, these changes presumably represent a very early cytoskeletal reorganization. The use of platelets in which this increased cross-linking of pre-existing actin filaments has already occurred can prove useful in experiments designed to identify components of the platelet membrane skeleton. Thus, even in platelets in which the cytoplasmic actin filaments remain sufficiently cross-linked to allow sedimentation at low g forces from lysates of unstimulated platelets, the skeleton separates from cytoplasmic actin and fragments upon centrifugation (1,18,19). The reason for this is not known. Perhaps cytoplasmic actin filaments are continuous with actin filaments of the membrane skeleton but are sheared during centrifugation; perhaps cytoplasmic actin filaments are associated with another protein in the membrane skeleton through an association that is sensitive to centrifugation-induced shear forces; or perhaps interactions between other membrane skeleton components are sensitive to shear.

Whatever the reason for the centrifugation-induced fragmentation of the membrane skeleton, it can be very useful in the identification and characterization of membrane skeleton proteins in platelets. As indicated in *Figure 1A*, cytoplasmic actin filaments can be sedimented at low g forces. The subsequent centrifugation of the low speed supernatant at high g forces sediments the membrane skeleton proteins. This approach of differential centrifugation has revealed that the membrane glycoproteins GPIb–IX and GPIa–IIa ($\alpha_1\beta_2$) (19) are selectively associated with the short actin filaments that sediment at these g forces. Additional proteins that co-isolate with the membrane skeleton are $\alpha_{IIb}\beta_3$, actin-binding protein, spectrin, talin, vinculin, dystrophin-related protein, and signalling molecules such as pp60[c-src], pp62[c-yes], and the p21[ras] GTPase activating protein (2) (*Figure 1A*).

As platelets are activated, there is an increased polymerization of actin, networks become more highly cross-linked as myosin associates with the filaments, and bundles of new filaments form in the extending filopodia. The resulting networks and bundles of cytoplasmic actin that form can be readily sedimented at low g forces from detergent lysed platelets. Proteins that associate with the cytoplasmic filaments co-sediment with the filaments at low g forces (*Figure 1B*). The membrane skeleton still fragments from the cytoplasmic filaments during centrifugation of the detergent lysates; this has allowed the detection of activation-induced changes to the components of the high speed, detergent insoluble fraction such as increased tyrosine phosphorylation of proteins in this fraction.

As platelets aggregate, additional cytoskeletal reorganizations are induced. As shown in *Figure 1C*, many of the proteins present in the high speed, detergent insoluble fraction redistribute to the low speed, detergent insoluble fraction. The redistribution of these proteins appears to result from $\alpha_{IIb}\beta_3$-

induced transmembrane signalling, since it does not occur in platelets from patients with Glanzmann's thrombasthenia. Additional proteins redistribute from the detergent soluble fraction to the low speed, detergent insoluble fraction in an $\alpha_{IIb}\beta_3$-dependent manner (*Figure 1C*). Based on the fact that the proteins that redistribute from the high speed to the low speed, detergent insoluble fraction all do so in a selective manner (other proteins that sediment at high *g* forces do not redistribute), that all of the proteins redistribute at the same rate, and that each of the proteins remains in the high speed, detergent insoluble fraction when thrombasthenic platelets are activated, it is thought that these proteins are all components of the membrane skeleton (2). The reason that these proteins all redistribute to the low speed, detergent insoluble fraction may be that $\alpha_{IIb}\beta_3$ is associated with one or more of these proteins, and that $\alpha_{IIb}\beta_3$-induced transmembrane signalling causes these membrane skeleton proteins to reorganize and become more tightly associated with the underlying cytoplasmic actin filaments such that they do not fragment during centrifugation of the detergent lysates. Methods for isolating detergent insoluble cytoskeletons (either total cytoskeletons by high speed centrifugation or separate cytoplasmic and membrane skeleton components by differential centrifugation of lysates) are described in *Protocol 1*.

Protocol 1. Isolation of proteins associated with the cytoskeleton in unstimulated platelets

Equipment and reagents

- Tyrode's buffer: 138 mM sodium chloride, 2.9 mM potassium chloride, 12 mM sodium bicarbonate, 0.36 mM sodium phosphate, 5.5 mM glucose, 1.8 mM calcium chloride, and 0.4 mM magnesium chloride pH 7.4
- Triton X-100 lysis buffer: 2% (v/v) Triton X-100, 10 mM EGTA, 2 mM phenyl methyl sulfonyl fluoride (PMSF), 2 mg/ml leupeptin, 100 mM benzamidine, 100 mM Tris–HCl pH 7.4—PMSF rapidly hydrolyses in aqueous solution and is therefore added immediately before the buffer is used
- Eppendorf Centrifuge (e.g. model number 5415C, Brinkman Instruments Inc.)

- 4 × SDS sample buffer: 40% glycerol, 8% SDS, 20% β-mercaptoethanol, 0.008% bromphenol blue, 250 mM Tris–HCl pH 6.8
- Ultracentrifuge: e.g. a Beckman L8–80 or L7–55 can be used with a 70.1 Ti or a 50 Ti rotor. These rotors accommodate tubes that hold 8 ml volumes (Beckman, Cat. No. 355603). It is generally not necessary to isolate platelet cytoskeletons from such a large volume of platelet lysate. However, the 8 ml polycarbonate ultracentrifuge tubes appear to survive centrifugation with volumes as small as 1.0 ml.

A. *Sedimentation of total cytoskeletons from detergent lysed platelets*

1. Pipette 500 μl of platelet suspension ($0.4–1.0 \times 10^9$ platelets/ml) into an 8 ml ultracentrifuge tube.

2. Add an equal volume of ice-cold Triton X-100 lysis buffer.

3. Mix contents of tube by inversion.

4. Immediately isolate cytoskeletons by centrifugation at 4°C for 2.5 h at 100 000 *g*.

Protocol 1. *Continued*

5. Carefully remove the supernatant with a Pasteur pipette, taking care not to disturb the small, translucent pellet of insoluble cytoskeleton.

6. Solubilize cytoskeletons by addition of 1 × SDS sample buffer (one part of 4 × SDS sample buffer plus three parts distilled water). The volume added should be the same as the volume of platelets from which the cytoskeleton originated. The cytoskeletons are very difficult to solubilize; one method is to dislodge the pellets from the centrifuge tube and break them into smaller pieces with a Pasteur pipette, heat to 90 °C for 10 min, and vortex vigorously. Considerable patience is needed to ensure that the cytoskeletons are completely solubilized in the SDS buffer.

7. Analyse the composition of the cytoskeleton by electrophoresis through polyacrylamide–SDS gels. The total amount of a platelet protein that co-sediments with the cytoskeleton should be assessed by preparing a sample of total platelet suspension for electrophoresis (300 μl of platelet suspension added to 100 μl of 4 × SDS buffer, heat at 90 °C for 10 min) and electrophoresing a volume of solubilized platelet suspension containing the same number of platelets as the cytoskeletons originated from. Electrophoresis of cytoskeletons originating from approximately 1×10^7–1×10^8 platelets is generally sufficient to detect cytoskeleton-associated proteins.

B. Separation of cytoskeletons into membrane skeleton and cytoplasmic actin filaments

1. Isolate platelets from plasma in the absence of PGI_2.[a] Resuspend platelets in Tyrode's buffer at ambient temperature.

2. Pipette 500 μl of platelet suspension (0.4–1.0 × 10^9 platelets/ml) into a microcentrifuge tube (1.5 ml, conical polypropylene).

3. Add an equal volume of ice-cold Triton X-100 lysis buffer.

4. Mix contents of tube by inversion.

5. Immediately isolate the network of cytoplasmic actin filaments by centrifugation in a microcentrifuge (15 600 *g*) at 4 °C for 4 min.

6. Carefully remove 800 μl of the supernatant; if extreme care is used not to disturb the pellet, this can be done directly from the microcentrifuge tube with an Eppendorf pipette. Alternatively, the supernatant can be removed with a Pasteur pipette and placed in an additional tube prior to measuring the 800 μl. In either case, remove the last few drops of supernatant from the microcentrifuge tube with extreme care (a Q-tip can be used). Solubilize the pellets by addition of a 1 × SDS buffer (the volume should be the same as that from which the cytoskeletons originated).

7. Place the 800 μl of supernatant (low speed supernatant) into an ultra-centrifuge tube. Centrifuge at 4°C, 100 000 *g*, for 2.5 h.

8. Carefully remove the high speed supernatant into one-third volume of 4 × SDS buffer. Solubilize the high speed pellet in 1 × SDS buffer as described in part A.

9. Analyse the detergent insoluble and detergent soluble fractions from comparable volumes of platelets on SDS gels as described in part A.

[a] Omission of PGI₂ appears to result in platelets in which the cytoplasmic actin filaments are sufficiently cross-linked that they can be sedimented at low *g* forces from otherwise un-activated platelets.

2.2.1 Identification of cytoskeletal proteins

Proteins that co-sediment with the detergent insoluble fractions are typically identified by Western blotting of the detergent insoluble fractions. In some cases, it may be necessary to separate a protein of interest from the rest of the detergent insoluble proteins, for example, to determine whether the protein that co-isolates with the cytoskeleton is phosphorylated differently from the component of the protein that remains in the detergent soluble fraction of the cell. To do this the detergent insoluble fractions can be solubilized in RIPA buffer and the solubilized proteins immunoprecipitated from this buffer for further analysis. This approach has been used successfully to show that pp60^{c-src} that associates with the cytoskeleton in activated platelets is phosphorylated on tyrosine 416, whereas the component that is recovered in the detergent soluble fraction is not (17). Procedures for solubilizing detergent insoluble fractions in RIPA buffer and for immunoprecipitating proteins from the solubilized fractions are described elsewhere in this volume (see Chapter 10).

2.2.2 Demonstration that a detergent insoluble protein is associated with the cytoskeleton

Once a protein has been shown to co-sediment with the detergent insoluble fractions from platelets, it is always important to determine whether this sedimentation occurs because the protein is associated with the cytoskeleton. Since many of the proteins in the 100 000 *g* pellet may be present in this pellet simply because they are inherently insoluble in detergent, it is particularly important to provide evidence other than detergent insolubility for these proteins being components of the cytoskeleton. A number of possible approaches can be taken. The membrane skeleton does not fragment but remains associated with the cytoplasmic actin filaments in detergent lysates of platelets in which α$_{IIb}$β$_3$-induced signalling has been induced (2). Thus, if a protein redistributes from the high speed, detergent insoluble fraction to the low speed, detergent insoluble fraction under the same conditions (e.g. it would not redistribute in thrombasthenic platelets) and at the same rate as proteins known by other means (see Section 2.3) to be components of the membrane skeleton (e.g. spectrin, $\alpha_{IIb}\beta_3$), it can be taken as an indication that the protein is a component of the membrane skeleton. The redistribution of membrane skeleton proteins to the low speed, detergent insoluble fractions of aggregating platelets appears to be selective in that other proteins do not redistribute in this way (2).

Another approach to determining whether a protein that is present in the detergent insoluble fractions of unstimulated platelets is there because it is associated with the cytoskeleton is to depolymerize the actin filaments and to determine whether this is accompanied by solubilization of the protein of interest (19). Depolymerization of actin filaments in detergent lysates can be accomplished by two methods. In one, Ca^{2+} is present in the lysis buffer. Under these conditions, gelsolin, a Ca^{2+}-dependent protein present in platelets, is active. Gelsolin depolymerizes cytoplasmic actin filaments, but the filaments of the membrane skeleton appear to be resistant to depolymerization by this protein. Thus, a different method is used to determine whether a protein present in the high g force, detergent insoluble fraction is there because it is associated with the membrane skeleton. In this method, DNase I is added to the lysis buffer (because this enzyme is active only in the presence of Ca^{2+}, Ca^{2+} must also be present in the lysis buffer). DNase I acts by binding to monomeric actin and shifting the equilibrium between monomeric and filamentous actin, so it depolymerizes both cytoplasmic actin filaments and those of the membrane skeleton. The methods for depolymerizing actin filaments in lysates of platelets are described in *Protocol 2*.

While the finding that a protein that is present in detergent insoluble fractions is solubilized when actin is depolymerized is highly suggestive of the protein being a cytoskeletal protein, the ideal way of showing that a protein is associated with the cytoskeleton is to use a morphological approach. Methods have been developed for labelling detergent insoluble cytoskeletons with antibodies and determining by thin section electron microscopy whether the protein of interest is associated with this structure (18). An appropriate method is described in *Protocol 3*.

Protocol 2. Depolymerization of detergent insoluble actin filaments

Equipment and reagents
- See *Protocol 1*

- DNase I, 2 mg/ml (Boehringer Mannheim,

A. Ca^{2+}-containing lysis buffers

1. Follow *Protocol 1* but omit EGTA from the Triton X-100 lysis buffer.

B. DNase I-containing lysis buffers

1. Follow *Protocol 1*, but omit EGTA from the lysis buffer and include 2 mg/ml DNase I in the buffer.

2. Incubate lysates at 4°C for 1 h prior to centrifugation.[a]

3. Isolate detergent insoluble fractions by centrifugation,[b] solubilize the pellets in 1 × SDS, and determine whether decreased amounts of the protein of interest are recovered in the detergent insoluble fractions when the amount of actin is decreased.

[a] Depolymerization of actin filaments by DNase I occurs in a time-dependent manner as the equilibrium between monomeric and filamentous actin is shifted. Thus, the extent of actin filament depolymerization will depend upon the length of time the lysate is left prior to centrifugation.
[b] Either low speed or high speed centrifugation, depending on whether proteins of the membrane skeleton, cytoplasmic network, or total cytoskeleton are under study.

Protocol 3. EM of platelet cytoskeletons

Equipment and reagents

- Triton X-100 lysis buffer (see *Protocol 1*)
- Protein A coupled to 15 nm diameter gold beads (Amersham, RPN 439)
- Freshly made 0.4 M glutaraldehyde in 0.06 M cacodylate pH 7.4 (Electron Microscopy Science, 16120)
- 0.08 M L-lysine in 0.06 M sodium cacodylate buffer pH 7.4[a]
- 0.1 M cacodylate–HCl buffer pH 7.6
- 0.05 M osmium tetroxide in 0.1 M cacodylate buffer
- 0.05 M uranyl acetate in water
- Epon 812 (Polysciences)
- Reynold's lead citrate
- Microcentrifuge

Method

1. Place 100 μl of platelet suspension in a microcentrifuge tube.

2. Add 100 μl of ice-cold Triton X-100 lysis buffer (see *Protocol 1*).

3. Add approx. 10 μg/ml of an affinity purified antibody against the protein of interest.

4. Add 200 μl of protein A coupled to 15 nm diameter gold beads.

5. Incubate lysates at 37°C for 60 min.

6. Mix the glutaraldehyde and lysine solutions in a 1 : 1 ratio and immediately add 2 ml of this fixative to the platelet lysate.

7. Incubate samples at ambient temperatures for approx. 1 h.

8. Centrifuge in a swing-out microcentrifuge for 15 min at 4°C.

9. Wash the fixed pellets two times in ice-cold cacodylate buffer pH 7.6.

10. Expose samples to 0.05 M osmium tetroxide at 4°C for from 15 min to overnight.

Protocol 3. *Continued*

11. Rinse pellets three times in ice-cold distilled water.

12. Stain samples overnight at 4°C in 0.05 M uranyl acetate in the dark.

13. Dehydrate fixed material in acetone and embed in Epon 812.

14. Cut thick (0.2 μm) sections, stain for 10–15 min with Reynold's lead citrate and uranyl acetate, and view by electron microscopy.

---

[a] The free base forms of lysine and cacodylic acid are used rather than the chloride salt in order to minimize the total amount of salts in the solution.

2.3 Identification of proteins associated with the cytoskeleton in intact platelets

A number of approaches can be used to determine whether an interaction detected in detergent lysates exists in the intact cell. One is a morphological approach. In other cell types co-localization of proteins with the cytoskeleton can be detected by immunofluorescence. In platelets, the small size of the cell makes this more difficult. However, when taken together with additional information such as co-sedimentation of a protein with the cytoskeleton from detergent lysates, immunofluoresence experiments can strengthen the conclusion that a protein is associated with the cytoskeleton. For example, the observation by immunofluorescence that myosin co-localizes with centralizing actin filaments in thrombin-activated or spreading cells (21–23), together with the finding that myosin co-isolates with cytoplasmic actin filaments from thrombin-activated platelets (24), provides convincing evidence that this protein associates with the cytoskeleton in activated platelets. Similarly, the finding that α-actinin, tropomyosin, and actin-binding protein all sediment with the cytoplasmic actin filaments from detergent lysed platelets (18) and co-localize with bundles of actin filaments in filopodia of activated platelets (22) supports the idea that these proteins are associated with cytoplasmic actin filaments in platelets.

A more convincing method for showing that a protein is associated with the cytoskeleton is to utilize electron microscopy. The cytoplasm of platelets is very dense, making it difficult to visualize actin filaments by conventional electron microscopy. One method that has been devised to allow removal of the dense soluble material but retention of actin filaments is to lyse the platelets with detergent while simultaneously fixing the detergent insoluble cytoskeleton (25). The fixative used in this protocol contains lysine, which prevents the damage to actin filaments that is induced by osmium in samples fixed with conventional fixatives (26). This protocol allows the retention of the networks of actin filaments and of the membrane skeleton at the periphery. However, because the fixative can prevent the subsequent labelling of specimens with antibodies, it has not been possible to use this method for demonstrating that other proteins are associated with the actin filaments. One approach to overcoming this obstacle has been to use the technique of simultaneously lysing and fixing platelets but to use phallacidin to stabilize actin filaments and to use a high resolution, quick freeze, deep etch approach to visualize the fixed cytoskeletons (20). The cytoskeletons isolated by this method contain a very dense membrane skeleton that does not allow visualization of individual molecules or labelling of the interior of the cytoskeleton. However, by varying the concentrations of fixative and phallacidin, Hartwig and DeSisto (20) have isolated cytoskeletons in which the membrane skeleton has fragmented and opened up to various extents. In these preparations, individual molecules can be clearly seen and identified by immunogold labelling. For example, strands 210 to 240 nm in length were detected in the membrane skeleton and shown by immunogold labelling to be spectrin. Immunogold labelling also revealed the presence of myosin, GPIb–IX, and actin-binding protein with the membrane skeleton. This approach should prove useful in the future in providing a detailed description of the proteins that are associated with the cytoskeleton and of the way that they are assembled in the intact cell.

Yet another approach for assessing whether a protein is associated with the cytoskeleton in intact cells is to ablate the interaction between the cytoskeleton and the protein of interest and to determine whether the function of the protein is altered. This approach has been used in cultured cells, in which antibodies or peptides have been injected or mutated forms of a protein have been expressed and the effects of the injections or mutations on the association of the protein with the cytoskeleton correlated with changes in the functional activity of the protein. For example, various mutant forms of pp60^{v-src} have been expressed in fibroblasts and a correlation demonstrated between the recovery of the expressed mutants with the detergent insoluble cytoskeleton and the activity of the enzyme within the cell (27). In platelets, it is not yet possible to express mutated forms of a protein, nor is injection of antibodies or protein fragments routinely performed. However, it is possible to modify the organization of the cytoskeleton and to determine whether this has a functional effect on the protein of interest. The way in which the cytoskeletal organization can be altered is to incubate the platelets with cytochalasins. Typically cytochalasin E or D is used. Concentrations in the 10^{-6} M range markedly inhibit the agonist-induced polymerization of new actin filaments. Concentrations of 10^{-5} M or 10^{-4} M also depolymerize the actin filaments that already exist in unstimulated platelets. Cytochalasin B is much less effective in decreasing the actin filament content than are the other two cytochalasins. Cytochalasins are added to platelets in dimethyl sulfoxide, which should be at a final concentration of no higher than 0.2%. Pre-incubation of cytochalasin with platelet suspensions for 15–30 min is sufficient to induce depolymerization of actin filaments. The use of cytochalasins in this way has allowed the demonstration that the activation of both pp125^{FAK} and calpain require the presence of an intact cytoskeleton (6,10). Together with the observation from cultured cells that these signalling enzymes co-localize with focal contacts (28,29), the findings obtained with cytochalasins suggest that the proteins may associate with the cytoskeleton in intact platelets. Similar experiments could potentially be performed with other proteins of known function that have been shown to co-isolate with cytoskeletal proteins from detergent lysed platelets.

3. Summary

Considerable information is now available on the organization of the platelet cytoskeleton, and it is becoming increasingly apparent that the cytoskeleton rapidly reorganizes to induce shape change and contractile events. In addition, it appears to provide a scaffolding for binding signalling molecules and their substrates, localizing them in appropriate locations within the cell. As platelets adhere and aggregate, the cytoskeleton responds to signals transmitted through the adhesion receptors, changing its organization and recruiting and activating additional signalling molecules such that the motile and contractile events that are required following adhesion and aggregation can be induced.

The primary method that has been used to identify the components of the cytoskeleton and the signalling molecules that associate with it has been to identify proteins that co-sediment with detergent insoluble actin filaments from lysed preparations. Provided that care is taken to address the question of specificity, this is a useful method of assessing the possibility that a protein is associated with the cytoskeleton. Morphological and functional approaches are also available for assessing the possibility that a protein is associated with the cytoskeleton. Ideally, one or more of these methods should be used in addition to detergent insolubility to provide more definitive evidence that a protein is indeed associated with the cytoskeleton in the intact cell. It is anticipated that an understanding of the signalling molecules that associate with the cytoskeleton and the way in which this association regulates the activity of the molecules will significantly increase our understanding of the role of the cytoskeleton in coming years.

References

1. Fox, J. E. B. (1993). *Thromb. Haemost.*, **70,** 884.
2. Fox, J. E. B., Lipfert, L., Clark, E. A., Reynolds, C. C., Austin, C. D., and Brugge, J. S. (1993). *J. Biol. Chem.*, **268,** 25973.
3. Clark, E. A. and Brugge, J. S. (1993). *Trends Cardiovasc. Med.*, **3,** 218.
4. Fox, J. E. B., Shattil, S. J., Kinlough-Rathbone, R. L., Richardson, M., Packham, M. A., and Sanan, D. A. *J. Biol. Chem.*, (submitted).
5. Haimovich, B., Lipfert, L., Brugge, J. S., and Shattil, S. J. (1993). *J. Biol. Chem.*, **268,** 15868.

6. Lipfert, L., Haimovich, B., Schaller, M. D., Cobb, B. S., Parsons, J. T., and Brugge, J. S. (1992). *J. Cell Biol.*, **119,** 905.
7. Kouns, W. C., Fox, C. F., Lamoreaux, W. J., Coons, L. B., and Jennings, L. K. (1991). *J. Biol. Chem.*, **266,** 13891.
8. Jackson, S. P., Schoenwaelder, S. M., Yuan, Y., Rabinowitz, I., Salem, H. H., and Mitchell, C. A. (1994). *J. Biol. Chem.*, **269,** 27093.
9. Zhang, J., Fry, M. J., Waterfield, M. D., Jaken, S., Liao, L., Fox, J. E. B., *et al.* (1992). *J. Biol. Chem.*, **267,** 4686.
10. Fox, J. E. B., Santos, G., Zuerbig, S., and Saido, T. C. (1995). *XVth Congress of the International Soc. on Thromb Haemost.* (Abstract).
11. Grondin, P., Plantavid, M., Sultan, C., Breton, M., Mauco, G., and Chap, H. (1991). *J. Biol. Chem.*, **266,** 15705.
12. Horvath, A. R., Muszbek, L., and Kellie, S. (1992). *EMBO. J.*, **11,** 855.
13. Huang, M.-M., Lipfert, L., Cunningham, M., Brugge, J. S., Ginsberg, M. H., and Shattil, S. J. (1993). *J. Cell Biol.*, **122,** 473.
14. Clark, E. A., Trikha, M., Markland, F. S., and Brugge, J. S. (1994). *J. Biol. Chem.*, **269,** 21940.
15. Shattil, S. J., Haimovich, B., Cunningham, M., Lipfert, L., Parsons, J. T., Ginsberg, M. H., *et al.* (1994). *J. Biol. Chem.*, **269,** 14738.
16. Fox, J. E. B., Taylor, R. G., Taffarel, M., Boyles, J. K., and Goll, D. E. (1993). *J. Cell Biol.*, **120,** 1501.
17. Clark, E. A. and Brugge, J. S. (1993). *Mol. Cell. Biol.*, **13,** 1863.
18. Fox, J. E. B., Boyles, J. K., Berndt, M. C., Steffen, P. K., and Anderson, L. A. (1988). *J. Cell Biol.*, **106,** 1525
19. Fox, J. E. B. (1985). *J. Clin. Invest.*, **76,** 1673.
20. Hartwig, J. H. and DeSisto, M. (1991). *J. Cell Biol.*, **112,** 407.
21. Pollard, T. D., Fujiwara, K., Handin, R., and Weiss, G. (1977). *Ann. N. Y. Acad. Sci.*, **283,** 218.
22. Debus, E., Weber, K., and Osborn, M. (1981). *Eur. J. Cell Biol.*, **24,** 45.
23. Painter, R. G. and Ginsberg, M. H. (1984). *Exp. Cell Res.*, **155,** 198.
24. Fox, J. E. B. and Phillips, D. R. (1982). *J. Biol. Chem.*, **257,** 4120.
25. Boyles, J., Fox, J. E. B., Phillips, D. R., and Stenberg, P. E. (1985). *J. Cell Biol.*, **101,** 1463.
26. Boyles, J., Anderson, L., and Hutcherson, P. (1985). *J. Histochem. Cytochem.*, **33,** 1116.
27. Fukui, Y., O'Brien, M. C., and Hanafusa, H. (1991). *Mol. Cell. Biol.*, **11,** 1207.
28. Kornberg, L., Earp, H. S., Parsons, J. T., Schaller, M., and Juliano, R. L. (1992). *J. Biol. Chem.*, **267,** 23439.
29. Beckerle, M. C., Burridge, K., DeMartino, G. N., and Croall, D. E. (1987). *Cell*, **51,** 569.

12

Methods for measuring agonist-induced phospholipid metabolism in intact human platelets

BRUCE J. HOLUB and STEVE P. WATSON

1. Introduction

Stimulation of platelets by agonists causes marked alterations in phospholipid metabolism (1,2). The activation of phospholipase C results in the degradation of phosphoinositides, noteably phosphatidylinositol 4,5-bisphosphate (PI $4,5$-P_2), resulting in the production of the second messengers diacylglycerol (DG) and inositol 1,4,5-trisphosphate (Ins 1,4,5-P_3) (3,4). DG is further metabolized to phosphatidic acid (PA) via DG kinase. In addition to PI 4,5-P_2 hydrolysis via phospholipase C with agonist stimulation, phosphatidylinositol (PI) is sequentially phosphorylated upon receptor occupancy to phosphatidylinositol 4-phosphate (PI 4-P) and PI 4,5-P_2 via PI and PI 4-P kinase activities, respectively (5). Recently, novel phosphorylated phosphoinositide compounds, namely phosphatidylinositol 3,4-bisphosphate (PI 3,4-P_2) and phosphatidylinositol 3,4,5-trisphosphate (PI 3,4,5-P_3), have been identified in stimulated platelets (5). The activation of phospholipase A_2 following agonist stimulation of platelets cleaves platelet membrane phospholipids, including PI, phosphatidylcholine (PC), phosphatidylethanolamine (PE), and phosphatidylserine (PS), at the *sn*-2 position producing the corresponding 1-acyl lysophospholipids and releasing predominately arachidonic acid (AA, 20 : 4n-6) (1,6). AA is further metabolized via cyclo-oxygenase to thromboxane A_2 (TxA_2), a potent potentiator of platelet activation (6). Plasmenyl-ethanolamine (alkenylacyl PI), which represents a considerable reservoir of AA in human platelets, is hydrolysed via phospholipase A_2 to lysoplasmenylethanolamine plus AA. Activation of platelets, from subjects who have consumed fish or fish oil, also releases the fatty acid eicosapentaenoic acid (EPA, 20 : 5n-3) from membrane phospholipids which is further metabolized to the weakly aggregatory product, TxA_3 (7). In addition to the above metabolic pathways for phospholipid metabolism, the degradation of PC and/or PE via phospholipase D (resulting in PA formation) in stimulated platelets has been documented (8,9).

Agonist-induced phospholipid metabolism via the enzyme pathways mentioned above can be assessed by monitoring levels (decreases) of precursors and/or the generated lipid products of the enzyme reactions in stimulated versus resting platelets. The two methods generally employed are mass studies and radiolabelling studies, where measurements of the mass and radio-activity, respectively, of the phospholipids in question are (or their derivatives) determined. This chapter will focus on some of the various techniques employed in the analysis of phospholipid metabolism in stimulated platelets.

2. Common techniques used in analysis of phospholipids in platelets

In order to study changes in platelet phospholipids with agonist stimulation, the following procedures are generally performed:

(a) Isolation of platelets from whole blood.

(b) Incubation of platelets with agonist.

(c) Extraction of phospholipids from platelets.

(d) Separation of the various phospholipids via thin-layer chromatography (TLC).

(e) Quantitation of phospholipids via lipid phosphorus measurements, gas–liquid chromatography (GLC) of their fatty acid residues, or via liquid scintillation counting (after pre-labelling).

Several different methods have been utilized for the isolation of platelets from whole blood. A method using Tris/saline buffer and cold temperatures (4°C) has been employed for platelet isolation and phospholipid quantitation using lipid phosphorus determinations (10). This method may not be appropriate when sensitive aggregation studies are performed due to the presence of EDTA in the buffer to bind calcium. The isolation of platelets using a Tyrode's buffer and warm temperatures (37°C) has often been employed (11) (see *Protocol 1*). The presence of physiological levels of calcium in this buffer make it appropriate for use in aggregation studies or when certain agonists, such as collagen or ADP, are employed. The concentration of apyrase in the first, second, and third platelet suspensions are 60, 30, and 3 µg/ml, respectively. The first platelet suspension also contains 50 U/ml heparin and 5 mM Hepes. Routine collection of 150–175 ml blood/subject yields an average total of 5×10^9 platelets/50 ml blood drawn.

Protocol 1. Isolation of platelets from whole blood and preparation of a washed platelet suspension (11)

Equipment and reagents

- ACD anticoagulant: 2.5% (w/v) trisodium citrate, 1.4% (w/v) citric acid, 2.0% (w/v) dextrose pH 4.5[a]
- Stock solution I: 16% (w/v) NaCl, 0.4% (w/v) KCl, 2.0% (w/v) NaHCO$_3$, 0.116% (w/v) NaH$_2$PO$_4$.H$_2$O[b]
- Stock solution II: 2.03% (w/v) MgCl$_2$.6H$_2$O
- Stock solution III: 2.19% (w/v) CaCl$_2$.6H$_2$O
- Glucose solution: 10% (w/v) glucose
- Hepes (1 M)
- Heparin (20 U/ml)

- 3.5% (w/v) fatty acid-free bovine serum albumin (BSA)[c](Boehringer Mannheim)
- Apyrase (3 mg/ml)[d]
- Siliconized glass bottle (450 ml capacity) with a vacuum established
- Conical-shaped polypropylene centrifuge tubes with caps (Fisher Scientific Co.)
- Siliconized Pasteur pipettes
- Centrifuge
- Coulter counter (Coulter Electronics)
- pH meter

Method

1. Draw blood from the antecubital vein of subjects (who have denied taking anti-inflammatory drugs for the past ten days) into a siliconized bottle,[e] which has had a vacuum established, containing ACD anticoagulant at 37°C (one part ACD/six parts blood) (12).

2. Distribute the blood from the bottle into large (50 ml capacity) polypropylene centrifuge tubes (25 ml blood/tube).

3. Centrifuge the tubes at 120 *g* for 15 min at 37°C to separate the red blood cells from the plasma.

4. During this spin:

    (a) Label small (15 ml capacity) polypropylene tubes for platelet-rich plasma (PRP), platelet sample I (PSI), and PSII (one tube each/ 50 ml of blood drawn). Label one large polypropylene tube for PSIII.

    (b) Add 25 µl heparin (20 U/ml) and 50 µl Hepes (1 M) to the PSI tubes.

    (c) Add 200 µl and 100 µl apyrase (3 mg/ml) to the PSI and PSII tubes, respectively.

5. Using siliconized Pasteur pipettes,[e] carefully transfer the PRP on top of the red blood cells to tubes labelled PRP (one tube PRP/50 ml of blood drawn) and place in a water-bath at 37°C to keep warm.[f]

6. Centrifuge the PRP tubes at 1100 *g* for 15 min at 37°C to pellet the platelets.

7. During this spin, make up the Tyrode's buffer:

    (a) Add the following to a 500 ml volumetric flask:
        - 300 ml distilled water

Protocol 1. *Continued*

- 25 ml stock solution I
- 5 ml stock solution II
- 10 ml stock solution III
- 50 ml BSA solution
- 5 ml dextrose solution

(b) Mix and add distilled water to 500 ml total volume.

(c) Take about 400 ml of the buffer and adjust the pH to 7.35.[g]

(d) Put the Tyrode's buffer in a stock bottle and cap.[h]

(e) Add 10 ml Tyrode's buffer to each PSI tube, cap, and place in a water-bath at 37 °C.

8. Pour off the platelet-poor plasma (discard) from the PRP tubes and resuspend the platelets as follows:

   (a) Take 1–2 ml of buffer in PSI tube and gently add to the platelet pellet.

   (b) Using a siliconized Pasteur pipette, resuspend the platelets thoroughly by repeatedly drawing up and expelling the buffer on to the platelet pellet. Resuspended platelets will appear to swirl in the buffer.

   (c) Transfer the platelet suspension (1–2 ml) to the PSI tube containing the rest of the buffer and repeat step (b).

9. Cap the PSI tubes and place in a water-bath at 37 °C for 15 min and shake at slow speed. During this time, periodically resuspend the platelets as described in step 8(b).[f]

10. Centrifuge the PSI tubes at 950 *g* for 10 min at 37 °C to pellet the platelets.

11. During this spin, add 10 ml Tyrode's buffer to the PSII tubes, cap, and warm to 37 °C.

12. Pour off the buffer from the PSI tubes and resuspend the platelets (as described in step 8) using the buffer from the PSII tubes.

13. Cap the PSII tubes and place in a water-bath at 37 °C for 10 min and shake at slow speed.

14. Centrifuge the PSII tubes at 950 *g* for 10 min at 37 °C.

15. During this spin, add apyrase to the remaining Tyrode's in the stock bottle (1 mg apyrase/ml buffer). Add this buffer to the PSIII tube (about 7 ml/50 ml blood drawn).

16. Pour off the buffer from the PSII tubes and resuspend the platelets (as described in step 8) using the buffer from the PSIII tubes.

17. Using an aliquot of the PSIII, determine the concentration of platelets

238

using a Coulter counter and adjust the concentration to 5×10^8 platelets/ml using the apyrase-containing Tyrode's buffer.

[a] Make all solutions in advance and store at 4°C.
[b] Make up stock solution I fresh every two weeks.
[c] Store BSA in the freezer (−20°C).
[d] Apyrase can be purchased (Sigma Chemical Co.) or isolated from potatoes according to the method of Molnar and Lorand (13), modified by dialysing the final material against 0.9% (w/v) NaCl. Store apyrase in aliquots at −80°C.
[e] Siliconization of bottles and Pasteur pipettes is by coating of these glass objects with 10% (v/v) Surfasil (Terochem Laboratories) in petroleum ether, followed by a drying period of 24 h. Alternatively, polypropylene pipettes and bottles may be used.
[f] During radiolabelling studies, incubate platelets in either PRP or PSI with the radiolabel for 2 h.
[g] Add the minimum of HCl or NaOH (two to four drops is usually sufficient) so that the osmolarity of the buffer is not affected. If the pH is over-adjusted, add some of the extra buffer to readjust the pH.
[h] Keep all the containers of Tyrode's buffer (including the polypropylene tubes) capped to maintain a pH of 7.35.

Once the platelets are isolated and a platelet suspension obtained, the platelets can be stimulated with an agonist (see *Protocol 2*). Several different platelet agonists can be used, such as thrombin (0.02–4 U/ml), collagen (1–20 μg/ml), or U-46619 (TxA$_2$ analogue, 1–20 μM). In some experiments, platelets may be incubated with specific platelet inhibitors (see *Table 1*) prior to the addition of agonist (see *Protocol 2*, step 3). Reactions are terminated by quenching and extraction of phospholipids.

A normal (neutral) Bligh and Dyer (20) extraction is sufficient to extract the major phospholipids and neutral lipids such as DG. For more polar/water soluble phospholipids, such as polyphosphoinositides and lysophospholipids, an acidified extraction as described by Allan and Michell (21) may be more appropriate (see *Protocol 3*). Vickers (22) has very recently reported on a two-step extraction (neutral Bligh and Dyer followed by an acidified extraction) which gave a 30% better yield of platelet PI 4,5-P$_2$ than a one-step

Table 1. Examples of inhibitors of the action of phospholipases and their products

Compound	Target	Concentration	Supplier	Reference
Arachidonyl tri-fluoromethyl ketone	Phospholipase A$_2$	10 μM	Biomol	14
BW755C	Cyclo-oxygenase/lipoxygenase	100 μM	Wellcome Foundation	15
Staurosporine	Serine/threonine and tyrosine kinases	1 μM	Calbiochem	16
Butanol	Phospholipase D	30 mM	–	17
SQ29548	Thromboxane receptor antagonist	0.5 μM	NEN/Dupont	18
Genistein	Tyrosine kinases	100 μM	Biomol	19

acidified extraction. Neutral followed by acidified extractions will also prevent the acid-induced hydrolysis of alkenylacyl PE which can occur when the acidic extraction is employed first.

Protocol 2.   Incubation of platelets with agonist

Equipment and reagents

- Agonist, e.g. thrombin (Parke-Davis), collagen (Hormon Chemie), U-46619 (Upjohn Scientific Co.)
- Platelet inhibitors (e.g. see *Table 1*)
- Chloroform/methanol (1 : 2, v/v)
- Siliconized cuvettes with siliconized stir rods
- Aggregometer (e.g. Payton Scientific Co.)
- Platelets (4–10 x 10^8/ml)

Method

1. Add 1.0 ml aliquot of platelet suspension to a siliconized cuvette containing a siliconized stir rod.

2. Place the cuvette in an aggregometer and pre-incubate with stirring (900 r.p.m.) at 37°C for 1 min.

3. Add the agonist to the cuvette and incubate for a specified time period.[a]

4. Stop the reaction by addition of chloroform/methanol (1 : 2, v/v).[b]

5. Repeat steps 1–4, except without agonist addition (unstimulated platelets).

[a] In some experiments, add a platelet inhibitor to the cuvette prior to agonist addition and incubate for a specified time period.
[b] This is the beginning of the extraction procedure (see *Protocol 3*).

Protocol 3.   Extraction of platelet phospholipids from a platelet suspension (20)

Equipment and reagents

- Chloroform/methanol (1 : 2, v/v)
- Chloroform
- 100 mM Na_2EDTA
- Chloroform/methanol (2 : 1, v/v)
- Screw-top glass test-tubes with caps
- Minivials with caps
- Heating block
- Pasteur pipette with bulb

Method

For each 1 ml platelet suspension in a tube:

1. Add 3.75 ml chloroform/methanol (1 : 2, v/v) to the tube, cap, and vortex for 60 sec.[a,b]

2. Add 1.25 ml chloroform to the tube, cap, and vortex for 60 sec.

3. Add 1.25 ml 100 mM Na$_2$EDTA to the tube, cap, and vortex for 30 sec.

4. Allow the two phases to separate (at 4°C) and remove the lower chloroform phase to a vial as follows:

    (a) Using a Pasteur pipette with bulb, expel the air in the pipette as it is lowered through the methanol/water phase to the chloroform phase.

    (b) Draw up the lower chloroform phase into the pipette and remove the pipette from the tube, being careful not to draw up any of the methanol/water phase.

5. If desired, re-extract the remaining upper phase. Add 2.5 ml chloroform to the tube, cap, and vortex for 30 sec. Repeat step 4 and combine the lower chloroform phases.

6. Place the vial in a heating block at 40°C in a fume-cupboard and evaporate the chloroform to dryness using a gentle stream of nitrogen gas.

7. Redissolve the lipid extract in about 25 ml chloroform/methanol (2 : 1, v/v).

8. Store the lipid extracts in the freezer until lipid separation via TLC.

---

[a] For an acidified extraction as described in ref. 21, add 3.75 ml chloroform/methanol/ concentrated HCl (20 : 40 : 1, by vol.) at this step instead of chloroform/methanol (1 : 2, v/v).
[b] If extracting lipids from a platelet suspension in an aggregometer cuvette, modify the extraction as follows:
(a) Add the chloroform/methanol (1 : 2, v/v) and let stir in the cuvette for 60 sec.
(b) Transfer the mixture in the cuvette to a screw-top test-tube.
(c) For step 2, add the chloroform to the cuvette to rinse it and then transfer to the test-tube.

The platelet lipids are then separated via one of the many TLC systems available, depending upon the phospholipids desired (see *Table 2*). A detailed description for the separation of the major phospholipids, PC, PE, PI, PS, and sphingomyelin (SPH), by one-dimensional TLC has been given elsewhere (23) (see *Figure 1*). Included herein is a two-dimensional TLC

Table 2. Thin-layer chromatography systems for separating platelet lipids

Lipids separated	Solvent systems	Figure
PC, PE, PS, PI, SPH	Chloroform/methanol/acetic acid/water (50 : 37.5 : 3.5 : 2, by vol.)	1
PC, PE, PS, PI, SPH, PA, lysoPC, lysoPE, lysoPS, lysoPI, free fatty acid	Chloroform/methanol/14.5% ammonium hydroxide (65 : 35 : 5.5, by vol.) Chloroform/methanol/88% formic acid/water (55 : 28 : 5 : 1, by vol.)	2
PI, lysoPI, PI 4-P, PI 4,5-P$_2$, PI 3,4-P$_2$	Chloroform/methanol/conc. NH$_4$OH/water (45 : 35 : 7 : 5, by vol.)	3

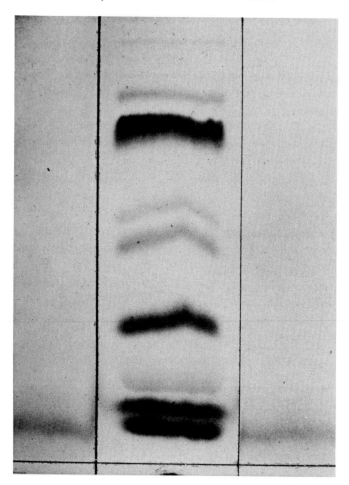

Figure 1. Thin-layer chromatographic separation of major phospholipids. A thin-layer chromatogram illustrating separation of phospholipids from rat liver by one-dimensional chromatography using the solvent described in *Table 2* is shown. Lipids were sprayed with 8-anilino-1-naphthalenesulfonic acid and visualized using ultraviolet light (366 nm). The following bands can be seen: sphingomyelin (R_f 0.06); phosphatidylcholine (R_f 0.10); phosphatidylserine (R_f 0.27); phosphatidylinositol (R_f 0.38); phosphatidylethanolamine (R_f 0.57); cardiolipin (R_f 0.73); neutral lipid (R_f 1.0).

method used in our laboratory for the separation of phospholipids, lysophospholipids, free fatty acid, and PA (see *Protocol 4* and *Figures 2* and *3*). Following their separation via TLC, the phospholipids are then quantitated via GLC (mass measurements of their fatty acid residues using a known amount of odd carbon saturated fatty acid, 15 : 0 or 17 : 0 as internal standard), or via liquid scintillation counting for radioactivity measurements.

Protocol 4. Two-dimensional thin-layer chromatographic separation of phospholipids, lysophospholipids, free fatty acids, and phosphatidic acid

Equipment and reagents

- Chloroform
- Methanol
- 14.8% ammonium hydroxide
- 88% formic acid
- 2',7'-dichlorofluorescein in methanol/water (1 : 1, v/v)
- Glass tanks with lids, 22 x 22 x 10 cm (Desaga)

- Merck silica gel 60 pre-coated 20 x 20 cm thin-layer plates (without fluorescein indicator) with 0.25 mm layer thickness (British Drug House Canada Ltd.)
- Whatman chromatography paper (0.18 mm thickness)
- Hamilton syringe

Method

1. Line a glass tank with Whatman chromatography paper.[a]

2. Make up 105.5 ml of chloroform/methanol/ammonium hydroxide (65 : 35 : 5.5, by vol.) and add to the lined tank. Replace the glass lid on the tank and allow the solvent mixture to run the entire height of the chromatography paper (approx. 45–60 min).

3. Add lysophospholipid (and PA, if desired) standards to the vials containing the platelet lipid extracts.[b]

4. Using a 25 ml Hamilton syringe, spot the lipid extract in the bottom, right corner of the pre-coated silica gel 60 plates, 2 cm from each edge.[c]

5. Place the plate as vertically as possible in the glass tank with the plate positioned so that the origin is in the bottom right corner. Allow the solvent to run up the plate (approx. 1.5 h).

6. When the solvent front has reached the top edge of the plate at the corners, remove the plate and let air dry for 10 min.

7. Place the plate in a nitrogen chamber[d] for 30 min. During this time, empty the tank, air dry for 5 min, rinse with distilled water, and thoroughly dry with paper towels.

8. Line the tank with chromatography paper, then make up and add 85 ml of chloroform/methanol/formic acid/water (55 : 28 : 5 : 1, by vol.) to the tank. Allow the solvent mixture to run up the paper.

9. After the 30 min time period in the nitrogen chamber, place the plate in the tank containing the new solvent mixture, with the plate positioned so that the previous origin is in the bottom, left corner. Allow the solvent to run up the plate (approx. 2 h).

10. When the solvent front is approximately 0.5 cm from the top edge of the plate at the corners, remove the plate and let air dry for 5–10 min.

Protocol 4. *Continued*

11. Using an atomizer with nitrogen gas flow, spray the surface of the plate with a saturated solution of 2′,7′-dichlorofluorescein in methanol/water (1 : 1, v/v).

12. Expose the plate to ammonia vapour by placing the plate in a raised bottom glass tank containing 50–100 ml of ammonium hydroxide.

13. View the lipid spots on the plate under ultraviolet light (wavelength of 366 nm).

[a] Use multiple tanks for multiple lipid extracts (one lipid extract per thin-layer plate and tank).
[b] The amount of platelet lipid extract spotted per plate is sufficient to detect the major phospholipids (and PA in stimulated platelet samples). For the analysis of lysophospholipids, lysophospholipid (Sigma Chemical Co.) standards are added to the lipid extract to aid in the detection of these lipids since their mass levels are generally too low for detection.
[c] Spot the extracts as a tight, single, circular spot not exceeding 4 mm diameter. Use a flow of nitrogen gas to aid the evaporation of the solvent.
[d] The nitrogen chamber is a box with a flow of nitrogen gas through it.

3. Mass measurements

3.1 Gas–liquid chromatography (GLC)

Following the separation of phospholipids via TLC, the individual phospholipids are prepared for derivatization and analysis of their fatty acids on the gas–liquid chromatograph. As little as 1–5 μg of total or individual phospholipid(s) can be quantified. The fatty acid components of the phospholipids are transmethylated, in the presence of a known amount of an internal fatty acid standard, to produce fatty acid methyl esters (FAMEs) (see *Protocol 5*). Appropriate gel blanks are simultaneously analysed with internal standard to allow for correction of minor extraneous GLC peaks. The FAMEs of each phospholipid are then analysed via GLC.

Protocol 5. Preparation of fatty acid methyl esters from phospholipids

Equipment and reagents

- 6% (v/v) concentrated H_2SO_4 in methanol
- Petroleum ether
- Hexane
- Monopentadecanoate (NuChek Prep)
- Screw-top test-tubes with Teflon-lined caps
- Razor blade
- Plastic funnel (to fit into test-tube)
- Heating block
- Vortex

Method

1. Add 3 ml of 6% (v/v) concentrated H_2SO_4 in methanol and 5–10 mg of monopentadecanoate, as an internal standard,[a] to several screw-top test-tubes.

2. With the aid of a razor blade and funnel, scrape the phospholipid spots or bands from the thin-layer plates into separate screw-top test-tubes containing the methylating reagent (see step 1).

3. Seal the tubes tightly using Teflon-lined caps to minimize evaporation of the methylating reagent.

4. Vortex the tubes for 60 sec and place in an oven at 80°C for 14 h.[b]

5. Remove the tubes from the oven and let cool to room temperature.

6. Add 2 ml petroleum ether and vortex each tube for 60 sec.

7. Add 1 ml water and vortex each tube for 30 sec.

8. Allow the phases to separate and transfer the upper petroleum ether phase, containing the fatty acid methyl ester, to 2 ml minivials.

9. Place the minivials in a sand-bath at 40°C and evaporate the petroleum ether to dryness under a gentle stream of nitrogen gas.

10. Immediately add 25 µl GLC grade hexane to the minivials to redissolve the fatty acid methyl esters.

11. Store the minivials containing the fatty acid methyl esters in the freezer until quantitation via GLC.

[a] The amount of 15 : 0 standard depends on the quantity of phospholipid being analysed and should approximate 20% of the total fatty acids in the phospholipid.
[b] Shorter methylating times of 3–6 h at 80°C are generally sufficient for methylating the fatty acids in PC, PE, PS, and PI.

A detailed description of the use of a megabore column installed on a Hewlett Packard 5890 gas–liquid chromatograph has been given by Holub and Skeaff (23). Identification of peaks is by comparison of retention data with known standards. By comparisons of the peak areas of the internal standard with those of the selected fatty acids, the mass (moles) of the individual fatty acids can be calculated. From this data, the phospholipid mass can be determined. Diacyl, ether-containing, lyso(monoacyl) phospholipids, and sphingomyelin contain molar ratios (fatty acid : phospholipid) of 2, 1, 1, and 1, respectively.

3.2 Methodologies for measuring alterations in major phospholipids and AA

The gas–liquid chromatograph can be utilized to determine the composition of the major phospholipids (PC, PE, PS, PI, and SPH) in platelets as well as the fatty acid composition within each phospholipid (24). Through the use of phospholipases A_1 and A_2, the positional distribution of the fatty acids in each phospholipid can be determined (24). In addition, the molecular species compositions (the *sn*-1 and *sn*-2 fatty acid pairs) in each phospholipid of resting (24) and stimulated platelets (25) can be assessed using additional

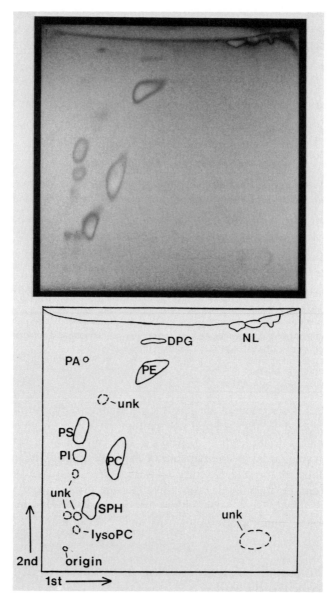

Figure 2. Two-dimensional thin-layer chromatographic separation of major phospholipids, lysophospholipids, and phosphatidic acid. A thin-layer chromatogram illustrating
separation of phospholipids and lysophospholipids from human platelets by two-dimensional chromatography using the solvents described in *Table 2* is shown. Lipids were
visualized using under ultraviolet light (366 nm) following spraying with 8-anilino-1-
naphthalenesulfonic acid. DPG: cardiolipin; lysoPC: lysophosphatidylcholine; NL: neutral
lipid; PA: phosphatidic acid; PC: phosphatidylcholine; PI: phosphatidylinositol; PS: phosphatidylserine; SPH: sphingomyelin; unk: unknown.

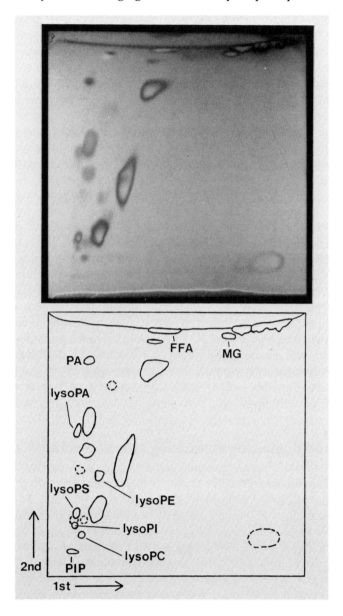

Figure 3. Two-dimensional thin-layer chromatographic separation of major phospholipids, lysophospholipids, and phosphatidic acid with added lipid standards. Conditions are as given in the legend of *Figure 2* with the exception that the following standards have been added: FFA: free fatty acid; lysoPA: lysophosphatidic acid; lysoPE: lysophosphatidylethanolamine; lysoPC: lysophosphatidylcholine; lysoPI: lysophosphatidylinositol; lysoPS: lysophosphatidylserine; MG: monoacylglycerol; PA: phosphatidic acid; PIP: phosphatidylinositol 4-phosphate.

methodologies. These include the phospholipase C-mediated hydrolysis of phospholipids to the corresponding diacylglycerols, acetylation of the diacyl-glycerols, and separation of the diacylglycerol acetates according to their degree of unsaturation via thin-layer argentation chromatography (25).

Thrombin-dependent mass changes in platelet PC, PE, PS, and PI have been determined via GLC by comparing the phospholipid mass levels from stimulated and resting platelets (25,27,28). Using a glycerol lysis technique (29), platelet plasma membranes can be isolated from agonist-stimulated as well as resting platelets and the component phospholipids (and inherent fatty acids) have been analysed by GLC as above (28). In addition, agonist-dependent changes in phospholipid fatty acid levels, particularly AA, can be assessed to determine the source of the released AA in stimulated platelets (27,28,30). The agonist-stimulated loss of AA and EPA mass from platelet phospholipids has also been measured following the isolation of platelets from subjects who have consumed a fish oil concentrate (31,32). Phospholipase A_2 inhibitors can be added to the platelet suspension prior to agonist addition to assess the phospholipase A_2-mediated degradation of phospholipids (30,31). The mass accumulation of free AA (and EPA) within stimulated platelets may be assessed through the use of the cyclo-oxygenase/lipoxygenase inhibitor, BW755C, which thereby blocks further metabolism via oxygenases of AA (and EPA) (31). Such an inhibitor will, of course, block the eicosanoid-dependent phospholipid degradations upon agonist exposure. Mass accumulation of thromboxane B_2, a stable but biologically inactive metabolite of TxA_2, can also be measured as an indirect monitor of phospholipase A_2 activation as described by McNicol (see Chapter 1).

3.3 Methodologies for measuring alterations in PA mass

The quantitation of PA in stimulated platelets (indicating activation of phospholipase C) is similar to that for the other major phospholipids. Several one-dimensional and two-dimensional TLC sytems have been developed to enable separation of PA (and lysoPA if needed) from other platelet phospholipids. A two-dimensional TLC system is described in *Protocol 4* and illustrated in *Figure 2*. A one-dimensional TLC system can also be used (23) (e.g. see *Figure 1*), following which the area containing PA is eluted and run in a second TLC system to isolate the PA (31); a simple and effective one-dimensional system which does not require further chromatography has also been described (17). The PA mass and the fatty acid masses within the PA can be assessed in stimulated platelets (30–32). In light of the recently demonstrated formation of PA from PC and/or PE in stimulated platelets (in addition to that derived from phosphoinositides), the major source of the newly-formed PA can be determined by analysis of the mass ratio of AA/EPA in the PA from platelets of fish oil consumers compared with the ratios in the individual resting platelet phospholipids (32).

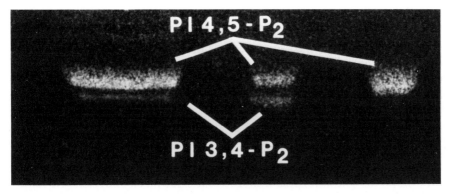

Figure 4. Autoradiograph of a thin-layer chromatographic separation of phosphoinositides. Platelet acidic extracts were separated by one-dimensional thin-layer chromatography using the solvent described in *Table 2*. Phosphoinositides were visualized under ultraviolet light following spraying with 8-anilino-1-naphthalenesulfonic acid. The figure shows a close-up of the region containing PI 4,5-P$_2$ and PI 3,4-P$_2$. Lane 1: platelets stimulated with the thromboxane mimetic, U46619 (2 μM, 3 min); lane 2: the eluted PI 3,4-P$_2$ band was re-chromatographed (there is approximately 4% contamination with PI 4,5-P$_2$); lane 3: PI 4,5-P$_2$ standard (Sigma Chemical Co.). The purity of the rechromatographed PI 3,4-P$_2$ band in lane 2, measured by HPLC, was essentially 100% (33). Reproduced with permission from Gaudette *et al.* (33).

3.4 Methodologies for measuring alteration in phosphoinositide mass levels

The mass levels of phosphoinositides can be determined by GLC following their separation via a phosphoinositide TLC system (33) (see *Table 2* and *Figure 4*). Phosphoinositides are typically visualized on the thin-layer plates following spraying with 0.1% ANS (8-anilino-1-naphthalenesulfonic acid) (34). The quantitation of phosphoinositides via GLC provides data on phosphoinositide amounts as well as fatty acid composition (33). Very short incubation times (10–15 sec) of agonist with platelets enables the assessment of phospholipase C activity on PI 4,5-P$_2$ (35), whereas longer incubations of agonist with platelets (2–3 min) provides for the assessment of phosphoinositide kinase activity on PI and PI 4-P (5,33). The phosphoinositide TLC system (shown in *Figure 4*) separates PI 4,5-P$_2$ from PI 3,4-P$_2$, allowing for the mass determination of each of these phosphoinositides in stimulated platelets (33).

4. Radiolabelling studies

4.1 Methodologies for measuring radioactive changes in platelet phospholipids

During the platelet isolation prodedure, platelets are incubated with the radiolabel in either PRP or the first washed platelet suspension (see *Protocol 1*, steps 5 and 9, respectively) for an extended time (usually two hours) to allow for the incorporation of the radiolabel into the platelet phospholipids. Longer times are required to approach equilibrium labelling for the ether-containing choline and ethanolamine phospholipids. Incorporation of the radiolabel is via *de novo* synthesis ([³H]glycerol, [³H]inositol, [³H]ethano-lamine), base exchange reactions for labelled bases ([¹⁴C]choline), deacyla-tion/reacylation plus *de novo* reactions (fatty acids, e.g. [³H]AA, [¹⁴C]stearic acid), futile cycling plus *de novo* reactions ([³²P]orthophosphate) (1). Platelets are isolated and their phospholipids extracted and separated by TLC. Radioactive phospholipids are prepared for counting as follows:

(a) Scrape the phospholipids from the thin-layer plates into separate scintil-lation vials.

(b) Add 1.5 ml water and 13.5 ml Aquasol-2 (New England Nuclear) to each vial and vortex for 30 sec.

The radioactivity associated with each phospholipid is determined using a scintillation counter. Agonist-stimulated changes in phospholipids can be determined by comparison of the phospholipid radioactivity (disintegra-tions/min or d.p.m.) in stimulated and resting platelets. Radiolabelling of platelet phospholipids may be utilized for one of several reasons:

(a) The mass of phospholipid being measured (e.g. lysophospholipid, phos-phoinositides) is too small to enable detection of agonist-stimulated mass changes.

(b) The alteration (e.g. decrease) in the phospholipid with agonist stimula-tion (e.g. PC, PE) is too small to be quantified via mass analysis.

(c) Low level agonist concentrations cause changes in phospholipids which are too small to be measured via mass analysis.

(d) Mass analysis via GLC is time-consuming, whereas radioactivity mea-surements are much quicker.

4.2 Use of [³H]glycerol or [³H]arachidonic acid to monitor alterations in PC, PE, PS, and PI

Labelling of platelets with [³H]glycerol can be achieved by the addition of the radiolabel to platelet-rich plasma. [³H]Glycerol labelling of platelets provides a means of labelling all the major phospholipids since glycerol is incorporated *de novo* into platelet phospholipids (1). Using [³H]glycerol, alterations in platelet phospholipid levels in agonist-stimulated platelets can be determined (36). The agonist-induced generation of lysophospholipids labelled with [³H]glycerol can also be assessed (36,37). Using the methodologies outlined in Section 3.2, changes in the molecular species of phospholipids with agonist stimulation can be measured to demonstrate selectivity for AA release (26,36).

Platelets labelled with [³H]AA incorporate the radiolabel into phospholipids via acyl transfer reactions as well as *de novo* biosynthesis. Sources of released AA in stimulated platelets can be determined by measuring alterations in [³H]AA radiolabelled phospholipids (26,38). Similarly, selectivity for phospholipase A₂-mediated AA release may be shown by the comparison of data from [³H]AA pre-labelled platelets with that of platelets pre-labelled with other fatty acids (26).

4.3 Use of [¹⁴C]stearic acid to monitor the generation of 1-acyl lysophospholipids

According to molecular species analyses of resting platelet phospholipids (24), the 1-stearoyl 2-arachidonoyl species predominate in both the AA-containing and the stearoyl-containing platelet phospholipids. For this reason, platelets can be pre-labelled with [¹⁴C]stearic acid (in the first washed platelet suspension) and the agonist-induced generation of 1-acyl lysophospholipids assessed as a measure of phospholipase A₂ activity releasing predominantly AA (39,40). This labelling method provides a unique method for assessing the source(s) of released AA in stimulated platelets. Platelet lysophospholipids can be separated by the two-dimensional TLC system described in *Protocol 4*.

4.4 Monitoring phosphatidic acid generation using radiolabelled platelets

In radiolabelling studies, the generation of PA can be monitored when using radiolabels that incorporate into phosphoinositides (with the exception of [³H]inositol). Agonist-stimulated PA formation can be measured in platelets pre-labelled with [³H]glycerol (36), since the label is incorporated into the backbone of phosphoinositides. In addition, since the 1-stearoyl 2-arachidonoyl species is the major molecular species of resting platelet phosphoinositides (24), PA generation in stimulated platelets can be assessed by pre-labelling platelets with [³H]AA (41) or [¹⁴C]stearic acid (39,40). The thin-layer chromatographic separation of PA from other platelet phospholipids may be achieved as described in Section 3.3.

4.5 Use of [³H]ethanolamine to monitor alterations in ethanolamine phospholipids

Platelets pre-labelled in a washed platelet suspension with [³H]ethanolamine incorporate the radiolabel into ethanolamine phospholipids, including diacyl PE and 1-alkenyl 2-acyl PE (alkenylacyl PE), via *de novo* synthetic pathways. Alkenylacyl PE (or plasmalogenic PE) is a major form of ethanolamine phospholipids and AA-containing phospholipid in resting platelets (42). Using platelets pre-labelled with [³H]ethanolamine, the phospholipase A-mediated degradation of diacyl PE and alkenylacyl PE can be measured along with the generation of their respective lyso forms, namely lyso(monoacyl) PE and lysoplasmenyl PE (1-alkenyl 2-lysoPE)(43,44). In order to separate these ethanolamine phospholipids from platelet extracts, a two-dimensional TLC system is employed (such as the one described in *Protocol 4*) with an acid hydrolysis step (45) between dimensions. Following the first dimension, the parent PE compounds co-migrate, as do their respective lyso forms. Exposure of these areas of the TLC plate to concentrated HCl fumes results in cleavage of the 1-alkenyl linkages. Alkenylacyl PE is cleaved to lyso(2-acyl) PE and lysoplasmenyl PE is cleaved to *sn*-glycero-3-phosphoethanolamine. The second dimension of the TLC system separates these components for subsequent scintillation counting.

4.6 Use of [^{3}H]inositol to monitor alterations in phosphoinositides and inositol phosphates

Platelets labelled with [^{3}H]inositol in the first washed platelet suspension incorporate the radiolabel into the various phosphoinositides. An approximate sevenfold increase in the amount of [^{3}H]inositol incorporated into phosphoinositides is achieved by replacing the 1 mM $MgCl_2$ and 5.6 mM glucose in the Tyrode's buffer with 2 mM $MnCl_2$ and 0.56 mM glucose, respectively (46). Decreasing the volume of the first washed platelet suspension for the radiolabelling incubation period can increase substantially the amount of radiolabel incorporated into phosphoinositides. However, the amount of radiolabel that can be incorporated in this way is relatively small compared to other tissues, which have a much higher rate of *de novo* synthesis of PI, or in cell lines, which can be radiolabelled over several days. This can be overcome to some extent by radiolabelling following electroporation thereby enabling increased uptake of [^{3}H]inositol (47).

Separation of the various phosphoinositides may be achieved using a one-dimensional TLC system (see *Table 2* and *Figure 4*). Agonist-stimulated decreases in phosphoinositides (PI and PI 4,5-P_2) can be measured in [^{3}H]inositol pre-labelled platelets, as well as the generation of lysoPI (48). In addition, the net accumulation of [^{3}H]inositol labelled PI 4-P, PI 4,5-P_2, and PI 3,4-P_2 in stimulated platelets due to phosphoinositide kinase reactions can be determined (5,48–50).

Agonist-stimulated formation of inositol phosphates can also be measured in [^{3}H]inositol pre-labelled platelets. The measurement of the Ca^{2+} releasing messenger, Ins 1,4,5-P_3, in this manner, however, is hindered by the low level of incorporation of [^{3}H]inositol (51,52) and the requirement for HPLC to enable separation from the inactive isomer, Ins 1,3,4-P_3 which is formed in much higher levels (53,54). Mass measurement of Ins 1,4,5-P_3 is therefore preferred and can be achieved through the use of a specific binding assay which exploits the selectivity of Ins 1,4,5-P_3 for its receptor (55). The assay can be purchased (e.g. Amersham International) or made using bovine adrenals (56).

There is, however, sufficient incorporation of radiolabel to enable routine measurement of 'total' [^{3}H]inositol phosphates, i.e. inositol mono-, bis- and trisphosphates. It is not necessary to include higher phosphorylated species of inositol in these measurements as their levels do not increase significantly on stimulation. The addition of LiCl (12 mM) to the Tyrode buffer prevents metabolism of [^{3}H]inositol monophosphates to [^{3}H]inositol with the result newly incorporated radioactivity into 'total' inositol phosphates becomes trapped (57); thus measurement of 'total' inositol phosphates in the presence of LiCl can be used to monitor phospholipase C activity over a period of time (58).

Protocol 6. Measurement of formation of 'total' [^{3}H]inositol phosphates

Equipment and reagents

- [^{3}H]Inositol (e.g. Amersham International, New England Nuclear)
- Dowex anion exchange resin (formate form; 100–200 mesh; 1 x 8) (Bio-Rad)
- Washed platelets resuspended in 1 ml per 50 ml of blood
- Tyrode's buffer (see *Protocol 1*)
- EGTA (100 mM)
- Prostacylin (100 µg/ml) (Wellcome Foundation)
- LiCl (150 mM)
- Water-bath
- Centrifuge

- Chloroform/methanol/HCl (50 : 100 : 2; by vol.)
- Chloroform
- Glass columns (capacity 10–20 ml) with collection rack
- 60 mM ammonium formate/5 mM sodium tetraborate
- 800 mM ammonium formate/100 mM formic acid
- Scintillation fluid capable of holding a large volume of fluid with high osmotic strength (e.g. liquiscint, National Diagnostics)
- Scintillation vials (20 ml)

Method

1. Incubate platelets with [^{3}H]inositol (30 µCi/ml of platelet suspension) in Tyrode buffer containing EGTA (1 mM) for 2–3 h at 37°C; resuspend the cells every 30–40 min by gentle agitation.

2. During this period, prepare Dowex anion exchange columns by addition of 1 ml of a 50% slurry of Dowex resin to a glass column containing a plug to prevent loss of resin, e.g. glass wool. Wash the resin with 2 x 10 ml of water and do not allow to dry.

3. Add prostacyclin (100 nM) and wash platelets by centrifugation at 950 *g* for 10 min.

4. Resuspend platelets in Tyrode buffer at 8×10^8/ml and leave for at least 30 min at 37°C to enable to the effects of prostacylin to decay.

5. Add LiCl (20 µl per 250 µl final volume) and incubate for 5 min before agonist addition. Terminate the reaction with 940 µl chloroform/methanol/HCl (50 : 100 : 2, by vol.) and leave for 5 min.

Protocol 6. *Continued*

6. Separate phases by addition of chloroform (310 µl) and water (310 µl) and leave to stand for at least 30 min.[a]

7. Remove 800 µl of the upper phase to Dowex anion exchange columns and allow to drain. Add 12 ml of 60 mM ammonium formate/5 mM sodium tetraborate and drain.

8. Add 6 ml of 800 mM ammonium formate/100 mM formic acid[b] and collect in 20 ml scintillation vials; add 10 ml of scintillation fluid.[c]

---

[a] Separation can be speeded up by centrifugation.
[b] Removes more than 90% of 'total' inositol phosphates (i.e. inositol mono-, bis-, and trisphosphates); columns can be reused by addition of a further 6 ml of 800 mM ammonium formate/100 mM formic acid followed by 2 × 10 ml water; columns should not be allowed to dry.
[c] The level of inositol phosphates in non-stimulated cells is in the order of 50–200 d.p.m. and a strong agonist, e.g. thrombin (1 U/ml), will increase this five- to tenfold during a 5 min incubation.

4.7 Use of butanol to monitor phospholipase D activity

The cleavage of phospholipids by phospholipase D generates PA and the corresponding head group of the lipid, e.g. choline. An essential step in this reaction is the introduction of a water molecule. Alcohols are preferably incorporated at this stage generating a product that is unique to this reaction, i.e. the corresponding phosphatidylalcohol (59). Butanol is the alcohol of choice for this reaction where it can also be introduced as radiolabel, e.g. [³H]butanol (17). However, the use of [³H]butanol is discouraged as it potentially volatile necessitating that the experiment is performed in a fume-cupboard and high levels are required because of the high concentration of butanol required to compete against water in this reaction. The alternative experiment, namely to radiolabel the lipid, e.g. with [³H]glycerol or [³H]fatty acid, is recommended. [³H]Phosphatidylbutanol is separated by TLC (17). Phospholipase D activity has been described in rabbit and human platelets (60,61).

4.8 Use of [³²P]orthophosphate to measure phospholipid metabolism

The use of [³²P]orthophosphate in the measurement of phospholipids has several advantages including its increased strength as a β-radiation emitter, thereby facilitating lipid detection by autoradiography, and because the same experimental sample (appropriately divided) can be used in the measurement of [³²P]protein phosphorylation. Labelling with [³²P]orthophosphate has a particular advantage in the labelling of all phosphoinositides apart from PI; the specific activity of the phosphate residues, with the exception of the 1-phosphate which can only be labelled with [³²P]orthophosphate by *de novo* synthesis, is close to that of cellular ATP, in part because of the futile cycling that occurs from PI to PI 4,5-P_2 and vice versa. A similar situation applies to formation of PA from 1,2-diacylglycerol. A one-dimensional TLC separation of [^{32}P]PA from other phospholipids is described (62). The labelling of platelets with [^{32}P]orthophosphate is described in Chapter 9.

Acknowledgements

S. P. W. is a Royal Society University Research Fellow.

References

1. Siess, W. (1989). *Physiol. Rev.*, **69**, 58.
2. Nozawa, Y., Nakashima, S., and Nagata, K. (1991). *Biochim. Biophys. Acta*, **1082**, 219.
3. Nishizuka, Y. (1984). *Nature*, **308**, 693.
4. Berridge, M. J. (1984). *Biochem. J.*, **220**, 345.
5. Thomas, L. M. and Holub, B. J. (1992). *Prog. Lipid Res.*, **31**, 399.
6. Arita, H., Nakano, T., and Hanasaki, K. (1989). *Prog. Lipid Res.*, **28**, 273.
7. Thomas, L. M. and Holub, B. J. (1993). In *Proceedings of the third international conference on essential fatty acids and eicosanoids* (ed. A. Sinclair and R. Gibson), pp. 303–7. American Oil Chemists Society, Champaign, IL.
8. Huang, R., Kucera, G. L., and Rittenhouse, S. E. (1991). *J. Biol. Chem.*, **266**, 1652.
9. Randall, R. W., Bonser, R. W., Thompson, N. T., and Garland, L. G. (1990). *FEBS Lett.*, **264**, 87.
10. McKean, M. L., Smith, J. B., and Silver, M. J. (1981). *J. Biol. Chem.*, **256**, 1522.
11. Mustard, J. F., Perry, D. W., Ardlie, N. G., and Packham, M. A. (1972). *Br. J. Haematol.*, **22**, 193.
12. Aster, R. H. and Jandl, J. H. (1964). *J. Clin. Invest.*, **43**, 843.
13. Molnar, J. and Lorand, L. (1961). *Arch. Biochem. Biophys.*, **93**, 353.
14. Riendeau, D., Guary, J., Weech, P. K., Laliberté, F., Yergey, J., Li, C., et al. (1994). *J. Biol. Chem.*, **269**, 15619.
15. Smith, J. B., Dangelmaier, C., and Mauco, G. (1985). *Biochim. Biophys. Acta*, **835**, 344.
16. Tamaoki, T., Nomoto, H., Takahashi, I., Kato, Y., Morimoto, M., and Tomita, F. (1986). *Biochem. Biophys. Res. Commun.*, **135**, 397.
17. Bonser, R. W. and Thompson, N. T. (1992). In *Signal transduction: a practical approach* (ed. G. Milligan), pp. 123–50. Oxford University Press, Oxford.
18. Watson, S. P. and Girdlestone, D. (1995). *Trends Pharmacol. Sci.*, **16**, 1S
19. Akiyama, T., Ishida, J., Nakagawa, S., Ogawara, H., Watanabe, S., Itoh, N., et al. (1987). *J. Biol. Chem.*, **262**, 5592.
20. Bligh, E. G. and Dyer, W. J. (1959). *Can. J. Biochem. Physiol.*, **37**, 911.
21. Allan, D. and Michell, R. H. (1978). *Biochim. Biophys. Acta*, **508**, 277.
22. Vickers, J. D. (1995). *Anal. Biochem.*, **224**, 449.
23. Holub, B. J. and Skeaff, C. M. (1987). In *Methods in enzymology* (ed. P. M. Conn and A. R. Means), Vol. 141, pp. 234–44. Academic Press, Orlando, FL.

24. Mahadevappa, V. G. and Holub, B. J. (1982). *Biochim. Biophys. Acta*, **713,** 73.
25. Takamura, H., Narita, H., Park, H. J., Tanaka, K., Matsuura, T., and Kito, M. (1987). *J. Biol. Chem.*, **262,** 2262.
26. Mahadevappa, V. G. and Holub, B. J. (1984). *J. Biol. Chem.*, **259,** 9369.
27. Broekman, M. J., Ward, J. W., and Marcus, A. J. (1981). *J. Biol. Chem.*, **256,** 8271.
28. Skeaff, C. M. and Holub, B. J. (1985). *Biochim. Biophys. Acta*, **834,** 164.
29. Barber, A. J. and Jamieson, G. A. (1970). *J. Biol. Chem.*, **245,** 6357.
30. Mahadevappa, V. G. and Holub, B. J. (1986). *Biochem. Biophys. Res. Commun.*, **134,** 1327.
31. Mahadevappa, V. G. and Holub, B. J. (1987). *J. Lipid Res.*, **28,** 1275.
32. Aukema, H. M. and Holub, B. J. (1989). In *Dietary omega-3 and omega-6 fatty acids* (ed. G. Galli and A. P. Simopoulos), pp. 81–90. Plenum Press, New York.
33. Gaudette, D. C., Aukema, H. M., Jolly, C. A., Chapkin, R. S., and Holub, B. J. (1993). *J. Biol. Chem.*, **268,** 13773.
34. Lynch, R. D. (1980). *Lipids*, **15,** 412.
35. Mauco, G., Dangelmaier, C. A., and Smith, J. B. (1984). *Biochem. J.*, **224,** 933.
36. Mahadevappa, V. G. and Holub, B. J. (1983). *J. Biol. Chem.*, **258,** 5337.
37. Imai, A., Hattori, H., Takahashi, M., and Nozawa, Y. (1983). *Biochem. Biophys. Res. Commun.*, **112,** 693.
38. Weaver, B. J. and Holub, B. J. (1987). *Biochem. Cell. Biol.*, **65,** 405.
39. Thomas, L. M. and Holub, B. J. (1991). *Biochim. Biophys. Acta*, **1081,** 92.
40. Thomas, L. M. and Holub, B. J. (1991). *Cell. Signal.*, **3,** 159.
41. Imai, A., Ishizuka, Y., Kawai, K., and Nozawa, Y. (1982). *Biochem. Biophys. Res. Commun.*, **108,** 752.
42. Mueller, H. W., Purdon, A. D., Smith, J. B., and Wykle, R. L. (1983). *Lipids*, **18,** 814.
43. Turini, M. E. and Holub, B. J. (1993). *Biochem. J.*, **289,** 641.
44. Turini, M. E. and Holub, B. J. (1994). *Biochim. Biophys. Acta*, **1213,** 21
45. Horrocks, L. A. (1968). *J. Lipid Res.*, **9,** 469.
46. Culty, M., Davidson, M. M. L., and Haslam, R. J. (1988). *Eur. J. Biochem.*, **171,** 523.
47. Authi, K. (1989). *FEBS Lett.*, **254,** 52.
48. Thomas, L. M. and Holub, B. J. (1991). *Lipids*, **26,** 689.
49. Gaudette, D. C. and Holub, B. J. (1990). *Biochem. Biophys. Res. Commun.*, **170,** 238.
50. Gaudette, D. C. and Holub, B. J. (1990). *Thromb. Res.*, **58,** 435.
51. Watson, S. P., McConnell, R. T., and Lapetina, E. G. (1984). *J. Biol. Chem.*, **259,** 13199.
52. Watson, S. P., Reep, B., McConnell, R. T., and Lapetina, E. G. (1985). *Biochem. J.*, **226,** 831.
53. Tarver, A. P., King, W. G., and Rittenhouse, S. E. (1987). *J. Biol. Chem.*, **262,** 17268.
54. Daniel, J. L., Dangelmaier, C. A., and Smith, J. B. (1987). *Biochem. J.*, **246,** 109.
55. Palmer, S., Hughes, K. T., Lee, D. Y., and Wakelam, M. J. O. (1989). *Cell. Signal.*, **1,** 147.
56. Godfrey, P. P. (1992). In *Signal transduction: a practical approach* (ed. G. Milligan), pp. 123–50. Oxford University Press, Oxford.
57. Berridge, M. J., Downes, C. P., and Hanley, M. (1982). *Biochem. J.*, **206,** 587.

58. Walker, T. and Watson, S. P. (1992). *Br. J. Pharmacol.*, **105,** 627.
59. Pai, J.-K., Siegel, M. I., Egan, R. W., and Billah, M. M. (1988). *J. Biol. Chem.*, **263,** 12472.
60. van der Meulen, J. and Haslam, R. J. (1990). *Biochem. J.*, **271,** 693.
61. Huang, R., Kucera, G. L., and Rittenhouse, S. E. (1991). *J. Biol. Chem.*, **266,** 1652.
62. Watson, S. P., Ganong, B. R., Bell, R. M., and Lapetina, E. G. (1984). *Biochem. Biophys. Res. Commun.*, **121,** 386.

13

Cyclic nucleotides: measurement and function

ELKE BUTT and ULRICH WALTER

1. Introduction

The activation of human platelets is inhibited by a variety of agents which exert their effects through distinct mechanisms. Examples include inhibitors of thromboxane A_2 generation (e.g. aspirin), inhibitors of thrombin (e.g. hirudin), scavengers of ADP (e.g. apyrase), and physiological and pharmacological cyclic nucleotide-elevating agents (1,2). Vascular endothelial cells, under basal conditions and in response to numerous vasoactive agents, synthesize and release prostacyclin (PGI_2) and endothelium-derived relaxing factor, nitric oxide (EDRF; or NO), two of the most important physiological platelet inhibitors. PGI_2 and EDRF/NO increase the intracellular messenger molecules cAMP and cGMP, respectively, in human platelets and other target cells. The inhibition of platelet activation caused by PGI_2 and EDRF/NO is mediated by cAMP- and cGMP-dependent protein kinases (cAMP-PK, cGMP-PK), respectively. As shown in *Table 1*, human platelets contain particularly high concentrations of cAMP-PK and cGMP-PK (3). The type III cGMP-inhibited phosphodiesterase (cGI-PDE) is an additional important target for cGMP. Elevation of cAMP mediated by cGMP inhibition of the cGI-PDE contributes to the well known synergism between cGMP- and cAMP-elevating platelet inhibitors (4). In human platelets, established cAMP-PK substrates include the small molecular weight G protein rap 1B, the β subunit of glycoprotein Ib (GPIbβ), the focal adhesion protein VASP, caldesmon, myosin light chain kinase (MLCK), cGI-PDE, and actin-binding protein (ABP) (2). Only the focal adhesion protein VASP is an established substrate for cGMP-PK in platelets although other substrates, perhaps also rap 1B and GPIbβ, may exist. The physiological effects of cyclic nucleotide-elevating platelet inhibitors are terminated by cyclic nucleotide-degrading phosphodiesterases (PDEs) and by protein phosphatases which dephosphorylate the cAMP-PK and cGMP-PK substrates. In human platelets, the major PDEs responsible for cAMP or cGMP hydrolysis are type III cGI-PDE and type V cGMP binding, cGMP-specific PDE (cGB-PDE), respectively (4,5).

Table 1. Concentration of cyclic nucleotides, cGMP-dependent protein kinase (cGMP-PK), and catalytic subunit of cAMP-dependent protein kinase (C subunit) in unstimulated washed human platelets[a]

Compound	Intracellular concentration (μM)	Molecules/platelet	Amount/10^9 platelets (pmol)	Protein (ng/μg)
cAMP	4.4	13 900	23.1	
cGMP	0.4	1200	2.0	
C subunit	3.1	9800	16.3	0.31
cGMP-PK	7.3	22 900	38.1	1.36

[a] See ref. 3 for further details. Additional data indicate that only small increases in platelet cAMP levels are required for the full activation of cAMP-PK. In contrast, the activation of platelet cGMP-PK is proportional to the level of cGMP elevation (3).

Platelet protein phosphatases have not been extensively investigated but include okadaic acid-sensitive protein phosphatases 1 and 2A. Stimulation of platelet cAMP-PK and cGMP-PK inhibits the response of platelet agonists at multiple sites including inhibition of phosphoinositide metabolism, Ca^{2+} mobilization, and subsequently inhibition of protein kinase C and fibrinogen receptor activation. Ultimately, this results in inhibition of platelet adhesion, aggregation, and secretion. *Figure 1* summarizes some aspects of cyclic nucleotide regulation and function in human platelets. The reader is referred to other sources for a comprehensive review of the cyclic nucleotide signal transduction system in human platelets (2,6).

2. Analysis of cAMP, cGMP, and cyclic nucleotide derivatives and metabolites by radioimmunoassay (RIA) and HPLC

Figure 1 provides a list of physiological and pharmacological agents which regulate platelet cAMP and cGMP levels. With intact human platelets, maximal increases (more than tenfold elevation of basal levels) in platelet cAMP are observed with 5–10 μM PGE_1, PGI_2, and the stable PGI_2 analogue Iloprost (Schering AG); threshold effects are observed with 1–10 nM of these stimuli (3,7,8). With respect to platelet cGMP levels, maximal effects (more than tenfold elevations compared to basal levels) are typically observed with 50–100 μM sodium nitroprusside (SNP) or morpholynosydnonimine hydrochloride (SIN-1), whereas threshold effects are observed with 0.1–1 μM of these two stimuli (3,7). In the absence of other cell types, nitrates such as nitroglycerin and isosorbiddinitrate only affect platelet cGMP levels at millimolar concentrations. When threshold concentrations of cAMP- and cGMP-elevating agents are used together, cGMP-elevating agents (e.g. 0.1 μM SNP or SIN-1) potentiate cAMP elevation by inhibition of cGI-PDE.

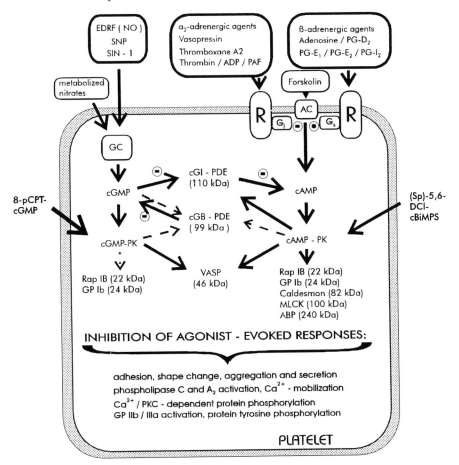

Figure 1. Regulation and action of cyclic nucleotides and cyclic nucleotide-dependent protein kinases in human platelets. The model summarizes the the regulaton (+ or no sign, activation; –, inhibition) of guanylyl cyclases (GC) or adenylyl cyclase (AC) by various vasoactive agents and drugs and the regulation of phosphodiesterases (PDE) and cAMP-/cGMP-dependent protein kinases (cGMP-PK, cAMP-PK). EDRF(NO), endothelium-derived relaxing factor (nitric oxide); SNP, sodium nitroprusside; SIN-1, morpholinosyd-nonimine hydrochloride; PAF, platelet activating factor; PG-D$_2$, PG-E$_1$, prostaglandin D$_2$, E$_1$ etc.; R, receptor; G$_i$, G$_s$, inhibitory and stimulatory G protein; cGI-PDE, cGB-PDE, cGMP-inhibited and cGMP binding PDE; Rap IB, a small molecular weight G protein; VASP, vasodilator-stimulated phosphoprotein; GP, glycoprotein; MLCK, myosin light chain kinase; ABP, actin-binding protein. Full arrows indicate a stimulatory (increased activity or phosphorylation) or (when indicated, –) an inhibitory effect. Dashed arrows indicate a possible effect which has not been unequivocally established in human platelets.

2.1 Extraction of cyclic nucleotides

Protocol 1. Extraction of platelet cAMP and cGMP from platelet-rich plasma (PRP)

Equipment and reagents

- Platelet-rich plasma (PRP) (1 × 10⁸ cells/ml) (see Chapter 1)ᵃ
- Water saturated diethyl ether
- 10% trichloroacetic acid, 4°C
- 50 mM Na acetate pH 5.8
- Bench-top centrifuge (e.g. Eppendorf 5415)
- Speed-Vac
- Eppendorf tubes (1.5 ml)

Method

1. Pipette 300 μl of PRP into an Eppendorf tube.

2. Centrifuge (8000 *g*, 10 sec) at room temperature.

3. Carefully remove and discard the supernatant. Resuspend the pellet in 300 μl of ice-cold 10% TCA.

4. Keep the TCA extract on ice for 30 min.

5. Centrifuge (8000 *g*, 4 min) at room temperature.

6. Remove the supernatant and discard the pellet.

7. Wash the supernatant four times with 5 vol. of water saturated diethyl ether, discarding the upper ether layer on each occasion.

8. Dry the remaining aqueous extract in a Speed-Vac at 30°C.

9. Dissolve the dried extract in 250 μl of 50 mM Na acetate buffer.

ᵃ The cell concentration can be adjusted with platelet-poor plasma to 1 × 10⁸ cells/ml. Washed or gel filtered platelets can also be used.

This protein-free platelet extract may be stored at –20°C until analysed by RIA. An important step in experiments with PRP platelets is the careful removal of the supernatant (platelet-poor plasma) in step 3 since plasma contains high levels of free cGMP which may interfere with the measurement of platelet-associated cGMP. When experiments with washed or gel filtered platelets are performed, an aliquot of the platelet suspension (e.g. 200 μl; 2.0 × 10⁸ cells) can be withdrawn from the incubation mixture and immediately mixed with an equal volume of ice-cold 20% TCA at the time point desired. The cyclic nucleotide extraction procedure is then continued at *Protocol 1*, step 4.

2.2 Radioimmunoassay

The RIA is based on the competition between unlabelled cAMP/cGMP and a fixed quantity of [¹²⁵I]cAMP/cGMP for the binding sites of a cAMP/cGMP-specific antibody. For the measurement of platelet cAMP we use a commercial RIA kit (Amersham) and the non-acetylated protocol as described in the manufacturer's instructions (sensitivity: 25–1600 fmol/100 µl sample volume). Platelet cGMP levels which are much lower than cAMP levels (*Table 1*) are measured by the more sensitive acetylation procedure (sensitivity 2–256 fmol/50 µl sample volume).

2.2.1 cAMP-RIA

For the quantitative determination of platelet cAMP, the [125I]cAMP assay system RPA 509 (Amersham) is used according to the manufacturer's instructions for the non-acetylation procedure. The reagents are sufficient for 100 samples. The equipment and reagents required are the same as described in the cGMP-RIA (*Protocol 2*). The protein-free extracts from *Protocol 1* are ready to be used in this assay system without further dilution. Antisera for cAMP are also available from other sources (e.g. Sigma, Biomol, Calbiochem).

2.2.2 cGMP RIA

Commercial cGMP antisera often overestimate the basal cGMP concentration in human platelets (3). This is most likely due to the low level of cGMP and presence of substances in platelet extracts which interfere with the cGMP RIA. In addition, partial cross-reactivity of the cGMP antiserum with cAMP and cyclic nucleotide metabolites has to be carefully evaluated since cGMP levels are usually much lower than cAMP levels (see also *Table 1*). In our hands, a non-commercial antiserum against cGMP could be successfully used for the determination of basal and stimulated platelet cGMP levels (3).

Protocol 2. cGMP radioimmunoassay

Equipment and reagents

- 100 mM Na acetate pH 6.0
- 130 mM NaCl, 4°C
- [125I]cGMP: 1 : 600 dilution in Na acetate buffer pH 6.0 (guanosine 3',5'-cyclic phosphoric acid 2'-O-succinyl [125I]iodotyrosine methyl ester) NEX-131 from NEN (1 µCi is sufficient for 400 samples)
- Non-immune rabbit IgG (e.g. Sigma, G-0261) dissolved (7 µg/µl) in Na acetate buffer—store in aliquots at –20°C
- Anti-rabbit IgG (e.g. from Sigma, R-5001) dissolved in 2 ml H$_2$O—store in aliquots at –20°C
- Rabbit cGMP antiserum (3) diluted 1/100 (v/v) in buffer A—store in aliquots at –20°C^a
- Buffer A: 100 mM Na acetate, 2.5% BSA RIA grade pH 6.0
- Buffer B: 50 mM Na acetate, 0.1 M NaCl, 0.01% NaN$_3$ pH 6.0

- Antiserum mixture: 2 vol. of a 1 : 100000 (v/v) diluted non-immune rabbit IgG in 130 mM NaCl; 1 vol. of a 1 : 50 (v/v) in buffer A diluted cGMP antiserum (final dilution 1 : 5000); 1 vol. of a 1 : 40 (v/v) in buffer B diluted anti-rabbit IgG (when commercial antisera are used, an antiserum dilution should be used which precipitates about 30–40% of the total [125I]cGMP under the conditions described below)
- 10 nM cGMP
- Acetylation reagent: acetic anhydride/triethylamine (1 : 2, v/v)
- Glass tubes (12 x 75 mm)
- Gamma radiation counter
- Bench-top centrifuge (e.g. Eppendorf 5415)
- Glass tube rack for decantation
- Parafilm

Protocol 2. *Continued*

Method

1. Prepare cGMP RIA standards in glass tubes as shown:

Tube	cGMP (μl)	Acetate buffer (μl)	Tube X (μl)	Final [cGMP] (fmol/50 μl)
A	128	122	–	256
B	–	125	A : 125	128
C	–	125	B : 125	64
D	–	125	C : 125	32
E	–	125	D : 125	16
F	–	125	E : 125	
G	–	125	F : 125	4
H	–	125	G : 125	2
Zero	–	125	–	0

2. Pipette 125 μl of cGMP standards or platelet extract into a glass tube. Add 6.25 μl of acetylation reagent and mix thoroughly.

3. cGMP RIA assay: Prepare duplicate tubes as shown below:

Sample	Acetate buffer	Buffer A	cGMP standards	Platelet	[^{125}I]cGMP	Antiserum mixture
Total	100 μl				50 μl	
Blank	87.5 μl	12.5 μl			50 μl	
cGMP standards			50 μl		50 μl	50 μl
Platelet extracts				50 μl	50 μl	50 μl

Mix and vortex thoroughly, cover with Parafilm, and incubate for 18–24 h at 4°C.

4. Pipette 1 ml of ice-cold 130 mM NaCl (do not vortex).

5. Centrifuge at 2000 *g* for 30 min at 4°C.

6. Place all tubes, except totals, into a decantation rack, pour off and discard supernatant (radioactive). Keep tubes inverted and place on a pad of absorbent tissues so as to allow the remaining fluid to drain (5 min).

7. Count all tubes (including totals) for 2 min in a gamma counter.

[a] Commercial rabbit cGMP antisera are available from several sources (e.g. Amersham, NEN, Calbiochem, Biomol, Sigma, Biotrend).

2.3 HPLC

For analysis of cyclic nucleotide derivatives and metabolites, an analytical method independent of antibodies is required. An effective system for sepa-

Table 2. HPLC conditions for separation of cyclic nucleotides

Compound	Solvent	Flow (ml/min)	λ_{max} (nM)	Retention time[a] (min)
cGMP	6% CH_3CN/5 mM TEAF	2	250	2 : 00
8-Br-cGMP	6 % CH_3CN/5 mM TEAF	2	260	4 : 00
	9% CH_3CN/25 mM TEAF	2	260	5 : 00
8-pCPT-cGMP	10% CH_3CN/10 mM TEAF	2.5	276	7 : 50
	40% CH_3CN/10 mM TEAF	1	276	15 : 00
(Rp)-8-pCPT-cGMPS	40% CH_3CN/10 mM TEAF	1	276	18 : 00
cAMP	6% CH_3CN/5 mM TEAF	2	258	3 : 00
8-Br-cAMP	6% CH_3CN/5 mM TEAF	2	264	6 : 00
(Sp)-5,6-DCl-cBiMPS	40% CH_3OH/5 mM TEAF	2	254	11 : 00

[a] The retention times were determined by reversed-phase HPLC using a 4 mm x 250 mm column containing LiChrosorb RP-18 (10 μm) material from Merck, Darmstadt.

ration of compounds with a hydrophobic purine base, a polar ribose moiety, and an ionic phosphate group is reversed-phase paired ion chromatography which offers high resolution with good recovery. The most widely used reversed-phase columns contain a packing material of very uniform silica beads (usually 5–10 μm diameter) coated with an 18 carbon alkyl chain (RP-18). The ion pairing agents most commonly used are 0.05–2% aqueous trifluoroacetic acid (TFA), phosphoric acid, and triethylamine phosphate. For preparative separation, the use of triethylamine formiate, a volatile ion pairing agent, is more convenient. Acetonitrile is the most commonly used organic solvent because it gives the best peak shape and highest resolution. Cyclic nucleotides may be eluted by isocratic conditions while complex cyclic nucleotide mixtures should be separated by gradients. Flow rates for analytical reversed-phase columns are 0.5–1.0 ml/min. Cyclic nucleotides are monitored by their absorbance in the 250–280 nm range. The sensitivity of the UV detection method is dependent on the extinction coefficient of the cyclic nucleotides and therefore limited to concentrations of 1–10 pmol. In *Table 2*, HPLC conditions for widely used cyclic nucleotides are summarized. In *Figure 2* a HPLC separation of cGMP and 5′GMP is shown.

3. Selective regulation of cAMP- and cGMP-dependent protein kinases in platelet extracts and intact platelets

3.1 cAMP- and cGMP-dependent protein kinase activators

The functional effects of platelet cAMP-PK or cGMP-PK may be examined in extracts, permeabilized, or intact human platelets. In platelet extracts and permeabilized cells, 1 μM cAMP or cGMP is usually sufficient for full and

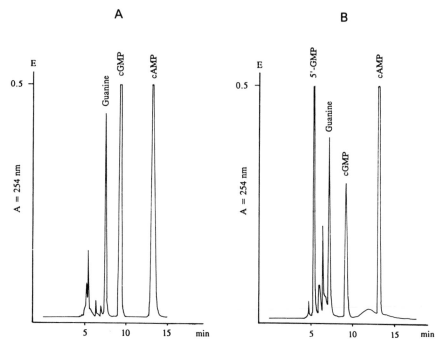

Figure 2. HPLC separation of cGMP, cAMP, and their metabolites. 10 μl of the supernatant from *Protocol 5* was applied to a Lichrosorb RP-18 column, 5 μm, 250 x 4 mm (Merck). The column was eluted with a 15 ml linear gradient from 6.5% acetonitrile/10 mM triethylammonium formiate to 50% acetonitrile/10 mM triethylammonium formiate at a flow rate of 0.5 ml/min. In comparison to the heat inactivated control cells in chromatogram A, chromatogram B shows a 50% hydrolysis of added cGMP to 5'GMP by the phosphodiesterases present in platelet homogenate after 15 min while very little added cAMP is degraded under these conditions.

selective activation of cAMP-PK or cGMP-PK, respectively (see *Table 3*). With intact human platelets, maximal and rapid (within 1–2 min) activation of the cAMP-PK can be obtained with 5–10 μM PGE$_1$, PGI$_2$, and Iloprost (a stable prostacyclin analogue).

Cyclic nucleotide analogues of cAMP and cGMP are widely used to investigate the biological role of cAMP-PK and cGMP-PK. A useful cAMP-PK or cGMP-PK activator should be hydrolysis-resistant and selective for the corresponding protein kinase. In studies with intact cells, a sufficient high lipophilicity of the nucleotide analogue is required to effectively penetrate the cell membrane and reach an intracellular concentration sufficient for cAMP-PK/cGMP-PK activation.

8-pCPT-cAMP is often used to investigate the functional role of the cAMP-PK. However, 8-pCPT-cAMP is a potent activator of both cAMP-PK and cGMP-PK (*Table 3*). In addition, the derivative is a potent inhibitor

Table 3. Some biological properties of cyclic nucleotides and their derivatives

Compound	K_a (μM)[a]		K_i (μM)[b]		Hydrolysis (V')[c]			Lipophilicity (log Kw)
	cAMP-PK	cGMP-PK	cAMP-PK	cGMP-PK	cGS-PDE	cGI-PDE	CaM-PDE	
cAMP	0.08	39			1.0	1.0	1.0	1.09
8-Br-cAMP	0.05	5.8			0.11	0.68	0.23	1.35
8-pCPT-cAMP	0.05	0.11			0.07	0.38	0.17	2.65
(Sp)-5,6-DCl-cBiMPS	0.03	10			0.008	None	None	2.99
Rp-cAMPS			3.7	53	None	None	None	1.21
cGMP	60	0.11			1.0	0.3	0.7	0.77
8-Br-cGMP	12	0.01			0.025	0.08	0.06	1.17
8-pCPT-cGMP	7	0.04			None	None	None	2.52
(Rp)-cGMPS			20	20	None	None	None	0.89
(Rp)-8-pCPT-cGMPS			8.3	0.5	None	None	None	2.60

[a] K_a, cyclic nucleotide concentration required for half-maximal activation.
[b] K_i, inhibition constant.
[c] Hydrolysis data are reported relative to cAMP hydrolysis taken as 1.0. See refs 7 and 8 for further details.
cAMP-PK, cAMP-dependent protein kinase; cGMP-PK, cGMP-dependent protein kinase; cGS, cGMP-stimulated phosphodiesterase; cGI-PDE, cGMP-inhibited phosphodiesterase; CaM-PDE, Ca^{2+}/calmodulin-dependent phosphodiesterase.

Table 4. Some chemical properties of cyclic nucleotide inhibitors and activators of cGMP- and cAMP-dependent protein kinase

Compound	Max. stock solution (water or buffer)[a]	Storage	M_r	λ_{max} (nm)	ε-Coefficient (pH 7)	Commercial sources
cAMP	50 mM	−20°C	329.2	258	15.000	Biolog, Sigma
8-Br-cAMP	10 mM	−20°C	408.2	264	15.700	Biolog, Sigma
(Sp)-5,6-DCl-cBiMPS	10 mM	−20°C	396.2	254	6.400	Biolog
(Rp)-cAMPS	20 mM	−20°C	345.3	258	15.000	Biolog, Boehringer
cGMP	50 mM	−20°C	345.3	252	13.600	Biolog, Sigma
8-Br-cGMP	50 mM	−20°C	446.1	261	15.100	Biolog, Sigma
8-pCPT-cGMP	60 mM	−20°C	487.9	276	21.500	Biolog
(Rp)-cGMPS	20 mM	−20°C	360.3	252	13.600	Biolog
(Rp)-8-pCPT-cGMPS	10 mM	−20°C	503.9	276	21.500	Biolog

[a] In case of incomplete solubility, place the tube in a water-bath of about 70°C for a short time. For longer storage periods (> two weeks), lyophilize the solution and freeze at −20°C to avoid degradation. Thiophosphates are unstable against oxidizing agents.

(IC_{50} = 0.9 μM) and substrate of the cGMP binding, cGMP-specific phosphodiesterase type V (cGB-PDE) (11). Therefore, 8-pCPT-cAMP is not a selective cAMP-PK activator. N^6,O^2-Dibutyryl-cAMP is a very poor cAMP-PK activator and needs to be metabolized by release of free butyrate to induce activation. Since this metabolism may differ from cell to cell and since the released free butyrate itself may have effects on the cell function, N^6,O^2-dibutyryl-cAMP cannot be considered as an ideal activator of cAMK-PK. Similar reasons can be advanced with respect to the use of N^6,O^2-dibutyryl-cGMP (10). 8-Br-cAMP, although a specific and potent cAMP-PK activator, has a relatively low lipophilicity and is also efficiently hydrolysed by at least four types of phosphodiesterases (*Table 3*). Selective activation of the cAMP-PK in intact human platelets bypassing adenylyl cyclases and phosphodiesterases was obtained with a newly designed, hydrolysis-resistant cAMP analogue, (Sp)-5,6-DCl-cBiMPS, at a concentration of 0.1–0.2 mM and and an incubation time of 10–30 min (9).

NO generating agents (nitrovasodilators) are believed to exert their effects via activation of the soluble guanylyl cyclase and subsequent formation of cGMP. Maximal and rapid (within 3–5 min) activation of the cGMP-PK can be obtained with 50–100 μM SNP or SIN-1 (both nitric oxide donors). However, NO donors also increase platelet cAMP levels under certain conditions mediated by cGMP inhibition of cGI-PDE (12). Therefore, selective activators of cGMP-PK, which do not affect other cGMP regulated proteins, e.g. cGMP regulated phosphodiesterases, are important tools to investigate the functional role of the cGMP-PK. As shown in *Table 3*, both 8-Br-cGMP and 8-pCPT-cGMP are potent and selective activators of the cGMP-PK. However, 8-Br-cGMP has a relatively low lipophilicity, is (at least to some extent) hydrolysed by PDEs and inhibits type III cGI-PDE at micromolar concentration. Therefore, 8-Br-cGMP is a useful cGMP-PK activator using cell extracts and more purified preparations whereas 8-pCPT-cGMP is the preferred analogue for activation of cGMP-PK in intact cells (10). Selective and potent activation of the cGMP-PK was demonstrated when intact human platelets were incubated for 10–30 min with 0.5–1.0 mM 8-pCPT-cGMP. *Tables 3* and *4* summarize the properties of a number of cAMP- and cGMP-derivatives often used for the regulation of platelet cAMP-PK and cGMP-PK (see also refs 9 and 10).

3.2 cAMP- and cGMP-dependent protein kinase inhibitors

In addition to selective protein kinase activators, specific protein kinase inhibitors are important tools to investigate the physiological functions of protein kinases. The heat stable inhibitor protein of cAMP-PK (PKI) (also known as Walsh inhibitor) and synthetic PKI peptides, containing the inhibitory pseudosubstrate region, are potent (K_i values in the nanomolar range) and highly selective inhibitors of the catalytic subunit of the cAMP-PK (13,14). Using platelet extracts, protein phosphorylation mediated by cAMP-PK can be selectively inhibited by 10 μM PKI peptide. However, PKI and PKI-derived peptides do not readily penetrate cell membranes and are therefore primarily used in experiments in which the peptides have a direct access to the cAMP-PK (e.g. cell extracts, membranes, permeabilized cells). Unfortunately, a similar inhibitory peptide for cGMP-PK does not exist. An antiserum and an affinity purified antibody against cGMP-PK potently and specifically inhibited cGMP-PK-mediated protein phosphorylation in platelet membranes (15).

Hidaka and co-workers developed a large series of protein kinase inhibitors (isoquinolinesulfonamides and derivatives, the so-called H-series), some of which are potent and somewhat selective inhibitors of cyclic nucleotide-dependent protein kinases (14). However, information concerning potency and selectivity of these H-series inhibitors using intact cells including intact human platelets is limited and needs to be examined in detail in future studies.

Another approach to inhibit cyclic nucleotide-dependent protein kinases is based on development of cAMP and cGMP stereoisomers. Earlier analogue studies suggested that the exocyclic oxygens of the cyclic phosphate are important for binding and activation of cyclic nucleotide-dependent protein kinases. Therefore (Rp)-derivatives with an equatorial sulfur have been synthesized and found to bind to the kinase but apparently not to cause the conformational change of the enzyme required for activation. These (Rp)-derivatives antagonize activation of cAMP-PK or cGMP-PK by cyclic nucleotides and activating analogues. We recently noted that a 30 min pre-incubation with 1 mM (Rp)-8-pCPT-cGMPS selectively inhibited the activation of platelet cGMP-PK by 0.2 mM 8-pCPT-cGMP (16). *Tables 3* and *4* summarize some properties of the available (Rp)-analogues of cAMP and cGMP. (Rp)-analogues, PKI, PKI-derived peptides, and many inhibitors of the H-series are commercially available (e.g. Sigma, Calbiochem, Biomol, Biolog).

4. Cyclic nucleotide-dependent protein phosphorylation

4.1 Measurement of protein phosphorylation

Platelet membranes of *Protocol 3*A contain high levels of endogeneous cGMP-PK and cAMP-PK and do not usually require the addition of cGMP-PK or C subunit of cAMP-PK to demonstrate the phosphorylation of cAMP-PK/cGMP-PK substrates.

Protocol 3. cAMP-PK- and cGMP-PK-mediated protein phosphorylation in platelet membranes

Equipment and reagents

- CCD buffer: 0.4 M Na citrate, 28 mM citric acid, 0.56 M glucose
- Membrane buffer: 113 mM NaCl, 4.3 mM KH_2PO_4, 4.3 mM Na_2HPO_4, 24.4 mM NaH_2PO_4, 5.5 mM glucose, 1.0 mM EDTA; adjust pH to 6.5
- Lysis buffer: 10 mM NaH_2PO_4, 2 mM EDTA, 2 mM EGTA, 1 mM fresh PMSF, 100 U/ml fresh aprotinin; adjust pH to 7.6
- Resuspension buffer: 20 mM NaH_2PO_4, 2 mM EDTA, 2 mM EGTA, 1 mM fresh PMSF, 100 U/ml aprotinin; adjust pH to 7.6
- Phosphorylation buffer: 100 mM Na–Hepes buffer, 50 mM $MgCl_2$, 10 mM dithioery-thriol (DTE), 2 mM EDTA; adjust to pH 7.6
- 20 μM cGMP or cAMP
- 40 μM [γ-^{32}P]ATP (22.000 c.p.m./pmol)
- PRP (see Chapter 1)

A. Preparation of platelet homogenate and membranes

Use plasticware throughout the entire preparation.

1. Collect blood or platelet concentrate into CCD anticoagulant (5 : 1, v/v) in 50 ml tubes.

2. Centrifuge at 300 *g* for 15–20 min at room temperature, and transfer supernatant (platelet-rich plasma) to a new 50 ml tube.

3. Centrifuge at 920 *g* for 20 min at room temperature, remove super-natant, and resuspend pellet in membrane buffer.

4. Centrifuge once more (920 *g*, 15 min) and discard supernatant.

5. Resuspend combined pellets in ice-cold lysis buffer to give 1×10^{10} cells/ml and store on ice for 10 min.

6. Freeze the lysed cells in liquid nitrogen. For analysis of PDE activity in platelet homogenate use the thawed homogenate.

7. Centrifuge the thawed cell homogenate at 100 000 *g* for 60 min at 4°C, remove the cytosol, and gently resuspend membranes in resuspen-sion buffer (40% of the starting volume). The membranes may be stored in aliquots at –80°C.

B. cAMP-/cGMP-dependent protein phosphorylation in platelet membranes

1. Pipette 2.5 μl of phosphorylation buffer, 2.5 μl of cGMP (or cAMP), and 2.5 μl of [γ-^{32}P]ATP into test-tube.

2. Adjust with H_2O to give a final volume of 25 μl after starting the re-action with platelet membranes.

3. Start the phosphorylation by adding 15 μg platelet membrane protein to the tube.

4. Incubate the sample 2.5 min at 30°C in a water-bath.

5. Stop the reaction by addition of a typical SDS-containing stop solution.

Protocol 3. *Continued*

6. Separate the proteins on a 9% SDS–PAGE.

7. Visualize the phosphorylated proteins by autoradiography.

Protocol 4. Analysis of cAMP-PK and cGMP-PK-mediated protein phosphorylation in intact human platelets

Equipment and reagents

- Citrate/EDTA buffer: 3.8% Na citrate, 30 mM EDTA pH 5.5
- Tyrode's buffer: 10 mM Hepes, 2.7 mM KCl, 137 mM NaCl, 5 mM glucose, 1 mM EDTA pH 7.4
- 2 mCi/ml [^{32}P]orthophosphate in HCl-free water (NEX 053, DuPont)
- 1 mM SNP or SIN-1
- 10 μM PGE$_1$
- SDS-containing stop solution[a]

A. Preparation of ^{32}P-labelled intact human platelets[b]

Use fresh plasticware throughout the entire preparation.

1. Collect 27 ml blood in 3 ml citrate/EDTA buffer.

2. Centrifuge at 300 *g* for 10 min at room temperature and transfer the supernatant (PRP) to a new tube.

3. Centrifuge at 400 *g* for 20 min at room temperature.

4. Discard supernatant and resuspend pellet in Tyrode's buffer to give 1×10^9 cells/ml (500 μl of this suspension are sufficient for ten assay points).

5. Incubate 500 μl of the platelet suspension with 500 μCi [^{32}P]orthophosphate for 1.5 h at 37°C.

6. Dilute the solution with 10 ml Tyrode's buffer, 1 mM EDTA and centrifuge at 300 *g* for 10 min at room temperature.

7. Discard radioactive supernatant and resuspend pellet in 500 μl Tyrode's buffer.

8. Leave for 15 min at room temperature before experiments are initiated. Platelets remain responsive for 1–2 h.

B. Activation of cAMP-PK or cGMP-PK in ^{32}P-labelled intact human platelets

1. Pipette 45 μl of the ^{32}P-labelled intact human platelet suspension (*Protocol 4*A) into a test-tube.

2. Start the reaction by adding 5 μl of the stimuli (e.g. SNP) (for more information see Sections 2, 3.1, and 3.2).

3. Stop the reaction by adding a typical SDS-containing stop solution.

4. Separate the proteins on a 9% SDS–PAGE.

5. Visualize the phosphorylated proteins by autoradiography (see *Figure 3*).

[a] See Chapter 9.
[b] A similar procedure using less radioactivity, is described in Chapter 9.

4.2 Substrates of cAMP- and cGMP-dependent protein kinase in human platelets

Activation of cAMP-PK in platelet extracts and intact human platelets leads to phosphorylation of several proteins with molecular masses of 22, 24, 50, 68, 130, and 240 kDa (*Figure 3*). Activation of cGMP-PK in platelet extracts and intact human platelets stimulates phosphorylation of a 46/50 kDa protein and occasionally proteins with molecular masses of 22 and 24 kDa. The identity and possible function of some of these proteins has been identified (2,4) (see *Table 5*).

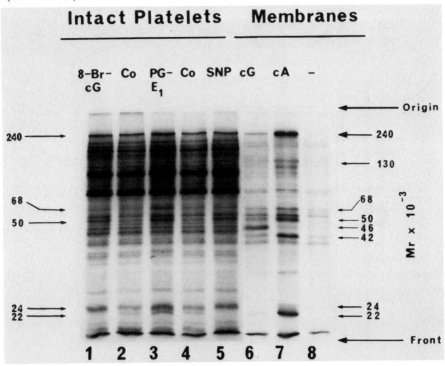

Figure 3. Protein phosphorylation in intact human platelets and platelet membranes. In intact human platelets, 100 μM SNP and 2 mM 8-Br-cGMP increased the phosphorylation of proteins with molecular weight (M_r) of 50 000 and 24 000, whereas 10 μM PGE$_1$ stimulated phosphorylation of proteins with M_r 240 000, 68 000, 50 000, 24 000, and 22 000. In platelet membranes, the phosphorylation of several proteins (e.g. proteins with M_r 240 000, 68 000, 50 000, 42 000, 24 000, and 22 000) was increased by 2 μM cAMP (cA). 2 μM cGMP (cG) stimulated the phosphorylation of proteins with M_r 50 000 and 46 000; (Co, control).

Table 5. Established substrates of cAMP- and cGMP-PK in human platelets

Protein kinase substrate	M_r (kDa in SDS gel)	Protein kinase	Phosphorylation	Phosphorylation site	Suggested effect of phosphorylation in platelets
Rap 1B	22	cAMP-PK (cGMP-PK)	In vitro and in vivo	Ser[179]	Possible regulation of PLC γ1
Glycoprotein 1b (GP1b)	24	cAMP-PK	In vitro and in vivo	Ser[166]	Inhibition of actin polymerization
Vasodilator stimulated phosphoprotein (VASP)	46	cAMP-PK cGMP-PK	In vitro and in vivo	Ser[157] Ser[239]	Inhibition of GPIIb/IIIa activation Inhibition of PLC activation and calcium mobilization
Caldesmon	82	cAMP-PK	In vitro and in vivo		Stabilization of the resting platelet cytoskeleton
Myosin light chain kinase (MLCK)	100	cAMP-PK cGMP-PK	In vitro	Ser	Not demonstrated in intact platelets
cGMP-inhibited phosphodiesterase (cGI-PDE)	110	cAMP-PK	In vitro and in vivo	Ser	Decrease of cAMP level
Actin-binding protein (ABP)	240	cAMP-PK	In vitro and in vivo	Ser	Inhibition of the cytoskeleton reorganization during activation

Many of these substrates can be detected by SDS–PAGE analysis and autoradiography in phosphorylation experiments (*Protocols 3* and *4*) with platelet membranes and intact human platelets (15,17,18). Some protein kinase substrates which are minor components of platelet proteins require more advanced detection methods. Such methods include 2D gels, immuno-precipitation, limited protease digestion, tryptic fingerprints, and microse-quencing (see ref. 19 as example). Protein phosphorylation in intact platelets can also be quantitatively analysed with antibodies which detect a phospho-rylation-induced change of the protein mobility in SDS–PAGE (7,18,19). The reader is also referred to the book *Protein phosphorylation: a practical approach*, published in this series. A full understanding of the functional role of cAMP-PK and cGMP-PK action in platelets requires identification of sub-strate proteins together with elucidation of the function and regulation by phosphorylation.

5. Analysis of activity and regulation of platelet cyclic nucleotide phosphodiesterases (cPDEs)

Hydrolysis of the 3′-phosphoester bond on cAMP and cGMP by phosphodi-esterases converts these second messengers to their inactive 5′-nucleotide metabolites. Different isozyme families of PDEs are known and exist in a wide variety of tissues and cell types. The predominant phosphodiesterase isozyme in human platelets is the cGI-PDE type III. This isozyme has a K_m for both cAMP and cGMP of about 0.4 µM and is inhibited by cGMP (IC$_{50}$ = 0.1 µM). Its activation is increased by a direct cAMP-PK catalysed phospho-rylation which increases the V_{max}. cGI-PDE represents more than 80% of the total high affinity cAMP phosphodiesterase activity and appears to mediate a negative feedback effect in platelet cAMP regulation. Selective inhibitors of cGI-PDE III have been demonstrated to inhibit platelet aggregation by increasing the concentration of cAMP. A cGMP-stimulated PDE type II (cGS-PDE), with similar properties to the well described enzyme from bovine adrenal gland, has been also demonstrated in platelets but appears to represent a minor PDE component. The cGB-PDE type V of human platelets is highly specific for cGMP (K_m of about 5 µM). Binding of cGMP to cGB-PDE allosterically affects the catalytic region and lowers the K_m for cGMP hydrolysis while leaving the V_{max} unchanged at 3–10 µmol/min/mg. The properties of the phosphodiesterases identified in human platelets are summarized in *Table 6*.

5.1 Assay for phosphodiesterase activity

Phosphodiesterase activities can be measured in human platelet homo-genates prepared as described in *Protocol 3A*. 80–90% of PDE activity is recovered in the cytosol. The presence of PDE isozymes can be probed with

Table 6. Some properties of cyclic nucleotide phosphodiesterases present in human platelets[a]

PDE isozyme	K_m (μM)	
	cAMP	cGMP
cGMP-stimulated PDE (type II)	36	11
cGMP-inhibited PDE (type III)	0.3	0.7
cGMP-specific PDE (type V)	150	5

[a] Quantitatively, PDEs type III and V are the most important cyclic nucleotide hydrolysing enzymes in human platelets. For further details see refs 22 and 24.

selective PDE inhibitors (see Section 5.2) using the assay described in *Protocol 5*. In addition, cyclic nucleotide hydrolysis can be measured using the standard radioligand assay (20) or non-radioactive phosphate release assay (21).

Protocol 5. Hydrolysis of cyclic nucleotides in platelet homogenate

Equipment and reagents
- Platelet homogenate, 1 x 10^{10} cells/ml (*Protocol 3*)
- 1 M Tris–HCl pH 7.6
- 0.1 M MgCl$_2$
- 10 mM cyclic nucleotides
- 3 mM guanine (standard)
- HPLC
- Eppendorf tubes (1.5 ml)

Method

1. To 10 μl of platelet homogenate in Eppendorf tubes add 5 μl of 1 M Tris–HCl pH 7.6, 10 μl of 0.1 mM MgCl$_2$, 65 μl of H$_2$O, and 10 μl of 10 mM cyclic nucleotide.
2. Incubate the sample at 30 °C in a water-bath.
3. Stop the incubation by heating for 10 min at 90 °C.[a]
4. Cool the sample and add 50 μl of 3 mM guanine (final concentration 1 mM) as internal standard for the HPLC analysis.
5. Pellet the homogenate at 6000 *g* for 2 min and collect the supernatant for direct HPLC analysis (see Section 2.3, *Table 2*, and *Figure 2*).[b]
6. For control experiments heat the sample 10 min at 90 °C before adding 10 μl 10 mM cyclic nucleotide. Continue at step 4.

[a] Under these conditions all tested cyclic nucleotides were stable.
[b] For the chromatograms shown in *Figure 2* we injected 10 μl of the supernatant.

Table 7. Selective inhibitors of specific phosphodiesterase isozymes present in human platelets[a]

Inhibitor	Phosphodiesterase isozyme family IC$_{50}$ (μM)			Commercial source
	II	III	V	
MEP-1	0.8	> 100	n.d.	– (see ref. 23)
Milrinone	150	0.3	110	Stirling Winthrop
Cilostamide	15	0.005	5.5	Biomol
Dipyridamol	8	40	0.9	Sigma, Biomol
Zaprinast	47	700	0.8	Sigma
Non-selective inhibitor				
IBMX	50	2	–	Sigma, Biomol

[a] For further details, see refs 22 and 24.

5.2 Phosphodiesterase inhibitors

A range of phosphodiesterase inhibitor agents of widely different chemical structures (mostly heterocyclic compounds) have been synthesized. Many of these compounds are used as cardiotonic and antithrombotic agents and as vasodilators (22). In *Table 7*, some properties of several commercially available PDE inhibitors are summarized. However, to date there are no PDE inhibitors which distinguish PDEs within a given PDE family.

Isobutylmethylxanthine (IBMX) appears to be relatively unspecific but is often useful to simultaneously inhibit the majority of phosphodiesterase activity in intact cells and cell extracts. The use of theophylline and caffeine as tools to examine the functional significance of PDE inhibition is limited because of their additional pharmacological activities including adenosine receptor antagonism and G_i protein inhibition. In our experiments with platelet homogenate (see *Protocol 3*), we used a final concentration of 10 μM dipyridamol as PDE V inhibitor, 50 μM milrinone as PDE III inhibitor, and 1 mM IBMX as unspecific inhibitor. For example, human platelet homogenate hydrolysed added cGMP to guanosine-5'-phosphate which was partially (> 50%) inhibited by 10 μM dipyridamol (*Figure 3*). With intact human platelets, inhibition of the cGI-PDE type III is observed with 10 μM milrinone, whereas inhibition of cGB-PDE type V requires 50 μM dipyridamole.

Acknowledgements

Our laboratory is supported by the Deutsche Forschungsgemeinschaft. The authors thank Dr M. Eigenthaler for constructive criticism and S. Ebert for the preparation of the manuscript, figures, and tables.

References

1. Stein, B., Fuster, V., Israel, D. H., Cohen, M., Badimon, L., Badimon, J. J., *et al.* (1989). *J. Am. Coll. Cardiol.*, **14,** 813.
2. Halbrügge, M. and Walter, U. (1993). In *Protein kinases in blood cell function* (ed. C.-K. Huang and R.I. Sha'afi), pp. 245–98. CRC Press, Boca Raton.
3. Eigenthaler, M., Nolte, C., Halbrügge, M., and Walter, U. (1992). *Eur. J. Biochem.*, **205,** 471.
4. Macphee, C. H., Reifsnyder, D. H., Moore, T. A., Lerea, K. M., and Beavo, J. A. (1988). *J. Biol. Chem.*, **263,** 10353.
5. Hamet, P., Coquil, J.-F., Bousseau-Lafortune, S., Franks, D. J., and Tremblay, J. (1984). *Adv. Cyclic Nucleotide Protein Phosphorylation Res.*, **16,** 119.
6. Butt, E. and Walter, U. (1994). In *The platelet* (ed. E. Lapetina). Advances in Molecular and Cell Biology (In press).
7. Halbrügge, M., Friedrich, C., Eigenthaler, M., Schanzenbächer, P., and Walter, U. (1990). *J. Biol. Chem.*, **265,** 3088.
8. Nolte, C., Eigenthaler, M., Schanzenbächer, P., and Walter, U. (1992). *Biochem. Pharmacol.*, **42,** 253.
9. Sandberg, M., Butt, E., Nolte, C., Fischer, L., Halbrügge, M., Beltmann, J., *et al.* (1991). *Biochem. J.*, **279,** 521.
10. Butt, E., Nolte, C., Schulz, S., Beltman, J., Beavo, J. A., Jastorff, B., *et al.* (1992). *Biochem. Pharmacol.*, **43,** 2591.
11. Connolly, B. J., Willits, P. B., Warrington, B. H., and Murray, K. J. (1992). *Biochem. Pharmacol.*, **44,** 2303.
12. Bowen, R. and Haslam, R. T. (1991). *J. Cardiovasc. Pharmacol.*, **17,** 424.
13. Kemp, B. E., Pearson, R. B., and House, C. M. (1991). In *Methods in enzymology* (ed. T. Hunter and B. M. Sefton), Vol. 201, pp. 287–304. Academic Press.
14. Hidaka, H. and Kobayashi, R. (1992). *Annu. Rev. Pharmacol. Toxicol.*, **32,** 377.
15. Waldmann, R., Bauer, S., Göbel, C., Hofmann, F., Jakobs, K. H., and Walter, U. (1986). *Eur. J. Biochem.*, **167,** 441.
16. Butt, E., Eigenthaler, M., and Genieser, H.-G. (1994). *Eur. J. Pharmacol.*, **269,** 265.
17. Waldmann, R., Nieberding, M., and Walter, U. (1987). *Eur. J. Biochem.*, **167,** 441.
18. Halbrügge, M. and Walter, U. (1989). *Eur. J. Biochem.*, **185,** 41.
19. Butt, E., Abel, K., Krieger, M., Palm, D., Hoppe, V., Hoppe, J., *et al.* (1994). *J. Biol. Chem.*, **269,** 14059.
20. Martins, T. J., Mumby, M. C., and Beavo, J. A. (1982). *J. Biol. Chem.*, **257,** 1973.
21. Gillespie, P. G. and Beavo, J. A. (1989). *Mol. Pharmacol.*, **36,** 773.
22. Nicholson, C. C., Challiss, R. A. J., and Shahid, M. (1991). *Trends Pharmacol. Sci.*, **12,** 19.
23. Podzuweit, T. and Müller, A. (1993). *Lancet*, **341,** 760.
24. Beavo, J. A. (1988). In *Advances in second messenger and phosphoprotein research* (ed. P. Greengard and G. A. Robinson), Vol. 22, pp. 1–38. Raven Press, New York.

Immunocytochemical and electron microscopic studies of platelets

SARA J. ISRAELS and JON M. GERRARD

1. Introduction

Although platelets were one of the first types of cells to be studied using the electron microscope, a clear understanding of normal platelet architecture using electron microscopy had to await improved techniques for the isolation, preservation, and fixation of these cells. Similarly, an understanding of the changes in blood platelet fine structure during clotting required improvements in preparative techniques. The preservation and fixation of certain platelet subcellular structures, notably dense granules and contractile filaments, have presented particular challenges. In this chapter, we describe basic fixation procedures for platelet transmission electron microscopy, and for immunofluorescent and immunoelectron microscopic studies, while providing a brief overview of some other aspects of platelet electron microscopic studies.

2. Basic electron microscopic studies

The cutting of ultrathin plastic sections for transmission electron microscopy is a skill best learned by example. Preparation of specimens, however, can be undertaken in most laboratories.

2.1 Fixation procedures

General fixation and staining procedures will be described followed by a modification for optimizing the preservation of specific ultrastructural features (*Figure 1*). For optimum preservation, platelets, either in plasma or physiological buffer, should be initially fixed in suspension at 37°C. Resting and stimulated platelets are treated in the same manner.

2.1.1 Fixation of platelets and resin embedding

Protocol 1. Fixation and embedding

Equipment and reagents

- White's solution A: dissolve 14 g NaCl (2.4 M), 0.75 g KCl (0.1 M), 0.55 g MgSO₄ (46 mM), 1.5 g Ca(NO₃)₂.4H₂O (64 mM) in 100 ml ddH₂O, and correct pH to 7.4—store at 4°C
- White's solution B: dissolve 1.1 g NaHCO₃ (0.13 M), 0.22 g Na₂HPO₄.7H₂O (8.4 mM), 0.05 g anhydrous KH₂PO₄ (3.8 mM), 0.01 g phenol red in 100 ml ddH₂O, and correct pH to 7.4—store at 4°C
- Glutaraldehyde (in White's saline): glutaraldehyde is used in a series of concentrations (see *Table 1*)—all concentrations > 1% should be made fresh before use
- 0.1% glutaraldehyde in White's saline (see *Table 1*)
- 3% glutaraldehyde in White's saline (see *Table 1*)
- Embedding resin (e.g. Epon/Araldite) (J. B. EM Services)
- 1% osmium tetroxide (in 1.5% potassium ferricyanide) (J. B. EM Services): mix 7.0 ml ddH₂O, 0.5 ml of 0.1 M CaCl₂ (5 mM), 0.15 g potassium ferricyanide, add 2.5 ml of 4% OsO₄—store at 4°C
- 3% aqueous uranyl acetate (J. B. EM Services): powder is dissolved in ddH₂O to appropriate concentration (it should be made fresh and kept from light)
- Ethanol (absolute)
- Propylene oxide (J. B. EM Services)
- ddH₂O
- Microcentrifuge tubes (Eppendorf)
- Bench-top microcentrifuge (Baxter)
- Magnetic stir plate
- Wooden applicator sticks
- Vacuum oven (60°C)
- Gelatin capsules or preformed embedding moulds (J. B. EM Services)

A. Fixation and dehydration

1. Fix platelets in suspension, in microcentrifuge tubes, by adding an equal volume of 0.1% glutaraldehyde in White's saline. Leave for at least 15 min at 37°C.

2. Spin to pellet platelets (15000 *g*) for 5 min at 25°C in a bench-top microcentrifuge.

3. Replace 0.1% glutaraldehyde with 3% glutaraldehyde, leave to fix for 1–2 h (platelets can be held in 3% glutaraldehyde for up to 24 h).

4. Replace 3% glutaraldehyde with 1% osmium tetroxide solution for 90 min at 4°C.

5. Remove osmium tetroxide and wash twice by gently breaking pellet using a wooden applicator in ddH₂O and re-pelleting.

6. For *en bloc* staining, remove ddH₂O and incubate pellet in 3% aqueous uranyl acetate for a minimum of 1 h at 4°C. Platelets can be left in this solution overnight.

7. Wash twice in ddH₂O (see step 5).

8. Remove ddH₂O and dehydrate in 50% ethanol for 15 min.

9. Remove 50% ethanol and dehydrate in 70% ethanol for 15 min.

10. Remove 70% ethanol and dehydrate in 90% ethanol for 15 min.

11. Remove 90% ethanol and dehydrate in two changes of 100% ethanol, each for 15 min.

12. Remove 100% ethanol and replace with two changes of propylene oxide, each for 5 min.

B. Embedding

1. Mix Epon/Araldite resin mixture as follows:

- Araldite   10 ml
- Epon 812   12.5 ml
- Hardener DDSA   30 ml
- Accelerator (DMP 30)   1 ml

Mix at slow speed using a magnetic stir plate for 20 min. Avoid introducing air bubbles. It may be used at once or drawn into syringes and stored at −20 °C for future use.

2. Replace propylene oxide (see part A, step 12) with 1 : 1 mixture of propylene oxide and resin. Leave for 1 h.

3. Replace mixture of propylene oxide and resin with complete resin and leave for 4 h.

4. To embed platelets in fresh resin, fill gelatin capsules or moulds with resin. Use a wooden applicator stick to transfer the pellet to the top of the resin and allow it to sink.

5. Polymerize the samples by incubating overnight at 60 °C in vacuum oven.

6. Once polymerized, sections are cut using an ultramicrotome. Sections should be 80–100 nm in thickness and mounted on copper grids.

Table 1. Glutaraldehyde in White's saline[a]

	Final concentration of glutaraldehyde				
	0.1%	1%	2%	3%	6%
White's solution A (ml)	0.5	0.25	0.25	0.25	0.25
White's solution B (ml)	0.5	0.25	0.25	0.25	0.25
Glutaraldehyde (25%) (ml)	0.04	0.20	0.40	0.60	1.20
ddH$_2$O (ml)	8.96	4.30	4.10	3.90	3.30
Total volume (ml)	10.0	5.0	5.0	5.0	5.0

[a] Correct pH to 7.4 (determined by phenol red indicator in White's saline).

2.1.2 Staining thin sections for electron microscopy (EM)

Staining of ultrathin EM sections improves contrast by increasing the electron density of the specimens. This is done by depositing heavy metals into or on to the tissue. Commonly used stains are salts of lead (lead citrate) and uranium (uranyl acetate), although other metal salts such as potassium permanganate or phosphotungstic acid can also be used. Double staining with a combination of uranyl acetate and lead citrate provides excellent contrast.

For all staining procedures use fresh double distilled water and keep all surfaces clean. Both lead and uranyl salts must be handled with appropriate precautions.

Protocol 2. Staining of thin sections

Equipment and reagents

- Uranyl acetate (J. B. EM Services): 50% solution in ethanol
- Ethanol
- No. 1 filter paper (Whatman)
- Lead citrate (J. B. EM Services)
- Sodium hydroxide pellets
- ddH$_2$O
- Petri dish
- Dental wax

A. Staining with uranyl acetate

This stain can be omitted if tissue has already been stained *en bloc* with uranyl acetate (see *Protocol 1*).

1. Make up a small volume of a saturated solution of uranyl acetate in 50% ethanol. Filter solution through a No. 1 filter paper into a clean tube. Wrap tube in foil to protect from light. This must be made fresh before use.

2. Place a drop of saturated uranyl acetate on to a piece of Parafilm and place the grid, section side down, on top of drop of uranyl acetate.

3. Cover with a box and leave in the dark for 10 min.

4. Wash the grid in several changes of ddH$_2$O, and touch grid with piece of filter paper to draw off excess moisture. Allow to dry.

B. Staining with lead citrate

1. Make up lead citrate as follows: mix 0.03 g lead citrate, 100 µl of 10 M NaOH, 10 ml ddH$_2$O, and shake to dissolve. Let sit for 5 min. Shake again and centrifuge at 2700 *g* for 10 min. Use only the top half of the solution.

2. Place sodium hydroxide pellets in the middle of a Petri dish filled with dental wax.

3. Place drops of lead citrate around the pellets.

---

4. Place the grid on drop of stain with the section side down, cover immediately with lid (avoid breathing on the lead citrate drops as this will cause stain deposit on the sections), and stain for 10 min.

5. Wash grids well with several changes of ddH$_2$O and blot dry on a piece of filter paper.

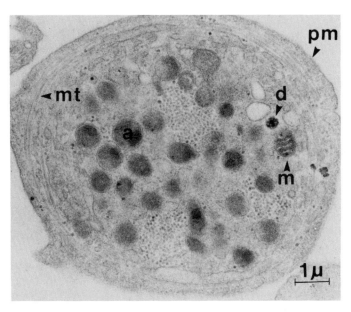

Figure 1. Resting platelet fixed in glutaraldehyde and osmium tetroxide and embedded in Epon/Araldite. Ultrastructural features include: plasma membrane (pm), microtubules (mt), alpha granules (a), dense granules (d), mitochondria (m).

2.1.3 Evaluation of dense granules

Dense granules contain 5-HT (serotonin), ATP, ADP, calcium, and pyrophosphate. The black appearance of rabbit dense granules is due to the presence of high concentrations of 5-HT which stains black when treated with glutaraldehyde and osmium (1). In contrast, human dense granules are inherently electron dense as a result of a high calcium content. The high concentration of calcium in the buffers used in *Protocol 1* gives optimum dense granule fixation in human platelets.

Rapid examination of platelet dense granules can be performed on platelet whole mounts. This is useful for assessing dense granule numbers, the normal range being four to eight per platelet (2,3).

Protocol 3. Preparation of platelet whole mounts

Equipment and reagents
- Formvar coated EM grids (see *Protocol 9*)
- Platelet-rich plasma
- 0.1% glutaraldehyde (see *Table 1*)
- ddH$_2$O
- Filter paper

Method

1. Place one drop of ddH$_2$O on a Formvar coated grid.

2. Place small amount (5–20 μl) of platelet-rich plasma on to water drop.

3. Let stand for 1 min to allow platelets to settle on to grid. Blot off with piece of filter paper.

4. Place grid in 0.1% glutaraldehyde in White's saline for 1 min.

5. Pass grid through ddH$_2$O and blot off by touching the edge of the grid with filter paper. Repeat.

6. Air dry.

2.1.4 Visualization of platelet membranes

The use of osmium ferricyanide described above (*Protocol 1*) enhances the preservation and appearance of platelet membranes. Various cytochemical approaches have been used to probe platelet structure and function.

(a) Surface connected canalicular system. Thorium dioxide and horse-radish peroxidase have been added in the external platelet milieu to enable the electron microscopic detection of the surface connected canalicular system (4,5). Such studies aid visualization of the pathway of platelet secretion.

(b) Dense tubular system. The dense tubular system can be visualized cytochemically using stains for endogenous peroxidase, or for glucose 6-phosphatase, such as a diaminobenzidine solution, which will distinguish the dense tubular system from other intracellular membrane systems (6).

(c) Platelet lysosomes. Stains for acid phosphatase and aryl sulfatase have been used to identify platelet lysosomes (7).

2.1.5 Visualization of platelet contractile proteins

A potential problem in using osmium tetroxide fixation, is damage to actin filaments. Such damage can be limited by the addition of lysine to the glutaraldehyde fixative (8,9). Full visualization of the actin filaments in platelets often requires additional steps such as the lysis of detergent soluble components using Triton X-100. The addition of detergent and fixative simultaneously appears optimum for visualization of platelet actin filaments (10).

2.2 Studies of platelet function using the electron microscope

Electron microscopy can be a powerful tool in the elucidation of platelet function when used appropriately.

2.2.1 Platelet adherence

Platelet adherence to an injured vessel wall can be studied using:

(a) Perfusion–fixation following an *in vivo* vessel injury (10).

(b) An everted vessel in which the endothelium has been removed and platelets perfused over the injured vessel (11,12).

2.2.2 Platelet granule centralization (internal contraction)

Platelets stimulated by a variety of agonists will undergo a change in shape and a calcium-mediated internal contraction in which the granules are moved toward the centre of single cells or toward the centre of a platelet clump (13). Optimum visualization of this process in single platelets requires the use of conditions in which most cells will remain single, either avoiding stirring, or employing inhibitors (e.g. RGD peptides) to block platelet–platelet attachment.

2.2.3 Granule labilization (membrane fusion)

During the process of platelet secretion the membranes of platelet granules fuse with each other, with the membranes of the surface connected canalicular system, and with the plasma membrane. Under conditions where internal contraction occurs, this process is difficult to follow because the morphological changes associated with the contraction (the centralization of the granules) masks the process of granule fusion. The use of conditions which allow selective activation of protein kinase C in platelets (for example using phorbol myristate acetate or oleoyl-acetylglycerol) without significantly increasing intracellular calcium provides for the visualization of granule membrane fusion (14).

2.2.4 Clot contraction

The association of platelets and fibrin strands within a clot can be studied by producing an isometrically contracted clot that results in linear alignment of fibrin strands and platelet pseudopods (15).

Protocol 4. Preparation of a platelet/fibrin clot

Equipment and reagents

- Tyrode buffer (10 ×): dissolve 160 g NaCl (2.7 M), 4 g KCl (54 mM), 20 g NaHCO$_3$ (238 mM), 8.2 g MgCl$_2$.6H$_2$O (40 mM), 1.3 g NaH$_2$PO$_4$ (9 mM) in 1 litre ddH$_2$O; store at 4°C—before use dilute to 1 x with ddH$_2$O, add 1 mg glucose/ml buffer, 1 mg BSA/ml buffer, and correct pH to 7.4
- Siliconized, open ended glass tubes (0.6 cm internal diameter)
- Tissue bath
- Tissue clamps
- Glutaraldehyde in White's saline (see *Table 1*)
- Thrombin
- Platelet-rich plasma
- Petri dishes
- Parafilm
- Thread

Method

1. Pour Tyrode buffer into Petri dishes, place on ice, and allow to cool.

2. Cover one end of the siliconized glass tube with Parafilm, add 1 U thrombin, then 1 ml of platelet-rich plasma to the glass tube. Cover with Parafilm, invert twice, and let stand for 10 min.

3. Remove Parafilm covers from the glass tube and shake the platelet/fibrin clot into the chilled Tyrode buffer.

4. Tie clot to tissue clamps and suspend in bath filled with chilled Tyrode buffer. Replace with 37°C Tyrode buffer under enough tension to straighten clot. The clot is allowed to contract (30–60 min).

5. Remove the buffer and replace with equal volumes of Tyrode buffer and 2% glutaraldehyde in White's saline. After 5 min replace with equal volumes of Tyrode buffer and 6% glutaraldehyde in White's saline. Fix clot for 30 min at 37°C.

6. Remove the clot, cut into smaller fragments, and fix for an additional 30 min in 3% glutaraldehyde in White's saline.

7. Transfer fragments to 1% osmium tetroxide in 1.5% potassium ferricyanide (see *Protocol 1*) for 90 min at 4°C.

8. Dehydrate in a graded series of ethanol concentrations (see *Protocol 1*).

9. Fragments are embedded for cutting by orientation along the direction of tension (longitudinal) or across the direction of tension (cross-section).

3. Immunofluorescent studies

Immuno- and affinity probes can be utilized for ultrastructural localization of surface receptors, membrane proteins, or the contents of organelles. Following activation, movement or redistribution of receptors, reorientation of components of the cytoskeleton, or secretion of granule contents can be followed microscopically. The relationship of two different molecules can be determined by double labelling procedures.

Platelets can be labelled in suspension and then placed on glass slides for viewing. Labelling of intact platelets will determine whether the antigen of interest is present on the platelet plasma membrane. Initial permeabilization of platelets before labelling will allow identification of intracellular antigens. Examination of platelets following activation can provide information regarding redistribution of antigens on or to the plasma membrane, or changes in the availability of antigens for the binding of probes. However, the small size of platelets and the limits of resolution of conventional light-based imaging procedures permits only general localization of molecules of interest. Ultrastructural localization requires use of electron microscopy.

3.1 Preparation of platelets for immunofluorescence studies

Protocol 5. Fixation of platelets for immunofluorescence studies

Equipment and reagents

- NH$_4$Cl/Tris-buffered saline (TBS): dissolve 3.6 g Tris (34 mM) and 8.0 g NaCl (120 mM) in 1 litre of ddH$_2$O and pH to 7.4 with HCl; add 26.7 g NH$_4$Cl (500 mM) and pH to 7.4
- Washed platelets
- Microcentrifuge

- 2% paraformaldehyde (PFA)/0.2% glutaraldehyde (GA) in cacodylate buffer (0.2 M): dissolve 0.428 g cacodylate [(CH$_3$)$_2$AsO$_2$ Na.3H$_2$O] in 7.25 ml ddH$_2$O; add 2.5 ml of 8% PFA and 0.25 ml of 8% GA
- Microcentrifuge tubes (Eppendorf)

Method

1. Add an equal volume of 2% PFA/0.2% GA in cacodylate to washed platelets. Fix for 1 h at room temperature.

2. Pellet platelets in microcentrifuge tubes for 5 min (25 °C).

3. Wash three times with TBS.

4. Wash three times with 0.1% bovine serum albumin (BSA) in TBS.

5. Resuspend pellet in 0.1% BSA in TBS in a microcentrifuge tube.

3.1.1 Permeabilization

If internalized proteins are to be detected, the cells must be permeabilized. A 0.1% Triton X-100 solution can be used as follows:

(a) Add a few drops of 0.1% Triton X-100 to a platelet pellet and resuspend.

(b) At 3 min stop the reaction by filling the microcentrifuge tube with TBS.

(c) Centrifuge the sample and wash the pellet three times with 0.1% BSA in TBS.

Saponin can also be used to permeabilize cells already settled on microscope slides (16).

3.2 Immunofluorescent labelling

Labelling may be performed with fluorochrome-conjugated antibody or as described below (*Protocol 6*) by using biotinylated antibody and fluorochrome-labelled avidin.

Protocol 6. Immunofluorescent labelling

Equipment and reagents

- Washed platelets
- Tris-buffered saline (TBS) (see *Protocol 5*)
- Bovine serum albumin (BSA)
- Primary antibody
- Biotinylated secondary antibody (Hyclone Lab)
- Fluorescein (FITC)/avidin (Vector Labs Inc.)
- Rhodamine (TRITC)/avidin (Vector Labs Inc.)
- Glycerol
- Microcentrifuge
- Microcentrifuge tubes (Eppendorf)
- Glass slides and coverslips

Method

1. Centrifuge platelets in microcentrifuge tubes to form a pellet and add primary antibody diluted in TBS.[a] Resuspend the pellet and incubate at room temperature for 30 min.

2. Wash three times with 0.1% BSA in TBS.

3. Pellet platelets and add biotinylated secondary antibody. Resuspend the pellet and incubate at room temperature for 30 min. The secondary antibody should be a biotin-conjugated antibody raised against the species of the primary antibody.

4. Wash three times with 0.1% BSA in TBS.

5. Add FITC/avidin diluted 1 : 3000 in TBS. Resuspend the pellet and incubate in darkness for 30 min at room temperature.

6. Wash three times with 0.1% BSA in TBS.[b]

7. Wash three times with TBS.

8. Resuspend in 10% glycerol in TBS.

9. Place aliquot on a glass slide, cover with a coverslip, and let platelets settle in darkness for 30 min before examination.

[a] A good starting point for dilution is 10 μg/ml but it will vary with each antibody.
[b] If localization experiments are to be done on two different proteins, a second primary antibody from a different host species can be added at this point. Different fluorochromes must be used for detection. Rhodamine (TRITC) is a good second label.

3.3 Immunofluorescence microscopy

Using a fluorescence microscope, fluorochrome-labelled antibodies can be excited with blue (for FITC) or green (for TRITC) radiation (filtered visible light) and re-emitted as green and red fluorescence respectively.

Since low level fluorescence does not last long, permanent photographic recordings are essential. This can be accomplished through the use of high speed (400 ASA or more) colour slide or black and white print film and the use of longer exposure times.

(a) Exposure times for the detection of punctate FITC-labelled platelets are usually in the range of 30 sec, while TRITC requires a 60 sec exposure time.

(b) Because the film is over-exposed the photographic paper must also be over-exposed during printing to achieve the original black background.

4. Immunoelectron microscopy studies

The availability of immuno- and high-affinity probes for electron microscopy allows identification and specific localization of a wide variety of molecules. This discussion will be limited to the use of colloidal gold probes and transmission EM, although elegant scanning EM and high voltage EM studies have also been carried out on platelets (17).

The basic approach is to stabilize the cells to preserve both antigenicity and ultrastructure followed by incubation with a probe (usually an antibody) and visualization using colloidal gold conjugates. Labelling may occur before or after the cells are embedded and sectioned.

(a) *Pre-embedding technique.* Immunoreagents are allowed to penetrate the partially fixed specimen allowing a three-dimensional distribution of the probe. This technique is most suitable for surface labelling as permeability of most probes is limited by the plasma membrane. Permeabilization techniques (as described in Section 3.1.1) can be used here but may disrupt ultrastructure and distribution of the antigen of interest. Following labelling, the tissue can be further fixed and processed as a conventional electron microscopy specimen (18) (*Protocols 1* and *2*).

(b) *Post-embedding technique.* The antibody is applied after processing and sectioning. The method of tissue preservation is, therefore, extremely important as it must provide maintenance of both ultrastructure and antigenicity. The following sections will discuss fixation and preparation of samples for post-embedding labelling.

4.1 Fixation of samples for immunoelectron microscopy

Fixation agents that are useful for preserving tissue for immunoelectron microscopy are:

- 8% paraformaldehyde
- 2% paraformaldehyde/0.2% glutaraldehyde
- 2% glutaraldehyde

8% paraformaldehyde is the best fixative for the preservation of antigenicity, but at the price of ultrastructural preservation.

Protocol 7. Fixation of platelets for immunoelectron microscopy

Equipment and reagents

- Phosphate-buffered saline (PBS): mix (1 : 4, v/v) Na_2HPO_4 (1.0 M) and NaH_2PO_4 (1.0 M) and pH to 7.4; store at 4°C
- Tyrode buffer (see *Protocol 4*)
- Washed platelets
- Paraformaldehyde and/or glutaraldehyde
- Microcentrifuge
- Microcentrifuge tubes (Eppendorf)

Method

1. Add an equal volume of fixative to platelets suspended in Tyrode buffer and let stand for 1 h at room temperature.
2. Pellet platelets and resuspend in fixative for 1 h.
3. Pellet platelets, wash three times with 0.1% BSA/0.1 M PBS.

Platelets are now ready to be labelled if pre-embedding techniques are going to be used, or to be embedded in immunocompatible resin.

4.2 Embedding in immunocompatible resins

A variety of resins formulated for immunocytochemical techniques are available. The important factors in choosing an embedding resin include: polarity, which preserves the orientation of tissue components, and hydrophilia, which determines the absorption of aqueous stains. Some examples of immunocompatible resins are: LR White (J. B. EM Services, London Resin Co.); the lowicryl resins (Polysciences); low acid glycolmethacrylate (SPI Supplies). A comparison of the resin specifications can be found in Bendayan *et al.* (19) and Stirling (18). The specific protocol for embedding and polymerization will depend on the resin chosen and detailed instructions are provided by the manufacturers.

4.3 Cryofixation

Cryofixation is an alternative to chemical preservation. This technique freezes cells or tissue rapidly while preventing ice crystal formation. The preparation of frozen cells is relatively easy and provides excellent preservation of epitopes. Frozen sections compare favourably for labelling efficiency with most of the available resins (19) but some ultrastructural details are often lost (*Figure 2*). A drawback is the expense of cryoultramicrotomy equipment for thin sectioning of the frozen tissue.

Protocol 8.   Preparation and storage of frozen cells

Equipment and reagents

- Microcentrifuge
- Magnetic stir plate
- Dissecting microscope
- Microscalpels (No. 7546 microunitome 45°, 3 mm) (Ingram and Bell Scientific)
- EM tweezers
- Parafilm
- Mounting pins for ultramicrotome
- Cryovials (Nalgene)

- Liquid nitrogen
- Washed fixed platelets (see *Protocol 7*)
- Paraformaldehyde (PF)
- Phosphate-buffered saline (PBS) (see *Protocol 7*)
- Na_2CO_3
- Poly(vinylpyrrolidone) (PVP) (Sigma)
- Sucrose

A. Preparation of cryoprotectant (20% PVP/1.84 M sucrose) (20)

1. Pour 80 ml of 2.3 M sucrose (in 0.1 M PBS) into 200 ml beaker. Add 4 ml of 1.1 M Na_2CO_3 and mix well.

2. Add 20 g of PVP. This will form a viscous solution. Cover with Parafilm and place on magnetic stirrer overnight.

3. The solution should become clear. Bring volume to 100 ml with 0.1 M PBS.[a]

B. Preparation of platelets for cryosectioning

1. Centrifuge fixed platelets in microcentrifuge tubes to form a pellet. Remove the supernatant and add 8% PF for 4 h at room temperature or overnight at 4°C.

2. Remove fixative. Cut the tip of the microcentrifuge tube and gently remove the pellet (it will have the consistency of tissue) into a Petri dish containing 0.1 M PBS.

3. Trim pellet into small blocks ($\approx$ 0.3 mm in diameter) in preparation for cryosectioning. This can be accomplished with the use of microscalpels and the aid of a dissecting microscope.

4. To prevent ice crystal damage immerse blocks in 20% PVP/1.84 M sucrose for approx. 4 h at room temperature. Infusion is complete when the blocks settle to the bottom of the microcentrifuge tube containing the PVP/sucrose mixture. In order start the infusion process, the tube should be shaken.

5. Mount the blocks on copper or aluminium mounting pins. The pins must be clean (with 70% ethanol), dry, and placed into a holder (a small piece of styrofoam will do). Under a dissecting microscope, retrieve a block from the cryoprotectant with fine EM tweezers and

---

Protocol 8. *Continued*

place on the top of the pin. Excess PVP/sucrose must be removed using the capillary action of the tweezers. There should only be a small well of cryoprotectant at the base to freeze the block to the pin. This must be done quickly because the molarity of the sucrose and the percentage of PVP rise rapidly which will hinder sectioning.

6. The sample is frozen by submerging the pin in liquid nitrogen. Samples are stored in capped cryovials in liquid nitrogen and sectioning may be completed at a later date.

a Variation in optimum cutting temperature may occur with each batch of PVP.

4.4 Cryoultramicrotomy

Cryoultramicrotomy is an art that is best learned by example. Companies that supply cryosectioning devices also provide seminars in methodology (Reichert-Jung, RMC). Detailed instructions are beyond the scope of this chapter (21). Grid preparation is, however, one important factor in maintaining the cryosection.

4.4.1 Preparation of coated grids

In order to support cryosections grids must be coated with Formvar and carbon. The metal surface is etched to allow adherence of the Formvar coating.

Protocol 9. Preparation of coated grids

Equipment and reagents

- Copper EM grids (J. B. EM Services)
- Glass slides
- ddH$_2$O
- HCl
- Formvar (J. B. EM Services)
- Acetone
- Dental wax
- Evaporator for carbon coating

Method

1. Place the copper grids in a beaker containing 30 ml ddH$_2$O and add a few drops of HCl. Pour off H$_2$O, add a few millilitres of acetone, remove the grids on to filter paper, and allow the grids to dry.

2. Dip clean glass slides into the Formvar solution (0.3% in ethylene dichloride) and allow to air dry. Scrape the sides of the slide and float the layer of dried Formvar off the slide and on to the water surface in a shallow tray.

3. Using tweezers, place dried grids on top of the floating Formvar. The grid/Formvar complex is picked up by slowly adhering dental wax to the free surface of the grids. The coated grids are allowed to dry.

4. A thin film of carbon is added to ionize the Formvar coat. Formvar alone is too hydrophobic to allow the cryosection to spread evenly. Settings for the evaporator should be approximately 100 millitorr with the filament adjusted to 60 KV for 60 sec.

4.5 Immunolabelling

The success of any immunolabelling technique depends on the primary antibody. Monoclonal antibodies have the advantage of being most specific. Polyclonal antibodies bind to more than one epitope and, therefore, usually give a higher density of labelling, but may also produce higher background.

4.5.1 Colloidal gold and conjugates

Colloidal gold is the particulate probe most often used for visualization because it is highly electron opaque and can be produced in a range of sizes (1–500 nm). 5–20 nm particles are the most useful for EM. Colloidal gold is produced by the reduction of tetrachloroauric acid and the size of the particles can be determined by the amount or type of reducing agent. Commercial colloidal gold conjugates are available (Janssen Pharmaceutica, UBI). A description of the preparation of colloidal gold, including sizing techniques can be found in Albrecht *et al.* (17). A wide range of substances will coat gold particles, therefore available probes include: staphylococcal protein A, streptococcal protein G, immunoglobulin, avidin, biotin, lectins, toxins, and enzymes.

(a) Proteins A and G bind with high affinity to the Fc portion of immunoglobulin and do not affect antigen–antibody binding. Reactivity with the primary antibody depends on species, immunoglobulin class, and subclass. Protein A has high affinity for rabbit, pig, and human IgG, but binds poorly to rat and mouse IgG, making it unsuitable for detection of monoclonal antibodies. Protein G–gold was introduced in the late 1980s and may have improved binding to mouse IgG as compared to protein A but its affinity may be dependent on its preparation (18).

(b) Immunoglobulins can be absorbed directly on to colloidal gold without loss of activity. It is possible to conjugate gold directly to the primary antibody, or to a secondary antibody to label a primary antibody (e.g. goat anti-mouse IgG–gold to label a primary mouse monoclonal antibody). IgG–gold may have a higher labelling density than protein A–gold but does have a tendency to cluster which may influence interpretation of distribution (22).

(c) Avidin and biotin form one of the strongest non-covalent bonds known. This reaction can be used in a multi-step approach with biotinylated antibody followed by avidin or streptavidin–gold. This multi-step approach produces amplification of labelling.

4.5.2 Non-specific binding

Background staining occurs as a result of non-specific binding of antibodies or gold probes. Strategies to decrease background include:

- reducing concentration of antibody and increasing incubation time
- pre-incubation with ovalbumin or immunoglobulin-free BSA (0.1–2.0%) or fish skin gelatin
- pre-treatment with dried or defatted milk
- Tween 20 (polyoxyethylene sorbitan monolaurate) (Sigma) prevents non-specific binding of gold probes
- the use of these agents is empirical and may be effective in combination depending on the antibody or gold conjugate being used

4.5.3 Immunogold labelling

All staining procedures are completed on a surface of Parafilm. Grids being stained with the same antibodies may be pooled, however 10 μl of diluted antibody is needed for each grid. During the staining steps a moist chamber should be set-up (a clear plastic cover enclosing the puddles) to prevent evaporation. Staining times vary with each antibody used, anywhere from ten minutes to a few hours at room temperature or even overnight at 4 °C.

For *Protocol 10*, immunogold labelling using a primary antibody and pro-

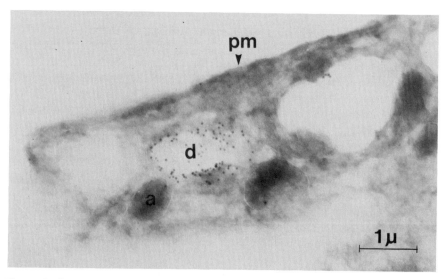

Figure 2. Cryosection of platelet showing immunogold labelling of a dense granule membrane protein. Dense granules lose their inherent density on cryopreservation. Primary antibody is visualized using protein A–gold (9 nm). Dense granule (d), alpha granule (a), plasma membrane (pm).

tein A–gold has been used as an example, but the method can be adapted to other colloidal gold conjugates.

Protocol 10. Immunolabelling with primary antibody and protein A–gold

Equipment and reagents

- Microcentrifuge
- Parafilm
- Anticapillary tweezers
- Filter paper (Whatman No. 50, hardened, ashless)
- 0.1 M PBS (see *Protocol 7*)
- 1% BSA in 0.1 M PBS
- 0.1% BSA in 0.1 M PBS
- 0.3% uranyl acetate (UA) in 2% poly(vinyl alcohol) (PVA) (10 000 M_r) (Sigma)
- Diluted antibodies and protein A–gold (all dilutions must be spun in a microcentrifuge for 5 min prior to use to remove IgG aggregates)

Method

1. Place grids, section down, on to puddles of 1% BSA in 0.1 M PBS for 15 min (to decrease non-specific binding). Wash grids three times in PBS (3 min each).

2. Place grids on a puddle of primary antibody appropriately diluted (in 0.1% BSA/TBS). Incubate grids for 30 min.

3. Wash grids five times in PBS (3 min each).

4. Place grids on a puddle of appropriately diluted protein A–gold (in 0.1% BSA/TBS). Incubate 30 min.

5. Wash grids five times in PBS (3 min each). Transfer grids through five puddles of ddH$_2$O (3 min each).

6. After all rinses, the sections must be counterstained with UA and embedded in PVA (20). Transfer the grids from ddH$_2$O to the UA/PVA and leave for 10 min.[a] Pick grids up with anticapillary tweezers and withdraw the excess mixture with filter paper.

[a] The PVA protects the sections from drying artefact. The final embedding mixture of UA and PVA must be made immediately before the embedding step.

4.5.4 Double labelling

Double labelling can detect two antigens simultaneously providing that the visualization markers are distinguishable and do not cross-react with both primary antibodies. The markers are usually gold particles of different sizes (e.g. 5 nm and 15 nm) that can be distinguished on electron micrographs. Resin embedded sections on uncoated grids may have each side of the section labelled separately with carbon coating of the first labelled face to protect it from contamination during labelling of the second side with a different antibody (23). If protein A–gold conjugates are being used as the markers, the second probe may contaminate still available sites on the first primary antibody. This may be prevented by saturating Fc sites on the first antibody with unconjugated protein A before labelling with the second primary antibody. IgG–gold conjugates may be a better choice for same face double labelling because they can be specific for primary antibodies of different species. An alternative is to have the primary antibodies directly conjugated to gold.

Acknowledgements

The authors wish to thank Ms E. McMillan and Ms C. Robertson for technical advice, and Ms B. Janz for preparation of the manuscript.

References

1. Gerrard, J. M., Rao, G. H. R., and White, J. G. (1977). *Am. J. Pathol.*, **87,** 633.
2. White, J. G. (1969). *Blood*, **33,** 598.
3. Witkop, C. J., Krumwiede, M., Sedano, H., and White, J. G. (1987). *Am. J. Hematol.*, **26,** 305.
4. White, J. G. (1973). *Ser. Haematol.*, **6,** 429.
5. White, J. G. (1974). *Prog. Hemostasis Thromb.*, **2,** 49.
6. Ebbeling, L., Robertson, C., McNicol, A., and Gerrard, J. M. (1992). *Blood*, **80,** 718.
7. Bentfield, M. E. and Bainton, D. F. (1975). *J. Clin. Invest.*, **56,** 1635.
8. Boyles, J., Anderson, L., and Hutcherson, P. (1985). *J. Histochem. Cytochem.*, **33,** 1116.
9. Boyles, J. K., Fox, J. E. B., Phillips, D. R., and Stenberg, P. (1985). *J. Cell Biol.*, **101,** 1463.
10. Baumgartner, H. R. (1973). *Microvasc. Res.*, **5,** 167.
11. Turitto, V. and Baumgartner, H. R. (1974). *Thromb. Diath. Haemorrh.*, **60,** 17.
12. Baumgartner, H. R. and Muggli, R. (1976). In *Platelets in biology and pathology* (ed. J. L. Gordon), pp. 23–60. Elsevier Science Publisher, Amsterdam.
13. Gerrard, J. M., Schollmeyer, J. V., Phillips, D. R., and White, J. G. (1979). *Am. J. Pathol.*, **94,** 509.
14. Friesen, L. L. and Gerrard, J. M. (1985). *Am. J. Pathol.*, **121,** 79.
15. Cohen, I., Gerrard, J. M., and White, J. G. (1982). *J. Cell Biol.*, **93,** 775.
16. Hattori, R., Hamilton, K. K., Fugate, R. D., McEver, R. P., and Sims, P. J. (1989). *J. Biol. Chem.*, **264,** 7768.
17. Albrecht, R. M., Olorundare, O. E., Simmons, S. R., Loftus, J. C., and Mosher, D. E. (1992). In *Methods in enzymology* (ed. J. J. Hawiger), Vol. 215, pp. 456–80. Academic Press, San Diego.
18. Stirling, J. W. (1990). *J. Histochem. Cytochem.*, **38,** 145.
19. Bendayan, M., Nanci, A., and Kan, F. W. K. (1987). *J. Histochem. Cytochem.*, **35,** 983.
20. Tokayasu, K. T. (1989). *Histochem. J.*, **21,** 163.

21. Griffiths, G., McDowall, A., Back, R., and Dubochet, J. (1984). *J. Ultrastruct. Res.*, **89,** 65.
22. Isenberg, W. M., McEver, R. P., Phillips, D. R., Shuman, M. A., and Bainton, D. F. (1987). *J. Cell Biol.*, **104,** 1655.
23. Bendayan, M. (1982). *J. Histochem. Cytochem.*, **30,** 81.

15

Clinical aspects of platelet function

KENNETH J. CLEMETSON

1. Introduction

Since the primary function of platelets is haemostasis, or stopping bleeding, platelet dysfunction is generally seen as an under- or over-expression of this, i.e. in bleeding problems or in various haemostatic or thrombotic disorders. The first task of the clinician faced with such symptoms is to eliminate the possibility of the disorder being produced by a lack or defect in plasma co-agulation factors such as factor VIII, von Willebrand factor, fibrinogen, factor IX, factor V, etc. which are commonly affected. Having shown that these lie within the normal range it is necessary to check for platelet-related problems. Basic parameters such as platelet count, platelet volume, and granulosity can be rapidly determined by flow cytometry. Thrombocytopenia, or low platelet count can clearly lead to bleeding problems though there is some controversy about what should be regarded as a threshold value. Normal values lie in the range 150 000–400 000 platelets/µl but bleeding problems may not appear until values below 10 000–20 000 platelets/µl are reached. There are many causes for thrombocytopenia which will be dealt with later. When necessary, basic treatment is intravenous platelet concentrates to try to restore platelet levels although the recent cloning of thrombopoietin may, when it becomes generally available, make this a preferred therapy. In principle the haemo-static quality of platelet concentrates should be checked before and after transfusion. While methods for estimating the overall haemostatic efficiency of platelets *in vitro* exist they are to a large extent still experimental and are not yet completely adapted to a clinical context. However, this situation is rapidly changing with development of these technologies. One method used now is bleeding time, the measure of the time to stop bleeding from a stan-dardized wound, but it is notoriously unreliable. Even when platelet counts are normal, changes in platelet volume may be indicative of problems. In cer-tain hereditary disorders the platelet size is affected for, as yet, unclear rea-sons. However, larger than normal platelets have been associated with myocardial infarctus and may reflect increased platelet turnover leading to abnormal platelet production from stressed megakaryocytes of a higher ploidy.

Basic aggregation tests are used to measure the response of platelet-rich plasma to agonists such as ADP, collagen, and ristocetin, or washed platelets to thrombin (see Chapter 1). Based on the pattern of results obtained here it is generally possible to make a rough classification of the problem so that more sophisticated, targeted methods can be applied to obtain a reliable diagnosis. Diagnostic criteria in platelet related disorders include:

(a) Platelet count:
   - normal
   - reduced
   - elevated

(b) Platelet size:
   - normal
   - increased

(c) Aggregation response normal, decreased, or increased:
   - ADP
   - collagen
   - arachidonic acid
   - thrombin
   - von Willebrand factor

(d) Normal or slightly decreased aggregation response in bleeding disorder linked to platelets—Thrombostat or equivalent measurement of adhesion. Possibility of granule defect.

(e) Granule function and morphology tested by measuring released products such as ATP, 5-HT, and proteins such as platelet factor 4, and by electron microscopy respectively.

(f) Where an abnormal immune response is suspected, the presence of antiplatelet antibodies and platelet binding of antibodies is tested for. In rare cases inhibition of platelet function may occur.

Many of the techniques used for platelet disorders are also used to investigate normal platelet function and have been dealt with in detail in earlier chapters so that the aim in this chapter will be to examine how these techniques can be applied to the rapid, accurate diagnosis of the platelet defect. It must be emphasized here that, as in other areas of haematology (or medicine), it is not yet possible to assign a molecular basis to all the disorders that may be encountered. For the practising haematologist, it is important to be able to diagnose those disorders for which such a basis is probable and, in other areas, to be able to classify a disorder into a broad likely category in the hope that a molecular diagnosis will be possible in the future and in order to apply a rational therapy. Acquired disorders may not have a molecular origin in the strictly biological sense but may nevertheless reflect the genetic composition of the patient.

2. Inherited bleeding disorders related to platelet membrane glycoproteins

Several well-known disorders affecting platelets are inherited and a history of bleeding problems within a family, possibly associated with a consanguinous marriage in earlier generations, suggests the possibility that one of these should be considered. A rapid classification can be made based on platelet aggregation responses together with some additional parameters.

2.1 Glanzmann's thrombasthenia

Glanzmann's thrombasthenia can be recognized by a prolonged bleeding time, normal platelet count and size, absent or reduced aggregation to ADP, arachidonic acid, collagen, and thrombin, decreased clot retraction, but normal response to ristocetin (1). The molecular basis is a mutation or deletion in the gene for GPIIb or IIIa leading either to absence or dysfunction of GPIIb–IIIa, the platelet fibrinogen receptor. Thus, platelets may, or may not show the absence or reduced expression of this complex. Flow cytometry or gel electrophoresis results showing the lack of, or a strong deficiency in, these glycoproteins in combination with the symptoms mentioned above can be regarded as diagnostic and used as the basis for molecular biology investigation to assign the genetic defect. However, there are increasing reports of rare cases where the glycoproteins are present in virtually normal amounts together with the above mentioned clinical symptoms and further investigations using sophisticated techniques are necessary to confirm the diagnosis. These may include studies of the Ca^{2+}-dependency of the GPIIb–IIIa complex or measuring the ability of the complex to be activated, using fibrinogen binding or binding of antibodies that recognize the activated conformation of the complex. It is even possible, in the future, that forms of Glanzmann's thrombasthenia will be found either affecting molecules involved in activation of the complex or where both activation of the complex and fibrinogen binding are normal and there is a defect in the later stages of signal transduction leading to receptor clustering. In such rare cases it will be necessary to keep an open mind in establishing a diagnosis and seeking a molecular origin. Molecular diagnosis follows a logical approach based upon assessing which gene is likely to be affected. In many cases this is simple since the corresponding glycoprotein is missing while the other(s) in a complex is(are) present in lower amounts. Generally, PCR is used to amplify residual platelet mRNA for sequencing to determine a mutation/deletion site (see Chapter 7). Where adequate mRNA is not available because of thrombocytopenia or degradation, alternative strategies involve amplification of individual exons of multiple exon genes and screening by techniques such as single-strand conformation polymorphism (SSCP) or denaturing gradient gel electrophoresis (DGGE) to detect mutations followed by sequencing of the mutant fragment (2).

2.2 Bernard–Soulier syndrome

Bernard–Soulier syndrome is an even rarer inherited bleeding disorder characterized by a prolonged bleeding time, larger than normal platelets ('giant'),
thrombocytopenia (as defined by platelet count), normal aggregation to
ADP, arachidonic acid, and collagen, but absent or reduced agglutination to
ristocetin, and a reduced response to low doses of thrombin. Clot retraction
is normal. The molecular basis is a mutation or deletion in the gene for one
of the components of the GPIb–V–IX complex though so far only defects in
GPIbα and GPIX have been found (3). In analogy with Glanzmann's thrombasthenia, in the classic form of this disorder all the subunits are absent (4).
Here also there are rarer forms where the subunits may be present in up to
normal amounts. Use of flow cytometry for diagnosis may therefore give mis-
leading results, depending on antibodies used. This is partially a consequence
of the low number of antibodies commercially available which are mostly
directed to the external N terminal domain of GPIbα. Some mutations seem
to lead to conformational changes causing rapid proteolysis and loss of this
region. Alternatively, the epitope for the antibody may be affected by a
mutation. This may then be interpreted as a complete lack of this subunit.
Thus, use of several antibodies is recommended in such cases. Examination
by gel electrophoresis coupled with Western blotting with suitable antibodies
can also be very informative if adequate amounts of platelets are available. A
major technical problem in Bernard–Soulier syndrome is the preparation of
adequate amounts of platelets to allow such studies. This is because of the
thrombocytopenia and also the size of the platelets. In fact it is the latter
problem that is the most critical since the actual total platelet mass may be
fairly normal. From a practical point of view separating the large platelets
from leucocytes and erythrocytes is difficult. Generally, leaving blood to
stand in tubes at 45° to the vertical for four hours so that the red and white
cells can sediment from the platelet-rich plasma is more effective and gentler
than centrifugation. Successive low speed centrifugations on a swing-out
rotor can then be used to remove residual erythrocytes and leucocytes from
the platelet-rich plasma and for washing. Alternatively, use of a Percoll gradient can be very effective.

2.3 Platelet-type, pseudo von Willebrand's disease

This is a very rare bleeding disorder caused by a mutation in platelet GPIb
leading to an enhanced interaction between platelets and normal plasma vWf
and, hence, both to depletion of the larger, more effective multimers of vWf
and to thrombocytopenia (5–7). The symptoms are very similar to those of
type 2B von Willebrand's disease where a mutation in the vWf leads to the
enhanced interaction with platelets. Differentiation between these two disorders is generally on the basis of stirred aggregometry in cross-mixing
experiments, normal platelets with patient's plasma, and vice versa.

2.4 Other platelet glycoprotein defects

A number of other defects in platelet GP leading to bleeding disorders have been described. One of the more interesting of these involved a defect in GPIa–IIa ($\alpha_2\beta_1$) which lead to a platelet adhesion defect (for assay see Chapter 7) and a specific aggregation defect in response to collagen (a defective response to wheat germ agglutinin was also reported in these patients) (8). Two similar cases were described (9) which appeared linked to hormone effects since they returned to normal after pregnancy, and the menopause, respectively. Such cases are very rare but the specific defect in collagen activation is a valuable pointer to this type of problem and confirmation of diagnosis can be obtained using flow cytometry with specific antibodies or by gel electrophoresis together with Western blotting.

Absence of CD36, a major platelet GP implicated in several receptor functions (collagen, thrombospondin, Plasmodium falciparum, oxidized LDL, neutrophil apoptosis) (10,11) is fairly common in certain populations but appears, nevertheless, to have no clinical consequences (12). Defects in other platelet GP that could be potential sources of pathological problems are those affecting receptors possibly belonging to the seven-transmembrane class. Patients have been described where the platelet ADP receptor was affected (13,14) and the platelet response to ADP and as a consequence to other agonists, such as collagen, where ADP has an important feedback function in activation, was strongly reduced. In the future it will be important to be able to differentiate between such rare, genetic disorders and similar symptoms produced by the thienopyridine class of antithrombotics (see below).

2.5 Detection of depletion/absence of platelet membrane glycoproteins in bleeding disorders

Although in simple cases it is possible to detect the absence of membrane glycoproteins by one-dimensional gel electrophoresis followed by Coomassie blue staining, the search for defects in rarer molecules as well as problems with staining lead to the use of various surface-specific labelling methods as well as the use of two-dimensional methods to give better resolution. Surface labelling methods have been mainly based upon protein labelling with [^{125}I] using mild oxidizing conditions with lactoperoxidase or Iodogen, or labelling carbohydrate with [^{3}H] using the periodate/borohydride method (*Figure 1*). Non-radioactive methods are gradually becoming more popular (15) but are limited by the efficiency of blotting of individual glycoproteins which is not always predictable. These methods can also be designed to be carbohydrate- or protein-specific depending on the glycoprotein of particular interest since labelling intensity depends upon the chemistry of the protein.

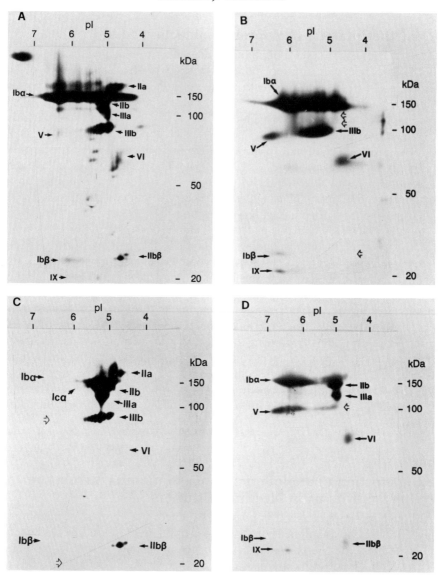

Figure 1. Detection of platelet glycoprotein defects by surface labelling with the perio-date/[³H]borohydride method. (A) Fluorogram of a two-dimensional, isoelectric focus-ing/gradient gel electrophoresis separation of platelets from a normal donor labelling by the periodate/[³H]borohydride method. The major membrane glycoproteins are indi-cated. (B) As (A) but platelets from a Glanzmann thrombasthenia patient. The missing glycoproteins GPIIbα, GPIIbβ, and GPIIIa are indicated by hollow arrows. (C) As (A) but platelets from a Bernard–Soulier syndrome patient. The missing/deficient glycoproteins GPIbα, GPIbβ, GPV, and GPIX are indicated by hollow/solid arrows, respectively. (D) As (A) but platelets from a patient with deficient GPIIIb (GPIV, CD36). The deficient glyco-protein GPIIIb is indicated by a hollow arrow.

Protocol 1. Biotin surface labelling of platelet proteins on carbohydrate

Equipment and reagents

- Washed platelets (see Chapter 1)
- 0.2 M NalO$_4$ (2 mM)
- Biotinamidocaproylhydrazide (Sigma)
- 20 mM NaHPO$_4$, 130 mM NaCl, 2 mM EDTA pH 6.5 and 7.0
- 0.63 M glycerol
- Pipette tips
- Plastic tubes (10 ml)
- Plastic Pasteur pipettes
- Bench-top centrifuge

Method

1. Prepare washed platelets and suspend at 5 × 10^9/ml in 20 mM NaHPO$_4$, 130 mM NaCl, 2 mM EDTA pH 6.5.

2. Add 0.2 M NalO$_4$ (2 mM) to the platelet suspension and cool to 4°C. Incubate in the dark for 10 min.

3. Stop reaction by adding 0.2 ml of 0.63 M glycerol per millilitre of platelet suspension.

4. Bring the platelet suspension gradually to room temperature and wash twice with the phosphate, saline, EDTA buffer pH 6.5 by centrifuging for 10 min at 1100 *g*. Resuspend in the same buffer at pH 7.0.

5. Add biotinamidocaproylhydrazide (0.5 mg/ml platelet suspension) dissolved in the same buffer. Leave the platelet suspension for 15 min at room temperature.

6. Wash the platelets with phosphate, saline, EDTA buffer pH 6.5, and solubilize the final pellet for gel electrophoresis.

Protocol 2. Biotin surface labelling platelet proteins on protein

Equipment and reagents

- Washed platelets (see Chapter 1)
- *N*-Hydroxysuccinimidobiotin (Sigma) (2 mg/ml in dimethyl formamide)
- 20 mM NaHPO$_4$, 130 mM NaCl, 2 mM EDTA pH 8
- Pipette tips
- Plastic tubes (10 ml)
- Plastic Pasteur pipettes
- Rocker-type shaker
- Bench-top centrifuge

Method

1. Prepare washed platelets and suspend at 5 × 10^9/ml in 20 mM NaHPO$_4$, 130 mM NaCl, 2 mM EDTA pH 8.

2. Add *N*-hydroxysuccinimidobiotin (2 mg/ml in dimethyl formamide), 10 μl per millilitre platelet suspension, leave for 1 h at room temperature gently mixing on a rocker-type shaker.

Protocol 2. *Continued*

3. Wash platelets four times with phosphate, saline, EDTA buffer pH 6.5, and solubilize the final pellet for gel electrophoresis.

Protocol 3. Detection of biotin labelled platelet proteins

Equipment and reagents

- Nitrocellulose (Schleicher & Schuell) or polyvinylidene fluoride (DuPont NEN) blotting membranes
- Polystyrol trays of a suitable size for incubation and washing membranes after blotting
- 20 mM NaHPO$_4$, 130 mM NaCl, 2 mM EDTA pH 7.5
- 20 mM NaHPO$_4$, 130 mM NaCl, 2 mM EDTA, 0.1% Tween 20 (Sigma) pH 7.5
- Phosphatase buffer: 0.1 M NaHCO$_3$, 1 mM MgCl$_2$ pH 9.8

- 2% bovine serum albumin in 20 mM NaHPO$_4$, 130 mM NaCl, 2 mM EDTA pH 7.5
- Streptavidin coupled with alkaline phosphatase (Sigma) (1 µg/ml) in 0.3% BSA, 20 mM NaHPO$_4$, 130 mM NaCl, 2 mM EDTA pH 7.5
- 5-Bromo-4-chloro-3-indolyl phosphate (Sigma) (stock 15 mg/ml in dimethyl sulfoxide)
- Nitrotetrazolium blue (Sigma) (stock 30 mg/ml in 70% dimethyl sulfoxide)
- Rocker-type shaker

Method

1. Use standard techniques for gel electrophoresis (one- and two-dimensional) and electrophoretic transfer to membranes (semi-dry method) throughout (see Chapter 7).

2. Perform all washings and incubations in polystyrol trays on a rocking shaker.

3. Wash the membrane (nitrocellulose or polyvinylidene fluoride) in 20 mM NaHPO$_4$, 130 mM NaCl, 2 mM EDTA pH 7.5, and block free protein binding sites with 2% bovine serum albumin (BSA) for at least 1.5 h (or overnight).

4. Incubate with streptavidin coupled with alkaline phosphatase (1 µg/ml) added in fresh buffer (0.3% BSA, 20 mM NaHPO$_4$, 130 mM NaCl, 2 mM EDTA pH 7.5) for 30 min.[a]

5. Wash the membrane four times for 5 min each with 20 mM NaHPO$_4$, 130 mM NaCl, 2 mM EDTA, 0.1% Tween 20 pH 7.5, once with 20 mM NaHPO$_4$, 130 mM NaCl pH 7.5, and once with phosphatase buffer (0.1 M NaHCO$_3$, 1 mM MgCl$_2$ pH 9.8).

6. Detect the bound phosphatase using 5-bromo-4-chloro-3-indolyl phosphate and nitrotetrazolium blue (stock 30 mg/ml in 70% dimethyl sulfoxide); 10 µl of each stock solution is added.

7. Stop the colour reaction when the desired bands/spots are clearly visible, by removing the staining solution and rinsing with water.

8. Dry the stained membranes between filter papers and store protected from light.

a Peroxidase-based detection may also be used and as alternative to staining reactions, several commercially available chemiluminescence methods may be used to detect and preserve the labelling pattern.

3. Hereditary defects in platelet granules

These are a very heterogeneous class of defects that cause bleeding disorders due to lack of important feedback factors coming from storage granules. Several rare subgroups have been somewhat better characterized. Overall, related problems may be fairly common but diagnosis remains difficult. In patients with a long bleeding time but with normal plasma factors and normal platelet aggregation parameters, possible granule defects should be considered. Since many different components are involved in the development, filling and exocytosis of α granules, dense granules, and lyzosomes, as well as in the signal transduction involved in triggering release, there are a multitude of candidate molecules that could lead to problems (16,17). Some varieties have been better characterized and a more precise diagnosis can be established, even if the molecular origin is not always clear.

In most of these granule deficiency disorders, with some exceptions, the *in vitro* aggregation responses to all agonists is virtually normal. This implies that it is adhesion that is primarily affected by the lack of granule contents and, indeed, these platelets do show reduced binding in adhesion assays. It is also interesting to note in this context that inhibition of ADP receptors (18) by thienopyridines (Ticlopidine, Clopidogrel) causes platelets to show a reduced response to shear activation (19). Probably, 5-HT and Ca^{2+} also have important roles in platelet adhesion function.

3.1 α Granule defects

These include Gray Platelet syndrome where the contents of the α granules are missing (20). The gray as opposed to normal beige colour of the platelets is a diagnostic criterion caused by the lack of the granule contents. Several different families have been described but a molecular origin has not yet been established. Apparently the membranes of the α granules are still present and typical α granule membrane proteins, such as P-selectin, can be detected in the remnant membranes by histochemical techniques but the contents are absent, implying a problem with intracellular trafficking, as soluble and integral proteins are under different trafficking control (21).

3.2 Dense granule defects

The second class of granule defects are those where dense granules are affected (22). These include Hermansky–Pudlak syndrome which is associated with partial or complete albinism, indicating that not only platelets are affected by this defect (23). There is recent evidence for a lack of a granule membrane protein in this disorder, called granulophysin, related to a protein, synaptophysin, involved in vesicle traffic in neural synapses (24). Chediak–Higashi syndrome has some symptoms in common with Hermansky–Pudlak syndrome and is thought to be also related to abnormal dense granules (25–27). Granulophysin was present in abnormally low amounts but was not completely absent.

Recently, a new variety of dense granule defect was described in which the granule membrane is present but the contents are missing (28). This has been called 'empty sack syndrome' and implies that in this case it is the trafficking of the soluble proteins and not the integral ones that are affected.

3.3 Other granule defects

Granule defects have been described that fall into none of these classes and have heterogeneous symptoms. These include the αδ group, where both the α and dense granules are affected (22).

4. Congenital thrombocytopenia

There is a large heterogeneous class of congenital thrombocytopenias, often involving larger than normal platelets, with often only mild bleeding symptoms where, in most cases, no clear biochemical defect has been demonstrated. These include the well-characterized disorder, Bernard–Soulier syndrome, dealt with above, Montreal syndrome (29), May–Egglin syndrome (30), characterized by the presence of Dohl bodies in the leucocytes, Alport's disease (31), and Wiskott–Aldrich disease (32).

Several acquired disorders of platelet function are known, generally linked to cancer-like states including myoproliferative disorders.

5. Paroxysmal nocturnal haemoglobinuria

A well-known haematological disorder affecting platelets as well as other blood cells, is paroxysmal nocturnal haemoglobinuria (PNH). This is known to be caused by the lack of synthesis of glycosylphosphatidylinositol anchors, necessary for the association of a group of glycoproteins (33) with the cell membrane. These glycoproteins are critical for protection against complement and their absence or low level of expression on platelets leads to lysis and hence to thrombocytopenia and bleeding. The disorder is clonal in nature and goes through cycles when most stem cells yielding blood cells are affected or when most are normal.

6. Immune thrombocytopenia

A common clinical problem affecting platelets is immune thrombocytopenia where the platelet destruction is caused by the development of antibodies against platelet membrane glycoproteins. These antibodies can be either allo- or auto- and can also be induced by certain treatments such as heparin or antimalarials like quinine. Allo-antibodies are induced by blood transfusions containing platelets or by transfusions with platelet concentrates where there is a polymorphic or other difference in the sequence of one of the glyco-proteins. This epitope is recognized as foreign and with repeated transfusion may lead to dangerous levels of antibodies causing platelet activation, aggregation, and destruction. Generally, such aggregates are removed by the spleen so that splenectomy is a common treatment to reduce thrombocytopenia. Intravenous gamma globulin is often as effective a treatment but is less aggressive. This involves intravenous treatment with gamma globulin isolated and purified from plasma from a large number of donors. Although the mechanism of action of this treatment is not yet established, it has been proposed that it acts through anti-idiotype antibodies present in the wide mixture affecting the balance of antibody production by acting directly on the B lymphocytes. Treatment with steroids is also often effective. The most common target of these antibodies is GPIIb–IIIa followed by GPIb–V–IX and GPIa–IIa (34).

In autoimmune thrombocytopenia it is clear that the problem is not due to polymorphism but that somehow the immune system is misled into producing antibodies against self molecules. This may be due to a problem with the process by which lymphocytes producing anti-self antibodies are eliminated during development or may be due to poorly understood side-effects of viral infections, as may well be the case in the acute immunocytopenia occurring in children.

Progress has been made in understanding some of the immune disorders induced as side-effects during treatment with various substances. For example, heparin-associated immunocytopenia is now known to be related to antibodies formed against complexes of heparin and the platelet α granule component, platelet factor 4 (35–37). This is a major problem since heparin is an effective form of prophylaxis against thrombosis during major surgery and is very commonly used. Presumably, these antibodies can bind to heparinoids on the platelet surface and induce both activation via the Fc receptor and complement activation.

Similarly, quinine or quinidine treatment for malaria may result in immune thrombocytopenia due to binding of quinine or quinidine to platelet glyco-proteins leading to neoantigens and production of antibodies (38). These recognize only the complex and therefore only bind to platelets in the presence of the alkaloids.

More recently antibodies against plasma glycoproteins, such as β_2-

microglobin 1, which bind to negatively charged phospholipids normally only exposed on cells activated and involved in procoagulant activity (such as platelets and erythrocytes) have been implicated in some forms of lupus (39).

7. Alterations in lipid content and distribution and in membrane deformability

There has been considerable interest over the years in changes in the composition of blood cell membranes and the way in which this may reflect both the state of health of the patient and, perhaps, provide a criterion for estimating risk of disease. The effect of dietary fat on a tendence to cardiovascular disease is still one that arouses passions on both sides of the argument. Comparing relative risks in different countries and among people who have immigrated to, and adopted the life-style of, countries with populations at higher/lower risk shows clearly that diet and life-style factors are very important items in determining relative risk. Of course, within a population, hereditary factors also play a role. However, differences in the types of fatty acids in the diet are incorporated into differences in the lipids forming the membrane and cleavage of these membrane lipids forms second messengers that participate in several signal transduction and feedback mechanisms. Thus, there is evidence that specific polyunsaturated fatty acids influence platelets to make them less easily activated, while cholesterol, which makes the membrane more rigid, tends to make platelet receptors more sensitive (40), perhaps by increasing coupling. On the other hand, some statistics indicate that polyunsaturated fatty acids cause a higher rate of cancer. Are platelets also implicated in this? Certainly there is accumulating evidence that integrins can play a role in metastasis and it is also possible that platelets which can be activated by, and bind to, many types of tumour cells, are involved in some of these processes. It is interesting to note that antithrombotic agents are also being investigated for auxiliary treatment of some types of experimental cancer.

Changes in platelet membrane fluidity have also been reported in other disorders such as Alzheimer's disease (increase) and seem to be characteristic (41). The origin and significance of these changes, however, remain obscure. Platelet α granules also contain the precursor of the β amyloid protein involved in this disorder and it is modified by thrombin treatment establishing another link (42). Again the significance is far from clear.

8. Other disorders implicating platelets

Platelets seem also either to be affected or to be linked to the problem in depression and migraine where 5-HT and both its transport and receptors are known to play a role. These changes are also paralleled in the platelets of the patient following an attack and may provide important clues to the development of the disorder.

Platelet sensitivity to activation appears to be one of the characteristics of diabetes and the presence of small platelet aggregates in the blood vessels of the retina is a fairly reliable non-invasive criterion of the disease state. Indeed it is this increased tendency to thrombosis which is responsible for many of the destructive side-effects of diabetes such as loss of limb extremities and blindness. Despite this the causes of the increased platelet activity are still unknown. It has been suggested that non-enzymatic glycosylation of platelet receptors by the elevated levels of glucose might be involved but as yet there is no hard evidence for such effects. Changes in signal transduction inside the platelets induced by side-effects of diabetes can also not be excluded.

It was already noted above that the size of platelets may provide important information about the state of health of the subject (43,44). However, we still know very little about the connection between the two. Nevertheless, the ability to measure such parameters may allow the necessary correlations to be made.

9. Detection of activation of platelets occurring *in vivo*

Methods of detection of platelet activation *in vivo* based on flow cytometry methods are described elsewhere in this volume and are undoubtedly very sensitive and flexible. There are, however, other methods of detecting platelet activation that were developed earlier. These are based on the fact that strongly activated platelets release the contents of granules and that some of these constituents are specific, or at least relatively specific for platelets. These are α granule constituents such as platelet factor 4, platelet basic protein and its proteolytic fragments, generally classed as β-thromboglobulin, and also thrombospondin for which platelets are a major although not unique source. Platelet factor 4 released from platelets binds to heparin and related molecules on the endothelial surface from which it can be flushed by heparin (hence the immune problems encountered). Most of the thrombospondin apparently binds back directly to the surface of activated platelets since it is not found free in the circulation. It can be assayed in this way. The half-life in the circulation of nine hours found for injected thrombospondin is therefore irrelevant to release from activated platelets *in vivo*. Thus, β-thromboglobulin is the only practical marker of this class and has been used fairly successfully in several studies to follow platelet activation in clinical studies and has been compared with the results from flow cytometry studies. Several effective commercial RIA or ELISA assays are available.

In various clinical conditions platelets may be exposed to products from the activation of other cells where they are possibly not activated themselves or only marginally activated. One example of such a situation might occur in inflammatory situations where platelets are exposed to enzymes from activated phagocytic cells such as neutrophils. One consequence of such exposure might be that surface glycoproteins are degraded, reducing the platelet reponse to agonists and exposing new sites. Other diseases where changes in platelet glycoproteins have been reported include liver cirrhosis (45) and myoproliferative disorders. These include changes in platelet glycoprotein glycosylation. Diagnostic methods are based upon flow cytometry with specific antibodies and/or lectins as well as various methods of gel electrophoresis using detection methods based upon blotting with specific antibodies or lectins or, alternatively, labelling methods specific either for protein or carbohydrate.

10. Assessment of platelet function in clinical trials of platelet and coagulation inhibitors and fibrinolytic agents

Over the last decade there has been a great increase in interest in the discovery, development, and testing of inhibitors of either coagulation or platelet function as a method of preventing thrombotic problems. In the short-term this is aimed at acute situations but in the long-term the goal is prophylaxis. Since thrombosis can be regarded as a pathological variant of haemostasis there is always a narrow margin between inhibiting the excesses of thrombosis and going too far in the other direction and inhibiting the physiologically essential haemostasis with the danger of life-threatening bleeding episodes that could result. It is therefore essential to have good methods of measuring haemostatic function at all stages during use of platelet or coagulation inhibitors to know to what degree platelet function is inhibited. In the long run such data can give valuable information about the relative risks involved in treatment and the variability of the response, on the one hand, concerning the benefit to the patient and, on the other hand, concerning measurable *in vitro* parameters. In the past, one of the classic ways of testing platelet response was aggregometry which remains a simple, sensitive technique for measuring overall response. More recently, methods based upon flow cytometry have shown much promise for monitoring platelet activation parameters and are dealt with in other chapters. Methods based on measurement of the kinetics of cytoplasm Ca^{2+} release are also gaining in popularity but require relatively sophisticated equipment. Since the main targets of therapeutic pharmacology have been thrombin and platelet GPIIb–IIIa, aggregometry and flow cytometry have been used fairly successfully to follow the effects of inhibitors *in vitro*. Displacement of more weakly bound, labelled GPIIb–IIIa inhibitors by the clinically used inhibitor has been proposed as an approach to measuring plasma levels. Interest also starts to turn towards inhibitors of platelet adhesion where these measurements may only poorly, if at all, reflect the *in vivo* effectiveness of the inhibitors.

There is, therefore, a demand for methods that can be used to measure this quickly and easily. Although some methods to measure adhesion have existed for some time they were complicated and labour-intensive. However, they have provided a great deal of high grade data on factors affecting platelet adhesion and how they can be modified. These include perfusion chamber methods which have been simplified and reduced in size over the years. Initial studies used everted, de-endothelized, arterial segments but these have now been replaced by collagen coated coverslips which have the advantage of being easier to standardize, to modify, and to quantitate. More recently, methods have been developed which measure platelet adhesion function together with aggregation function (46,47) and are therefore complementary to the aggregation method alone. They also have the advantage of being rapid and requiring relatively small whole blood samples. Typical methods involve passage of blood samples through either a small hole in a membrane or a capillary coated with collagen. In both cases, adhesion of platelets is dependent on the presence of vWf and the rate of adhesion is shear-dependent. Adhesion is followed by aggregation and the hole or capillary is blocked. The time to blockage can be measured and is related to both adhesion and aggregation. It is therefore possible to measure an *in vitro* equivalent to the bleeding time. The bleeding time, despite its notoriously poor reproducibility, is generally thought to be a representative indicator of platelet function *in vivo*. A more reliable *in vitro* version provides additional information about many aspects of platelet activity that aggregation measurements alone can not. For example, it is relatively easy to find out if a blood donor has taken aspirin or not by comparing the response in the absence and presence of ADP since this amplification factor is strongly reduced when thromboxane synthesis is blocked.

Protocol 4. *In vitro* 'bleeding time' measurement with the Thrombostat 4000/2

Equipment and reagents
- Thrombostat 4000/2 or similar (Dade International)
- Capillary adaptors (Dade)
- Membrane cartridges (Dade) (150 µl hole)
- Whole blood sample
- 10 mM ADP
- 37°C block or water-bath
- Collagen coated membrane

Method
1. Switch on the instrument (46,47) and allow the temperature in the 37°C block to stabilize. Test the gaskets seal until the gas-tight fit is reproducible.
2. Pre-warm to 37°C a whole blood sample, fresh or reconstituted, from a patient or a normal donor, and either incubate with inhibitors or

313

Protocol 4. *Continued*

  antibodies to be tested, or place directly in a measurement position in the instrument.

3. Attach a capillary to a cartridge containing a collagen coated membrane with a 150 μm hole. Add 40 μl of 10 mM ADP to the surface of the membrane and start the measurement. *Figure 2D* shows a diagram of the instrument and its principle of operation.

4. Measure occlusion time and volume for the sample with a control in the second measuring position. Repeat the measurement with the positions of the sample and control reversed in the instrument to compensate for any systematic errors between the two positions. Typical results are shown in *Figure 2*.

5. In the case of inhibitors, use serial dilutions to obtain a dose–response curve.

Another recently developed technique which has not yet seen much application to clinical problems is the use of a defined shear stress on a blood or platelet sample using various designs of viscometers. Such techniques may, in the future, be particularly useful for differentiating certain types of von Willebrand's disease, especially where there is a qualitative difference in the interaction between vWf and platelets, such as in type 2B and platelet-type, pseudo von Willebrand's disease. They are already showing promise for the analysis of signal transduction pathways induced by shear stress (47). It may not be too far-fetched to expect that rare bleeding disorders may involve defects in such pathways.

Fibrinolysis is a necessary step for removal of the clot causing stenosis by blocking a vessel. Several different enzymes have been used in this process and one approach is by activation of plasminogen to plasmin. As well as its fibrinolytic action plasmin is known to cleave platelet glycoproteins, affecting the platelet response (48,49). Several other enzymes used for such treatments may also have similar side-effects. Therefore, control of platelet function after such treatment is important. Of course, it is also important to be able to inhibit either platelets or thrombin during fibrinolysis in order to avoid rapid restenosis triggered by thrombin bound to fibrin and released to activate platelets during cleavage of fibrin. This is a primary target of platelet and thrombin inhibitors currently under development. However, at present, these would be delivered at the same time as the fibrinolytic treatment and are rapidly reversible so that the platelet response should also return quickly to normal. Good methods for testing platelet function both during and after such treatment will be increasingly in demand.

During development of platelet inhibitors, *in vitro* testing to give a better idea about desired *in vivo* properties will become more essential. At the moment such testing, followed by preclinical screening in animal models is

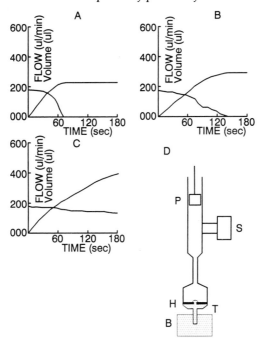

Figure 2. Inhibitor effects on platelets measured with the Thrombostat. In A–C the lower curve represents the flow rate through the hole in the membrane while the upper curve represents the total volume to have passed the hole. (A) Occlusion of membrane aperture by control whole blood. (B) Occlusion of membrane aperture by whole blood incubated with F(ab)′ fragments of rabbit anti-GPIb antibodies (50 µg/ml blood). (C) Occlusion of membrane aperture by whole blood incubated with F(ab)′ fragments of rabbit anti-GPIb antibodies (100 µg/ml blood). (D) Diagram of Thrombostat and principle of operation. B is blood sample. T is the capillary leading from the blood sample to the membrane aperture H. P is the piston drawing the blood through the hole, and S is the sensor holding the pressure constant and providing the feedback information and output.

not only expensive but also gives only a partial picture of the clinical situation. Improved *in vitro* studies should be able to both reduce and complement these. However, the cardiovascular system is complicated and it is always difficult to predict what effects supposedly specific inhibitors may have on their target (50) or on other parts of the body. While thrombin, for example, is an extremely important platelet activator and is critical for an efficient haemostasis, its role in regulation in many other tissues may also be more important than previously supposed. Thrombin receptors have been found on a wide range of cells including endothelial cells (51), fibroblasts (52), nerve cells (53), and T lymphocytes (54) suggesting a role in neural development and in immunology. Although brief treatments with thrombin inhibitors might be acceptable to prevent platelet activation during fibrinolysis, longer prophylactic treatments might have untoward consequences.

Generally, the person testing for platelet inhibitors knows that the patient is receiving such treatment. In the future it is conceivable that, when more people may be receiving antithrombotics on a longer-term basis, it will be necessary to be able to differentiate in the haematology laboratory between different categories of antithrombotics. Ideally patients will carry identity cards with such treatments indicated, and developments in this direction are under way, but in accidents such cards may be lost or mislaid and the patient may not be able to communicate with the doctor. What should be done when it is difficult to stop bleeding? Is the problem a hereditary disease or is the patient on some kind of antithrombotic? These are problems that are being actively discussed. Perhaps simply investigation of washed platelets will be enough to differentiate between these possibilities and, certainly, an analysis of the spectrum of responses can often provide valuable clues.

11.   Methodology

Clearly, most methods used for the diagnosis of functional and molecular defects in platelets involved in diseases are identical to those used for the investigation of these functions and molecules on normal platelets which are described extensively in other chapters. However, there are a few specialized methods which have been used, particularly, for well-known bleeding disorders, as well as methods which are being developed specifically for diagnosis of disease states or for evaluation of platelet function inhibitors (see protocols).

Acknowledgements

I thank Barbara Hügli and Susanne Weber for technical assistance with the methods described and Dr Jeannine M. Clemetson for reading and correcting the manuscript. I would also like to thank Ad de Waard, Dade AG, for the loan of the Thrombostat 4000/2, provision of membrane cartridges, and help with the use of the instrument. The supply of buffy coats from the Central Laboratory of the Swiss Red Cross Blood Transfusion Service is gratefully acknowledged. Work performed in the Theodor Kocher Institute was supported by grants from the Swiss National Science Foundation (current No. 31–32416.91).

References

1. George, J. N., Caen, J. P., and Nurden, A. T. (1990). *Blood*, **75**, 1383.
2. Jin, Y., Dietz, H. C., Nurden, A., and Bray, P. F. (1993). *Blood*, **82**, 2281.
3. Clemetson, K. J. and Clemetson, J. M. (1994). *Curr. Opin. Hematol.*, **1**, 388.
4. Clemetson, K. J., McGregor, J. L., James, E., Dechavanne, M., and Lüscher, E. F. (1982). *J. Clin. Invest.*, **70**, 304.

5. Miller, J. L. (1991). *Am. J. Clin. Pathol.*, **96,** 681.
6. Scott, J. P. and Montgomery, R. R. (1991). *Am. J. Clin. Pathol.*, **96,** 723.
7. Russell, S. D. and Roth, G. J. (1993). *Blood*, **81,** 1787.
8. Nieuwenhuis, H. K., Akkerman, J. W. N., Houdijk, W. P. M., and Sixma, J. J. (1985). *Nature*, **318,** 470.
9. Kehrel, B., Balleisen, L., Kokott, R., Mesters, R., Stenzinger, W., Clemetson, K. J., *et al.* (1988). *Blood*, **71,** 1074.
10. Tandon, N. N., Kralisz, U., and Jamieson, G. A. (1989). *J. Biol. Chem.*, **264,** 7576.
11. Barnwell, J. W., Asch, A. S., Nachman, R. L., Yamaya, M., Aikawa, M., and Ingravallo, P. (1989). *J. Clin. Invest.*, **84,** 765.
12. Yamamoto, N., Akamatsu, N., Yamazaki, H., and Tanoue, K. (1992). *Br. J. Haematol.*, **81,** 86.
13. Cattaneo, M., Lecchi, A., Randi, A. M., McGregor, J. L., and Mannucci, P. M. (1992). *Blood*, **80,** 2787.
14. Heilmann, E., Hourdillé, P., Humbert, M., Papanneau, A., Savi, P., Herbert, J.-M., *et al.* (1993). *Thromb. Haemost.*, **69,** 909.
15. Heilmann, E., Friese, P., Anderson, S., George, J. N., Hanson, S. R., Burstein, S. A., *et al.* (1993). *Br. J. Haematol.*, **85,** 729.
16. White, J. G. (1993). *Lab. Invest.*, **68,** 497.
17. Harrison, P. and Cramer, E. M. (1993). *Blood Rev.*, **7,** 52.
18. Cattaneo, M., Akkawat, B., Lecchi, A., Cimminiello, C., Capitanio, A. M., and Mannucci, P. M. (1991). *Thromb. Haemost.*, **66,** 694.
19. Cattaneo, M., Lombardi, R., Bettega, D., Lecchi, A., and Mannucci, P. M. (1993). *Arterioscler. Thromb.*, **13,** 393.
20. Nurden, A. T., Kunicki, T. J., Dupuis, D., Soria, C., and Caen, J. P. (1982). *Blood*, **59,** 709.
21. Milgram, S. L., Eipper, B. A., and Mains, R. E. (1994). *J. Cell Biol.*, **124,** 33.
22. Weiss, H. J., Lages, B., Vicic, W., Tsung, L. Y., and White, J. G. (1993). *Br. J. Haematol.*, **83,** 282.
23. White, J. G. and Gerrard, J. M. (1976). *Am. J. Pathol.*, **83,** 590.
24. Gerrard, J. M., Lint, D., Sims, P. J., Wiedmer, T., Fugate, R. D., McMillan, E., *et al.* (1991). *Blood*, **77,** 101.
25. Gorius, J., Lebret, M., Klebanoff, C., Buriot, D., Griscelli, C., Levi-Toledano, S., *et al.* (1983). *Am. J. Pathol.*, **111,** 307.
26. Duque, P., Dangelmeier, C., and Holmsen, H. (1985). *Br. J. Haematol.*, **59,** 471.
27. Meyers, K. and Seachord, C. (1990). *Thromb. Haemost.*, **64,** 319.
28. McNicol, A., Israels, S. J., Robertson, C., and Gerrard, J. M. (1994). *Br. J. Haematol.*, **86,** 574.
29. Okita, J. R., Frojmovic, M. M., Kristopeit, S., Wong, T., and Kunicki, T. J. (1989). *Blood*, **74,** 715.
30. Djaldetti, M., Creter, D., Butanover, Y., and Elian, E. (1982). *Haematology*, **67,** 530.
31. Clare, N. M., Montiel, M. M., Lifschitz, M. D., and Bannayan, G. A. (1979). *Am. J. Clin. Pathol.*, **72,** 111.
32. Marone, G., Albini, F., di Martino, L., Quattrin, S., Poto, S., and Condorelli, M. (1986). *Br. J. Haematol.*, **62,** 737.
33. Polgar, J., Clemetson, J. M., Gegenbacher, D., and Clemetson, K. J. (1993). *FEBS Lett.*, **327,** 49.

34. Chong, B. H., Du, X., Berndt, M. C., Horn, S., and Chesterman, C. N. (1991). *Blood*, **77,** 2190.

35. Greinacher, A., Pötzsch, B., Amiral, J., Dummel, V., Eichner, A., and Müller-Eckhardt, C. (1994). *Thromb. Haemost.*, **71,** 247.

36. Kelton, J. G., Smith, J. W., Warkentin, T. E., Hayward, C. P. M., Denomme, G. A., and Horsewood, P. (1994). *Blood*, **83,** 3232.

37. Visentin, G. P., Ford, S. E., Scott, J. P., and Aster, R. H. (1994). *J. Clin. Invest.*, **93,** 81.

38. Visentin, G. P., Newman, P. J., and Aster, R. H. (1991). *Blood*, **77,** 2668.

39. Permpikul, P., Rao, L. V. M., and Rapaport, S. I. (1994). *Blood*, **83,** 2878.

40. Sorisky, A., Kucera, G. L., and Rittenhouse, S. E. (1990). *Biochem. J.*, **265,** 747.

41. Kukull, W. A., Hinds, T. R., Schellenberg, G. D., Van Belle, G., and Larson, E. B. (1992). *Neurology*, **42,** 607.

42. Li, Q.-X., Berndt, M. C., Bush, A. I., Rumble, B., Mackenzie, I., Friedhuber, A., *et al.* (1994). *Blood*, **84,** 133.

43. Toplak, H., Sagmeister, E., and Wascher, T. C. (1994). *Int. J. Obes.*, **18,** 355.

44. Weinberger, I., Fuchs, J., Davidson, E., and Rotenberg, Z. (1992). *Am. J. Cardiol.*, **70,** 981.

45. Sánchez Roig, M. J., Rivera, J., Moraleda, J. M., Martinez, I., and Vicente, V. (1994). *Eur. J. Haematol.*, **52,** 240.

46. Kratzer, M. A. A. and Born, G. V. R. (1985). *Haemostasis*, **15,** 357.

47. Razdan, K., Hellums, J. D., and Kroll, M. H. (1994). *Biochem. J.*, **302,** 681.

48. Hoffmann, J. J. M. L. and Janssen, W. C. M. (1992). *Thromb. Res.*, **67,** 711.

49. Pasche, B., Ouimet, H., Francis, S., and Loscalzo, J. (1994). *Blood*, **83,** 404.

50. Kouns, W. C., Kirchhofer, D., Hadvary, P., Edenhofer, A., Weller, T., Pfenninger, G., *et al.* (1992). *Blood*, **80,** 2539.

51. Lum, H., Andersen, T. T., Siflinger-Birnboim, A., Tiruppathi, C., Goligorsky, M. S., Fenton, J. W. II, *et al.* (1993). *J. Cell Biol.*, **120,** 1491.

52. Borich, S. M., Englebretsen, D., Harding, D. R. K., and Scott, G. K. (1994). *Cell Biol. Int.*, **18,** 639.

53. Suidan, H. S., Stone, S. R., Hemmings, B. A., and Monard, D. (1992). *Neuron*, **8,** 363.

54. Howells, G. L., Macey, M., Curtis, M. A., and Stone, S. R. (1993). *Br. J. Haematol.*, **84,** 156.

Platelet procoagulant activity and its measurement

EDOUARD M. BEVERS, PAUL COMFURIUS,
CHRIS P. M. REUTELINGSPERGER, and ROBERT F. A. ZWAAL

1. Introduction

Platelets serve an important function in the haemostatic process. Vessel wall injury causes exposure of subendothelial structures to the blood stream and initiates the process of platelet adhesion, aggregation, and release of granule contents resulting in formation of the primary haemostatic plug. Tissue thromboplastin, released by the damaged vessel wall, initiates activation of the coagulation pathway, leading to formation of thrombin. The action of thrombin on soluble plasma fibrinogen gives rise to deposition of an insoluble fibrin network which consolidates the primary haemostatic platelet plug to a stable thrombus. There exists a mutual interaction between thrombin formation and platelet activation: while thrombin is one of the most potent platelet activators, its formation is strongly enhanced in the presence of activated platelets. The latter is due to the exposure of procoagulant phospholipids at the surface of the platelet plasma membrane, known as the procoagulant response. In this chapter, we will describe two methods to measure this procoagulant response. One method concerns the direct measurement of a lipid-dependent coagulation reaction, i.e. the formation of thrombin by the enzyme complex factor Xa and factor Va, known as the prothrombinase reaction. The other method is based on the detection of surface exposed procoagulant lipid, i.e. phosphatidylserine (PS) by means of Annexin V, a protein with high affinity for anionic phospholipids.

1.1 Lipid-dependent coagulation reactions

Apart from the factor VIIa/tissue factor catalysed activation of factor X, two sequential reactions of the coagulation process are strongly enhanced by the presence of phospholipids. The first reaction involves the formation of factor Xa by the enzyme complex factor IXa–VIIIa, and the second the formation of thrombin by a complex of factor Xa–Va, referred to as 'tenase' and 'prothrombinase' reaction, respectively. The presence of an anionic phospholipid surface causes the K_m for both substrates of these reactions, factor X and prothrombin, to decrease to a value far below their respective plasma concentrations, allowing both reactions to proceed at rates approaching V_{max} conditions. Although a variety of anionic phospholipids may act as catalytic surface for both reactions, a strong preference exists for phosphatidylserine to serve as procoagulant phospholipid, as was shown recently (1–4). An excellent review on the pivotal role of lipids in the assembly of the enzyme–substrate complexes of the coagulation cascade is given in ref. 5.

1.2 The procoagulant response

The various phospholipids in the plasma membrane of platelets (as well as other blood cells) are distributed over both membrane leaflets in an asymmetric fashion: most importantly, choline-containing lipids predominate the outer membrane leaflet, whereas the aminophospholipids, in particular phosphatidylserine, are almost exclusively present in the cytoplasmic leaflet of the membrane. Therefore, the resting, non-stimulated platelet cannot serve well as catalytic surface for the tenase and prothrombinase reactions. Platelet activation may lead to loss of lipid asymmetry causing exposure of PS in the outer leaflet of the plasma membrane. The extent of PS exposure determines the level of the procoagulant response and is dependent on the type of platelet activator used. The mechanisms involved in maintenance and regulation of lipid asymmetry are topics of current research. For recent reviews on this topic, consult refs 6 and 7.

Formerly, the stimulating effect of platelets in the coagulation process was measured as shortening of the clotting time of plasma in the presence of Russell's viper venom, which activates factor X and V, known as the platelet factor 3 (PF3) assay. The observed shortening in clotting time, however, was shown to be due to a combined effect of exposed procoagulant phospholipids and released factor V. A more defined system to measure the platelet procoagulant activity is to assay for tenase or prothrombinase activity in a system using purified coagulation factors and washed platelets. Although both reactions allow estimation of the procoagulant response, the prothrombinase assay is more convenient because of the greater stability of factor Va in comparison to factor VIIIa. In the following, we will describe protocols for washing and activating platelets and measuring prothrombinase activity. Because factor Va required for the prothrombinase assay is not readily commercially available, whereas the coagulation factors Xa and prothrombin are, the protocol for purification of factor Va will be provided here as well.

2. Platelet isolation and activation procedures

2.1 Preparation of washed platelets

The best way to measure the platelet procoagulant response is to work with washed platelets in order to exclude any contribution of plasma factors other than the prothrombinase components or platelet activators required for the assay. Isolation of washed platelets is described in *Protocol 1*. It is of note, that the isolation procedure may be accompanied by minor platelet activation, affecting the procoagulant activity of the 'non-activated' platelets. The best results are obtained when isolation is performed using acidified washing buffers. Each washing step requires careful and gentle resuspension of the platelet pellet and it is recommendable to work quickly, in order to avoid prolonged presence of the platelets in acidified medium. After completion of the isolation procedure, the platelet suspension is allowed to stand for 10–15 minutes before starting experiments. One may judge the quality of the platelet preparation by the visual appearance of the Schlieren effect when the suspension is swirled. The presence of fatty acid-free (human) serum albumin in the washing buffers and in the final platelet suspension is essential to maintain a low 'basal' prothrombinase activity of platelets. Storage of washed platelets in buffers without albumin will give rise to gradual increase of procoagulant activity in time.

Protocol 1. Isolation of platelets

Equipment and reagents

- Buffer A (Hepes buffer pH 6.6): 137 mM NaCl, 2.68 mM KCl, 10 mM Hepes (Sigma, H0763), 1.7 mM $MgCl_2$, 25 mM glucose, 0.05 (w/v) fatty acid-free human serum albumin (Sigma), adjusted with HCl at pH 6.6
- Bench-top centrifuge
- Anticoagulant (acid–citrate–dextrose) (ACD): 0.052 M citric acid, 0.08 M trisodium citrate, 0.18 M glucose
- Buffer B (Hepes buffer pH 7.4): composition as described above, adjusted to pH 7.4
- Polystyrene tubes
- Coulter counter or spectrophotometer

Method

1. Collect blood on ACD, using 1 vol. anticoagulant for 5 vol. blood. Blood is collected into a polystyrene tube preferably by free flow from the forearm vein, using a lightly applied tourniquet. (The first few millilitres of blood are discarded.)

2. Centrifuge at 200 *g* for 15 min in bench-top centrifuge at room temperature (no brake).

3. Collect platelet-rich plasma (PRP) carefully to avoid contamination with red cells or leucocytes.

4. Centrifuge PRP at 1000 *g* for 15 min (room temperature).

5. Discard supernatant and resuspend pellet by adding a small volume (1–2 ml) of buffer A. Use a 1 ml micropipette to suspend the platelets. After resuspension, adjust volume to 14 ml and add 1 ml ACD.

6. Centrifuge at 1000 *g* for 15 min (room temperature).

7. Repeat steps 5 and 6 twice.

Protocol 1. *Continued*

8. After final wash, resuspend pellet in 0.5 ml buffer A and adjust volume to 5 ml with buffer B (Hepes pH 7.4). Do not add ACD in this step!

9. Allow platelets to 'recover' from isolation procedure by leaving them at room temperature for 5–15 min. Inspect swirling aspect of suspension.

10. Measure platelet count using a Coulter counter or determining optical density at 405 nm using buffer B as a blank (OD_{405} of 0.025 corresponds to 10^6 platelets/ml, a calibration curve of OD_{405} versus platelet number can be established with a Coulter counter).

2.2 Activation of platelets

A variety of physiological agonists are known to cause platelets to change shape, express fibrinogen binding sites with subsequent aggregation, and to cause secretion of granule contents. Only a few of these agonists can evoke a significant procoagulant response. Non-physiological compounds such as calcium ionophore and sulfhydryl reagents can also cause a procoagulant response. In all cases, the presence of extracellular Ca^{2+} during activation is essential for expression of procoagulant activity; some agonists also require stirring for maximal stimulation of the procoagulant response. For agonists that cause platelets to aggregate, it is recommended to perform platelet activation and measurement of the prothrombinase activity in the same incubation tube, i.e. to avoid subsampling procedures. For agonists which do not cause platelet aggregation, activation may be carried out at higher platelet concentrations, followed by subsampling to the prothrombinase system. *Protocol 2* describes the method for activation of platelets by collagen plus thrombin, which is the best physiological stimulus in evoking to the highest procoagulant response.

Protocol 2. Activation of platelets

Equipment and reagents

- Washed platelets at a concentration of 5 × 10^6/ml in buffer B
- Magnetic stirring bars (Teflon coated) 7 × 2 mm
- Polystyrene flat-bottom tubes
- $CaCl_2$ solution: 175 mM

- Collagen (Hormon Chemie) diluted to 250 µg/ml in buffer supplied by manufacturer
- Thrombin diluted in buffer B to a concentration of 200 nM
- Water-bath at 37 °C
- Magnetic stirrer

Method

1. Incubate 300 µl platelet suspension in flat-bottom tube for 3 min at 37 °C. Stir at approx. 300 revolutions/min using Teflon coated stirring bar.

2. Add 5.5 µl CaCl$_2$ solution.

3. Add 13 µl collagen, followed by 6.5 µl thrombin, and continue stirring for the desired time interval before measuring prothrombinase activity. Continue as in *Protocol 3*.

Alternatively, other stimulators may be used in step 3. Among these are:

(a) Ionophore A23187 (Sigma, C 7522) or ionomycin (Sigma, I 0634), added 1 : 200 from a stock solution in DMSO (dimethyl sulfoxide) at final concentrations of 1–2 µM. If other concentrations are to be tested, avoid DMSO concentrations above 0.5% (v/v). Stimulation with ionophore does not require stirring (except during mixing) to evoke maximal prothrombinase activity.

(b) Collagen alone, i.e. in absence of thrombin. This will result in a lower procoagulant response. However, it should be realized that thrombin formed in the prothrombinase assay will cause post-activation of the platelets, resulting in an overestimation of the effect caused by collagen alone.

(c) Sulfhydryl reagents such as diamide (Sigma, D 3648) used at a final concentration of 5 mM, or PDA (pyridyldithioethanolamine) (8) at a concentration of 1 mM.

(d) The complement membrane attack complex, C5b–9, also induces procoagulant activity. Since assembly of this pore *in vitro* requires not readily available complement proteins and a rather specific incubation procedure, this protocol is not supplied here. The reader is referred to the original papers by Sims and coworkers (9).

(e) Other agonists such as thrombin alone, platelet activating factor, ADP, and 5-HT are less potent in evoking the procoagulant response.

3. Measurement of platelet procoagulant response

3.1 The prothrombinase measurement

Subsequent to the above described platelet activation, the components of the prothrombinase complex are added to the same tube in which the activation took place. This will avoid the risk of unreliable subsampling from aggregated platelet suspensions. In order to monitor exposure of procoagulant lipids, the assay system requires saturating conditions for both enzyme and substrate. Moreover, thrombin formation must be linear with time at least to the moment when a sample is taken to analyse the amount of thrombin formed. It is advisable to check for this linearity by making a calibration curve with completely lysed platelets (see Section 3.2). Although a homologous system with human platelets requires coagulation factors of human origin, a prothrombinase assay with bovine coagulation proteins suffices for the determination of the procoagulant response.

Since activation of platelets, in particular with collagen plus thrombin, is subject to substantial variation, activation and subsequent prothrombinase measurement are best performed routinely in triplicate.

Protocol 3. Prothrombinase assay

Equipment and reagents

- Bovine coagulation proteins factor Xa, prothrombin, and thrombin can be obtained commercially (e.g. Sigma). Purification of factor Xa and prothrombin according to published methods (10,11) may be profitable when many assays are to be carried out.
- Tris/HSA buffer: 0.05 M Tris–HCl, 0.12 M NaCl, 0.5 mg/ml human serum albumin, essentially fatty acid free (Sigma, A 1887), pH 7.9. The presence of albumin in the prothrombinase assay is essential to prevent binding of the proteins of the prothrombinase complex to the surface of the tubes, which results in increased thrombin formation, even in the absence of platelets.
- Cuvette buffer: 0.05 M Tris–HCl, 0.12 M NaCl, 2 mM EDTA pH 7.5
- Thrombin-specific chromogenic substrate (e.g. S2238 from Chromogenix or Chromozym TH from Boehringer Mannheim) dissolved in water at a concentration of 3 mM
- Plastic tubes (2 ml)
- Disposable plastic cuvettes
- Spectrophotometer at 405 nm

- Factor Xa/Va: stock solutions of coagulation factors Xa (300 nM) and Va (600 nM) in Tris/HSA buffer are stored in small aliquots at –70°C. Working solution for prothrombinase assay is prepared freshly each day by mixing and diluting factor Xa and factor Va in Tris/HSA buffer to a final concentration of 30 nM and 60 nM, respectively. This reagent, referred to as 'factor Xa/Va mix' must be kept on ice. Although the functional prothrombinase complex consists of equimolar amounts of factors Xa and Va, in the assay, twice the concentration of factor Va is used compared to factor Xa. This will prevent any contribution to the observed rate of thrombin formation upon release (and subsequent activation) of factor V from the alpha granula of platelets stimulated with thrombin.
- Prothrombin: dissolved in Tris/HSA buffer at a concentration of 16 μM, supplemented with $CaCl_2$ at final concentration of 3 mM. The preparation is kept on ice, but a working solution (1 ml) for the assay is prewarmed at 37°C.

Prothrombinase activity is measured by adding the various components of the complex to the 325 μl platelet incubation mixture of *Protocol 2*. It is recommended to maintain stirring during the prothrombinase assay.

Method

1. Add 50 μl Xa/Va mixture (0°C) to platelet suspension and incubate for 1 min to allow assembly of the enzyme complex at available binding sites.

2. Add 125 μl prothrombin solution (37°C) to start the prothrombinase reaction.

3. Stop reaction at fixed time interval (see note) by transferring 25 μl aliquot to a disposable cuvette containing 1 ml cuvette buffer and mix carefully. This will arrest thrombin production due to complexation of Ca^{2+} ions by EDTA which causes dissociation of the prothrombinase complex.

4. Add 50 μl chromogenic substrate solution to cuvette and mix thoroughly (use Parafilm and shake well).

5. Place cuvette in spectrophotometer and monitor the rate of change in absorbance at 405 nm, resulting from production of *p*-nitroaniline.

6. Construct calibration curve by taking 25 µl aliquots from serial dilutions of a solution of thrombin of well defined concentration and proceed from step 4. Use calibration curve to read the concentration of thrombin in the 25 µl aliquot taken in step 3.

Note:

(a) Depending on the procoagulant activity of the platelet suspensions, thrombin formation is allowed for various periods of time. For suspensions of unstimulated platelets, at the prothrombinase conditions described in this protocol, it is recommendable to allow thrombin production for at least 2 min. For platelets which express maximal procoagulant activity (e.g. after stimulation with ionophore or using platelet lysates), thrombin formation for 1 min will be sufficient to obtain sufficiently high readings.

(b) In particular for the detection of the 'basal' procoagulant activity of non-activated platelets, it is important to correct prothrombinase activities for the rate of thrombin formation in absence of any phospholipid surface. This can be done by replacing 300 µl platelet suspension in *Protocol 2*, step 1 by 300 µl buffer B.

(c) Because of surface activity of coagulation proteins, all reactions are performed in disposable plastic tubes or cuvettes. The Teflon coated stirring bars are cleaned in a mixture of sulfuric acid : hydrogen peroxide (1 : 1, v/v) (caution!) for 15 min, and subsequently rinsed (five times) in distilled water, followed by 96% ethanol.

3.2 Quantitating procoagulant activity and correction for cell lysis

Procoagulant activity of platelets (or other cell membranes) is not exclusively dependent on the amount of surface exposed PS. Other lipids such as phosphatidylethanolamine and sphingomyelin have modulating effects. Therefore, quantitating procoagulant activity of platelets in terms of molar fractions PS being exposed is not feasible. In general, however, the rate of thrombin formation is proportional to the amount of PS exposed. Since lysis of platelets will cause exposure of PS present in the inner leaflet of the plasma membrane as well as the membranes of intracellular organelles, it is important to check for cell integrity under various conditions of platelet activation. Lysis can be quantified enzymatically by measuring lactate dehydrogenase according to standard procedures (12). Correction for the contribution of lysed cells to the procoagulant activity of a suspension of stimulated platelets can be made by measuring prothrombinase activities of serial dilutions of completely lysed platelets (obtained by freeze–thawing). It

Table 1. Prothrombinase activities of washed (stimulated) platelets

Platelet activator	Prothrombinase activity (nM thrombin/min)
None	34
ADP (10 µM)	36
Thrombin (4 nM)	40
Collagen (10 µg/ml)	98
Collagen plus thrombin	351
Diamide (5 mM)	356
A23187 (1 µM)	843

should be emphasized that right side out resealing of membranes from lysed cells may lead to an overestimation of the contribution of lysis in the procoagulant activity.

Table 1 shows a typical example of prothrombinase activities obtained following the above mentioned protocols. It should be noted that the activity of the unstimulated platelets may vary from one preparation to another. This could reflect individual differences between different donors or indicate different extents of either platelet lysis or activation due to the isolation procedure. In addition, minor differences in observed activities may arise from the use of different preparations of coagulation factors.

For rapid screening of various blood samples or when isolation of platelets is undesirable, for instance when platelets are hyperreactive (e.g. platelets from Bernard–Soulier patients), one may consider to use 1 : 30 or 1 : 50 diluted platelet-rich plasma to measure prothrombinase activity (13).

3.3 Purification of factor Va and determination of its activity

Protocol 4. Purification of factor V

Equipment and reagents

- Anticoagulant: 0.1 M Na oxalate, 50 mM benzamidine, 10^5 U/litre heparin—dissolve soybean trypsin inhibitor (1 g/litre) immediately before use
- PEG 6000: dissolve 500 g PEG 6000 in water to a final volume of 1 litre
- Buffer C: 0.02 M Tris, 0.1 M NaCl pH 7.5
- Buffer D: 0.02 M Tris, 0.2 M NaCl, 1 mM benzamidine pH 7.3
- Buffer E: 0.02 M Tris, 0.4 M NaCl, 10 mM benzamidine pH 7.5
- Oxalate–phosphate buffer: 0.02 M Tris, 0.15 M Na oxalate, 0.04 M K_2HPO_4, 0.04 M KH_2PO_4 pH 7.3
- 2 M $CaCl_2$
- 0.02 M Tris, 0.1 M NaCl, 5 mM $CaCl_2$ pH 7.5
- Ca oxalate elution buffer: 0.2 M K_2HPO_4, 0.2 M KH_2PO_4, 10 mM benzamidine pH 7.0
- 0.02 M Tris, 0.01 M benzamidine pH 7.4
- ACA column buffer: 0.05 M Tris, 0.4 M NaCl, 10 mM benzamidine pH 7.4
- 0.05 M Tris, 0.1 M NaCl pH 7.5
- Strong anion exchanger, QAE–Sephadex (Pharmacia LKB)
- Gel filtration medium, Ultrogel ACA-22 (Pharmacia LKB)
- $BaSO_4$

- Nylon cloth
- Bench-top centrifuge
- $(NH_4)_2SO_4$
- ACA-22 gel filtration column (5 x 90 cm)

Method

1. Collect bovine blood from the local slaughterhouse. Be sure to discard the first litre to avoid activation of clotting factors. Collect the blood in anticoagulant in a ratio of 9 vol. of blood to 1 vol. of anticoagulant.

2. Centrifuge the blood for 15 min at 1000 g at 4°C and collect plasma.

3. Add 75 g of solid $BaSO_4$ per litre to the plasma while continuously stirring. Continue stirring for 30 min at 4°C.

4. Slowly add 100 ml of PEG 6000 (50%, w/v) for each litre of $BaSO_4$–plasma while stirring. Stir for another 15 min at 4°C.

5. Remove the precipitate by centrifugation (at 4°C) for 15 min at 1000 g.

6. Swell QAE–Sephadex in buffer C one day before use. Replace the buffer once with fresh buffer. Add the QAE slurry to the supernatant obtained after $BaSO_4$–PEG adsorption and centrifugation of the plasma. For every litre of supernatant add an amount of slurry corresponding to 2.5 g of dry Sephadex powder.

7. Stir the mixture for 60 min at room temperature.

8. Allow the QAE–Sephadex to settle for 15 min before pouring it on to nylon cloth in a glass funnel (this allows most of the supernatant to run through the cloth before the flow rate decreases because of the Sephadex on the cloth). Transfer all the QAE–Sephadex to the funnel using buffer C.

9. Wash the QAE–Sephadex on the cloth with approx. 20 bed volumes of buffer C.

10. Resuspend the QAE–Sephadex in buffer C and pour into a wide bore column (*c.* 10 cm diameter).

11. Wash the column with buffer D until the green/blue colour is removed, leaving a yellowish column.

12. Elute the column with buffer E. Elution rates may vary from 0.1–0.2 ml/min/cm^2, so the actual rate depends on the width of the column. Collect fractions corresponding to about 5% of the bed volume. Pool the fractions containing factor V (determined as described in *Protocol 5*).

13. Mix the pooled fractions with an equal volume of oxalate–phosphate buffer, and add 2 M $CaCl_2$ slowly (under stirring, at room temperature) until a final concentration of 0.11 mM calcium is reached (58 ml/litre). Stir for 30 min.

14. Centrifuge at 1000 g for 20 min at 4°C to isolate the Ca oxalate precipitate which contains the bound factor V.

Protocol 4. *Continued*

15. After centrifugation wash the tubes with 0.02 M Tris, 0.1 M NaCl, 5 mM Ca^{2+} pH 7.5 without disturbing the pellet.

16. Resuspend the pellets in oxalate elution buffer to desorb factor V from the Ca oxalate precipitate. Stir for 30 min at 4°C.

17. Centrifuge for 15 min at 1000 *g* (4°C). Collect the supernatant and extract the pellet once more using the same procedure. Combine the supernatants.

18. Cool the supernatant on ice to 0°C and slowly add solid ammonium sulfate to 35% saturation (209 g $(NH_4)_2SO_4$/litre). Stir for 15 min at 0°C. If a precipitate forms, remove it by centrifugation (20 min, 1000 *g*, 4°C).

19. Add more ammonium sulfate to the supernatant, to reach 55% saturation (129 g/litre 35% supernatant).

20. Collect the precipitate by centrifugation (20 min, 1000 *g*, 4°C).

21. Dissolve the pellet in a minimal volume of 20 mM Tris, 10 mM benzamidine pH 7.4.

22. Remove insoluble material by centrifugation (10 min, 10000 *g*, 4°C).

23. Apply the solubilized precipitate to a ACA-22 gel filtration column, prepared and washed with ACA buffer (a column of 5 × 90 cm is sufficient for a sample of 40–50 ml). Elute the column with ACA buffer and collect fractions of about 0.5–1% of the bed volume. Check the collected fractions for OD_{280} and factor V activity (see *Protocol 6*).

24. Pool the fractions containing factor V and dialyse against 0.05 M Tris, 0.1 M NaCl pH 7.5.

25. After dialysis convert factor V into its active form, factor Va, by incubation for 15 min with 1 nM thrombin in the presence of 1 mM Ca^{2+}. Measure the concentration of the protein as described in *Protocol 6*. Bring to the desired concentration, and store the preparation at –70°C.

3.4 Determination of factor V concentration

After its purification, factor V is converted to factor Va by the action of thrombin as described in *Protocol 4*, step 25. Detection and standardization of factor V (Va) is based on prothrombinase activity measured in the presence of phospholipid vesicles and factor Xa. In this set-up, factor Va can be made rate limiting. Increasing amounts of factor Va will cause increased rates of thrombin formation until factor Xa becomes rate limiting. Given the concentration of factor Xa, the concentration of factor Va is determined based on a 1 : 1 stoichiometric complex of both proteins as described in the legend of *Figure 1*.

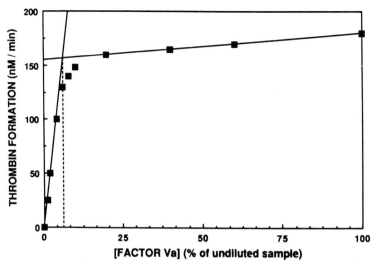

Figure 1. Determination of factor Va concentration. Relative concentration of factor Va is plotted against the thrombin formation rate. The projection on the *x* axis of the interception point of the two straight lines reflects the dilution (relative concentration) that is necessary to give a final concentration in the assay of 1 nM factor Va, i.e. equal to factor Xa. From this dilution, the actual Va concentration in the undiluted sample is calculated.

For the above mentioned prothrombinase assay, lipid vesicles composed of 80 mol% phosphatidylcholine (PC) and 20 mol% phosphatidylserine (PS) are used.

Protocol 5. Preparation of lipid vesicles

Equipment and reagents

- Phosphatidylcholine (PC) from egg yolk, dissolved in chloroform at 10 mg/ml
- Phosphatidylserine (PS) from bovine brain, dissolved in chloroform at 10 mg/ml
- Tris buffer: 0.05 M Tris, 0.12 M NaCl pH 7.5
- Tris/HSA buffer: 0.05 M Tris, 0.12 M NaCl, 0.5 mg/ml human serum albumin pH 7.5
- High speed centrifuge with 10 x 10 ml fixed-angle rotor
- Probe sonicator (7)

Method

1. Transfer 300 µl aliquot from PC stock and 75 µl aliquot from PS stock in chloroform to a glass tube to give a mixture containing 20 mol% PS and 80 mol% PC.

2. Evaporate the chloroform by a stream of nitrogen, leaving a thin film of the lipid mixture on the wall of the tube.

3. Add 5 ml Tris buffer *without* albumin to the tube. This will give a lipid concentration of about 1 mM.

Protocol 5. *Continued*

4. The lipids are dispersed by sonication (7). Use a probe-type sonicator. Sonicate at 150 W for 10 min. Cool the tube with tap-water (*c.* 15°C).

5. Centrifuge the sonicated preparation (10 min, 10 000 *g*) to remove large structures and metal particles.

6. Dilute the vesicle suspension to 0.5 µM with Tris/HSA buffer. Add CaCl$_2$ to a final concentration of 3 mM.

Protocol 6. Prothrombinase assay to measure factor Va concentration

1. Activate fractions to be tested (see *Protocol 4*) by incubation with 1 nM thrombin in the presence of 1 mM CaCl$_2$ for 15 min at 37°C to convert factor V into Va.

2. Make serial dilutions of the activated sample with Tris/HSA buffer.

3. Prepare phospholipid vesicles containing 20 mol% PS as described above.

4. Add 50 µl 10 nM factor Xa (final concentration 1 nM) and 10 µl of the dilutions of the fraction to be tested to 315 µl of the vesicle suspension.

5. Start the reaction by adding 125 µl prothrombin (final concentration 4 µM).

6. 1 min after addition of prothrombin transfer a sample of the incubation to a cuvette containing 1 ml of cuvette buffer, consisting of 120 mM NaCl, 50 mM Tris, 2 mM EDTA, adjusted at pH 7.9. The amount of thrombin formed is measured as described in the previous section on the prothrombinase assay.

7. Since factors Xa and Va are present in equimolar amounts in a functional prothrombinase complex, titrating factor Xa of a known concentration with different dilutions of an unknown Va sample allows determination of the concentration of factor Va in this sample (14). Briefly, prepare a curve by plotting the dilution factor (relative concentration) of the Va preparation versus the reaction rate, i.e. the amount of thrombin formed in 1 min (see *Figure 1*). Draw a line through the points at low Va concentration where the reaction velocity is linearly dependent on the amount of Va. Draw another line through the points of the curve where the Va concentration is high enough to make the reaction rate independent of the amount of Va. The intersection point of these lines corresponds to the dilution of the Va preparation which contains enough Va to saturate all Xa present, i.e. where Va and Xa are present in equimolar amounts. Since the Xa concentration is known, the Va concentration of the sample can be calculated.

4. Measurement of loss of platelet lipid asymmetry using Annexin V

4.1 Annexin V, a member of the multigene family of Annexins

Annexin V is a water soluble single chain protein of approximately 36 kDa. It belongs to a multigene family of proteins, the Annexins, that share structural and functional features (reviewed in refs 15–17). Annexins are defined by a repeated sequence motif, initially termed the endonexin loop (18), and a biological property to bind to phospholipids in a Ca^{2+}-dependent way.

Annexins belong to a class of amphipatic proteins, that localize intracellularly as well as in the extracellular space in mammals. In the absence of Ca^{2+} ions, they are water soluble whereas in the presence of Ca^{2+} ions they become membrane binding proteins. Annexin V was the first member with a resolved tertiary structure (19,20). In the absence of Ca^{2+} Annexin V shows abundant polar, charged amino acid residues on its surface. Annexin V can bind three Ca^{2+} ions at three distinct sites, which are believed to be directly involved in membrane binding. The interaction with the phospholipid membrane is postulated to occur through ligation of the Ca^{2+} ions with carboxyl and phosphoryl oxygens of amino acids and phospholipids, respectively (20). This type of interaction results in a binding of extrinsic nature and is completely reversed following removal of Ca^{2+} ions by for instance EDTA (21).

4.2 Annexin V binding to phosphatidylserine

In the presence of Ca^{2+} Annexin V binds with a high affinity ($K_d < 10^{-10}$ M) to synthetic phospholipid bilayers consisting of phosphatidylcholine and phosphatidylserine (PS) (22,23). The interaction of Annexin V with a PC/PS surface has a few unique characteristics.

(a) The Ca^{2+}-sensitivity is not an independent parameter of Annexin V but arises from the composition of the lipid surface. For instance the molar fraction of PS in the bilayer determines the Ca^{2+}-sensitivity of Annexin V binding (23). The higher the PS fraction, the lower the $[Ca^{2+}]$ required for maximal binding.

(b) During binding to the membrane Annexin V forms a two-dimensional lattice on the membrane surface (24). This phenomenon largely explains the high affinity of Annexin V towards a PS-containing surface and its competition with vitamin K-dependent coagulation factors for binding to the lipid surface.

The phospholipid binding of Annexin V is not restricted to PC surfaces comprising PS. Annexin V can also bind to PC surfaces which contain phosphatidylethanolamine (PE). However, the Ca^{2+}-sensitivity of binding to such surfaces is less than for binding to a PS-containing surface (23).

Annexin V appears to bind also to membranes of platelets, in which lipid asymmetry is lost in response to activation (25). The loss of lipid asymmetry is mainly characterized by an increase in surface exposed PS and PE. Binding of Annexin V to activated platelets may therefore occur to sites, which contain PS and/or PE. Several lines of evidence suggest that at Ca^{2+} levels below 2.5 mM, PS is the major site at the platelet surface to which Annexin V binds.

(a) The amount of Annexin V bound to activated platelets depends on the type of activator used in a similar way as the exposure of procoagulant phospholipids (25,26).

(b) Annexin V competes with factors Xa and Va for binding to the platelets (25,27) and thereby inhibits the activated platelet induced catalysis of prothrombin activation by these factors (24,27).

All these features make Annexin V an attractive tool to study the surface exposure of PS by platelets. This tool gains versatility and simplicity by the fact that Annexin V can be submitted to various conjugation procedures without impairing its phospholipid binding properties.

4.3 PS exposure by activated platelets as measured with Annexin V

4.3.1 Annexin V

Annexin V can either be purchased as a recombinant product from Bender Diagnostics or purified from human placenta.

A purification procedure of Annexin V is presented below. Considering purification it is noteworthy that Annexin V remains quite stable in homogenized tissues at physiological pH and temperatures below 25 °C. Loss of its phospholipid binding properties is observed at temperatures above 42 °C and at pH below 5.0. Freezing of the protein in acetate buffer of pH 5.2 will also destroy its phospholipid binding property.

The first purification steps take advantage of the Ca^{2+}-dependent phospholipid binding capacity to obtain a fraction enriched in Annexin V from placental homogenate. This fraction contains also other members of the Annexin family. These are separated from Annexin V by ion exchange chromatography.

Protocol 7. Purification of placental Annexin V

Equipment and reagents

- Buffer F: 50 mM Tris–HCl, 1 mM $CaCl_2$, 5 mM benzamidine, 100 µg/ml soybean trypsin inhibitor pH 7.9
- Buffer G: 15 mM Hepes–NaOH, 4 mM EDTA, 1 mM EGTA pH 7.5
- Buffer H: 50 mM Tris–HCl, 1 mM EDTA pH 7.8
- Buffer I: 50 mM Tris–HCl pH 7.8
- Buffer J: buffer I containing 1.0 M NaCl
- Buffer K: 25 mM Na acetate pH 5.2

- Buffer L: buffer K containing 0.5 M NaCl
- A fresh or frozen human placenta
- Braun MX32 mixer
- DEAE–Sepharose Fast Flow (Pharmacia Biotech)
- FPLC system and Mono Q and S column (Pharmacia Biotech)
- Centrifuge
- UV spectrophotometer

Method

1. Soak the placenta in ice-cold buffer F and remove the amnionic membrane and the umbilical cord. Cut the placenta with a pair of scissors in small pieces. Weigh 100 g of tissue pieces and homogenize these in 500 ml ice-cold buffer F with the Braun mixer for 15 min. Homogenize on ice.

2. Centrifuge the homogenate for 30 min at 20 000 g at 4 °C. Discard the supernatant and resuspend the pellet in 500 ml ice-cold buffer F using the Braun mixer.

3. Repeat step 2 three times. These washing steps remove proteins from the pellet that have no or weak interaction with the sedimenting structures during centrifugation.

4. Suspend the pellet of the last wash step in 100 ml ice-cold buffer G using the Braun mixer. Chelation of the Ca^{2+} ions by EDTA induces the release of the proteins, that bind Ca^{2+} dependently and reversibly to the pellet structures.

5. Centrifuge the suspension for 30 min at 20 000 g at 4 °C and keep the resulting supernatant. Resuspend the pellet in 100 ml of ice-cold buffer G using the Braun mixer and repeat the centrifugation step.

6. Combine both supernatants and dialyse overnight at 4–8 °C against 5 litres buffer H with continuous stirring. Change the buffer three times with intervals of at least 3 h.

7. From here on the steps are performed at ambient temperature unless indicated otherwise. During chromatography with the FPLC, ice is put in the fraction collector to chill the eluting fractions.

8. Wash 100 ml of DEAE–Sepharose at least ten times, with 200 ml of buffer I each time, in order to equilibrate the resin with this buffer. Add the dialysed solution of step 6 to the washed DEAE–Sepharose and swirl gently to mix. Continue mixing for 30 min. Pour the suspension of beads into a column with adaptors that can be connected to an FPLC system. Do this fractionwise and each time before the beads have settled completely in order to obtain a continuous packing.

9. Fill pump A and B with respectively buffer I and J and mount the column to the FPLC system. Start with 100% A at a flow of 2 ml/min and wash the column until the optical density at 280 nm reaches basal levels. Apply a linear gradient of 0.25% B/ml at a flow rate of

Protocol 7. *Continued*

2 ml/min. Start collecting fractions of 5 ml when 10% B elutes from the column. (Note that during the gradient the actual per cent B at the outlet of the column is different from the value indicated by your controller.) Annexin V elutes with 15% to 20% B from the column.

10. Pool the Annexin V-containing fractions and dialyse overnight at 4–8°C against buffer H. Determine roughly protein contents of the dialysed fraction by adsorption measurements at 280 nm.

11. The FPLC pumps are still filled with buffer I (pump A) and J (pump B). Equilibrate the Mono Q column with buffer I. Load maximally 20 mg of protein on the Mono Q column with a flow rate of 1 ml/min at 0% B. If the pressure exceeds the limit value for the Mono Q column, the flow rate should be decreased. Keep washing with 0% B until the optical density at 280 nm approaches basal values. Then apply a linear gradient of 2% B/ml. Start collecting fractions of 0.5 ml when 15% B is eluting from the column. Annexin V elutes with 17.5% to 19% B from the column.

12. Pool the Annexin V-containing fractions and dialyse overnight at 4–8°C against buffer K.

13. Fill pump A with buffer K and pump B with buffer L. Equilibrate the Mono S column with buffer K. Load the dialysed fraction on the Mono S column with a flow rate of 1 ml/min. Keep washing with 100% A until the optical density at 280 nm is back at the basal level. Then apply a gradient of 2% B/ml. Start collecting fractions of 0.5 ml when 15% B is eluting from the column. Annexin V elutes as a single peak around 20% B.

14. Pool the peak fractions. This peak is homogeneous for Annexin V, that appears as a single 32 kDa band with SDS–PAGE under reducing and non-reducing conditions. Under non-reducing conditions some dimer will be formed spontaneously in the presence of SDS.

15. The described procedure yields approx. 2 mg of Annexin V. If stored below −20°C in a buffer with a pH of 7–8 the protein will be stable for at least two years.

4.3.2 Annexin V–FITC

Annexin V can be tagged easily with isothiocyanate derivatized compounds. The protein contains 22 lysine residues, three of which are located within the three Ca^{2+} binding sites that are directly involved in phospholipid binding.

Conjugation of Annexin V with isothiocyanate derivatized compounds at pH 9.0, however, does not result in detectable loss of its phospholipid binding property, indicating that these three lysine residues are not readily accessible to the isothiocyanate compounds. *Protocol 8* outlines a simple procedure to obtain Annexin V–FITC.

Protocol 8. Conjugation of Annexin V with fluorescein

Equipment and reagents

- Buffer M: 50 mM sodium borate–NaOH, 150 mM NaCl, 1 mM EDTA pH 9.0
- Buffer O: 50 mM Tris–HCl, 80 mM NaCl, 1 mM EDTA pH 8.0
- FPLC system and a Mono Q column (Pharmacia Biotech)
- Fluorescein isothiocyanate (FITC) isomer I (F-7250, Sigma)
- Buffer N: 1 M glycine in water
- Micro BCA protein determination kit (Pierce Chemicals bv)
- Recombinant or human placental Annexin V (*Protocol 7*)
- Amber coloured microcentrifuge tubes (Biozym)

Method

1. Dialyse 5 ml of 1.8 mg Annexin V/ml overnight against buffer M at 4–8°C.

2. Dissolve 8 mg FITC in 10 ml buffer M. Add 125 μl of this solution to the 5 ml of dialysed Annexin V solution. Incubate the mixture for 2 h at 37°C. The isothiocyanate group reacts under this condition with primary amino groups of Annexin V to yield a covalent bond between Annexin V and fluorescein.

3. Add 50 μl of buffer N to stop the coupling reaction and to neutralize the unreacted FITC.

4. Dialyse the sample overnight against buffer O at 4–8°C.

5. Fill pump A and B of the FPLC system with buffer I and J (see *Protocol 7*) respectively. Equilibrate the Mono Q column with buffer I.

6. Apply the dialysed sample to the Mono Q column with a flow rate of 1 ml/min at 0% B. Wash with 5 ml at 0% B. Apply a gradient of 2% B/ml. Unconjugated Annexin V elutes around 18% B. The conjugated forms of Annexin V elute with higher per cent B.

7. Analyse the eluted peaks by protein determination according to the suppliers protocol of the micro BCA kit, and by absorption measurement in a 1 cm cuvette at 492 nm. Calculate the fluorescein concentration by using the extinction coefficient of 78 000/M/cm. These analyses give the stoichiometry of the Annexin V–FITC complex. The peak eluting around 22% B and immediately following the peak with unconjugated Annexin V contains the 1 : 1 complex.

8. Pool the peak fractions and dialyse overnight against buffer P. Determine protein contents by the micro BCA method. Divide the dialysed sample in portions, which contain enough material for one set of experiments and store in the amber coloured microcentrifuge tubes at −20°C. Repeated thawing–freezing will cause loss of activity.

4.3.3 Flow cytometry

The binding of Annexin V–FITC to the platelet surface can be easily assessed by means of flow cytometry. Any microparticles formed during the activation procedure can also be evaluated for Annexin V–FITC binding. It should be emphasized once more that Annexin V binding to a particle not necessarily implies PS exposure. Annexin V has also an affinity for PE (see Section 4.2). Hence, increased binding of Annexin V to platelets and microparticles may arise from increased exposure of PE as well. The affinity of Annexin V for a specific phospholipid species depends on the Ca^{2+} ion concentration. Variation of the Ca^{2+} ion level, thus, offers the possibility to tune Annexin V's preferences of binding. At less then 2.5 mM Ca^{2+}, indirect evidence indicates a preferential binding of Annexin V to surface exposed PS. However, under these conditions binding to PE has not been fully excluded as yet. *Protocol 9* describes a method in the presence of 1.8 mM Ca^{2+} ions. At this level Annexin V binding correlates very well with the expression of procoagulant sites as function of the type of activator.

Protocol 9 outlines in detail a method using the FACSort apparatus of Becton Dickinson. The presented settings are therefore specific to this apparatus and should be adjusted for other flow cytometers. The reader is referred to Chapter 6 of this book and ref. 28 for comprehensive treatises of the technique of flow cytometry.

Protocol 9. Flow cytometric analysis of Annexin V binding to platelets and microparticles

Equipment and reagents

- Washed platelets (*Protocol 1*) suspended at 10^8/ml
- Annexin V–FITC 312 µg/ml (*Protocol 8*)
- Mouse anti-CD42b (GPIb) conjugated to phycoerythrine (PhE) (Dako-CD42b, AN51) (Dako)
- Polystyrene tubes (Falcon 2058, Becton Dickinson)
- Buffer P: 10 mM Hepes–NaOH, 150 mM NaCl, 1.8 mM $CaCl_2$, 5 mM KCl, 1 mM $MgCl_2$, 5 mM dextrose pH 7.4
- FACSort (Becton Dickinson)
- Collagen (1 mg/ml) (Horm)
- Human alpha thrombin (200 nM)
- Ca^{2+} ionophore A23187 (250 µM)

Method

1. Activation of the FACSort for data acquisition. Turn both the FACSort and the computer on. The FACSort is at stand-by. Make sure that the left container has sufficient sheath fluid and that the right waste container is empty. Load the Lysys II program. Activate ACQ (acquisition) under Lys. Open 4 small boxes under Format, and Detectors and Parameters under Instr-Ctrl. Set in the window FACSort Detectors thresholds for FSC-H and FL2-H at respectively 20 and 180, FSC at E01, SSC at 425, and both FL1 and FL2 at 550. Choose in the window

FACSort Parameters the logarthimic scales for FSC-H, SSC-H, FL1-H, and FL2-H. Open Show Protocol under Protocol. Define ID and file name of the experiment. Set the number of events at 10 000 counts.

2. Preparation of the platelet sample. Dilute 10 µl of the washed platelets with 480 µl buffer P. Add 10 µl buffer P or 10 µl activators (5 µl collagen plus 5 µl thrombin or 10 µl ionophore) and stir the suspension. After 10 min of activation add 2 µl of anti-CD42b-PhE and incubate for 10 min in the dark at room temperature. Then add 8 µl Annexin V–FITC, continue the incubation for another 10 min in the dark at room temperature.

3. FL2 threshold setting. The anti-CD42b-PhE is added in order to be able to set a threshold value so as to collect and store events for off line analysis that contain GPIb above a certain level. The position of the threshold is very important because it determines which events are stored or ignored. The investigator can choose for another platelet surface antigen as a discriminator to collect or ignore events for off line analysis.

   Switch the FACSort to run position and choose the low rate option. Transfer a suspension of unactivated platelets (see step 2) to a polystryrene tube and position it under the needle of the FACSort. Double click Begin in acquire box and increase and decrease the FL2 threshold within the FACSort Parameter window continuously. Observe the FL1-H versus FL2-H box. Two clouds of events become distinguishable. A cloud of events with low FL2 signal and one with high FL2 signal. Position the threshold such that the top part of the first cloud remains visible. Hence, the threshold value is arbitrary and may vary for each set of experiments. Choose within the 4 boxes window acq mode normal. Begin acquisition.

4. Analysis of the data. Activate LYS (analysis) under Lys. Open region tools and Gates Specs under gates. Create window and get histogram FL2-H of the file with data of the unactivated platelets. Define the region GP1b positive (G1) by positioning the left limit at the start of the peak and the right limit at the right end of the abscissa. Create window and get histogram FL1-H of the file with data of the unactivated platelets. Define the region Annexin V positive (G2) by positioning the left limit at the end of the peak and the right limit at the right end of the abscissa. Having defined regions G1 and G2 the data of the files can be analysed for Annexin V binding to particles with either none/low GP1b or high GP1b expression. *Figure 2* illustrates an analysis of an experiment in which unactivated platelets, collagen plus thrombin activated platelets, and Ca^{2+} ionophore-stimulated platelets measured by flow cytometry according to this protocol.

SELECTED PREFERENCES: Arithmetic/Linear

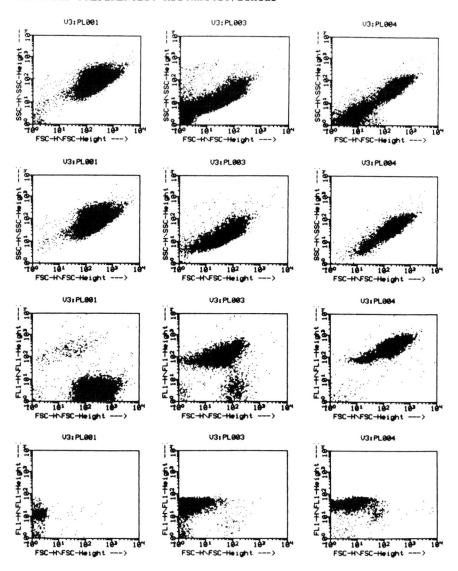

Figure 2. Analysis of flow cytometric data of platelets, that were either unactivated (left column), collagen plus thrombin stimulated (middle column), or Ca^{2+} ionophore stimulated (right column). The first row shows the forward and side scatter of ungated particles. Collagen plus thrombin and Ca^{2+} ionophore stimulation induced the formation of particles with low forward and side scatter (microparticles). The second row shows the forward and side scatter of the G1 gated particles. It can be seen that most of the microparticles have disappeared by this gating procedure, indicating that they contain no or low amounts of GP1b. The third row shows forward scatter and Annexin V–FITC of G1 gated particles. Most unactivated platelets bind no or low amounts of Annexin V. Collagen plus thrombin and Ca^{2+} ionophore stimulation increase the binding of Annexin V. Increased binding is observed for the platelets and the microparticles. The fourth row shows forward scatter and Annexin V–FITC of the 'not G1' particles. Most microparticles with no or low GP1b bind Annexin V. With region statistics the mean fluorescence intensity data of the various regions can be retrieved. *Table 2* shows the statistics of the experiment illustrated by *Figure 2*.

Table 2. Statistical analysis of the data from the experiment of *Figure 2*

Platelet sample	Gate	Annexin V positive population (G2)		Annexin V negative population (not G2)	
		Mean population fluorescence	Per cent of total gated events	Mean population fluorescence	Per cent of total gated events
Control	G1	519	3	3.3	97
Coll + IIa	G1	160	89	7.2	11
A23187	G1	380	99	3.8	1
Control	Not G1	20	48	4.4	52
Coll + IIa	Not G1	35	82	3.6	18
A23187	Not G1	41	92	3.1	8

References

1. Rosing, J., Tans, G., Govers-Riemslag, J. W. P., Zwaal, R. F. A., and Hemker, H. C. (1980). *J. Biol. Chem.*, **255**, 274.
2. Nesheim, M. E., Taswell, J. B., and Mann, K. G. (1979). *J. Biol. Chem.*, **254**, 10952.
3. Gilbert, G. E. and Drinkwater, D. (1993). *Biochemistry*, **32**, 9577.
4. Comfurius, P., Smeets, E. F., Willems, G. M., Bevers, E. M., and Zwaal, R. F. A. (1994). *Biochemistry*, **33**, 10319.
5. Mann, K. G., Nesheim, M. E., Church, W. R., Haley, P., and Krishnaswamy, S. (1990). *Blood*, **76**, 1.
6. Schroit, A. J. and Zwaal, R. F. A. (1991). *Biochim. Biophys. Acta*, **1071**, 313.
7. Devaux, P. F. (1991). *Biochemistry*, **30**, 1163.
8. Connor, J. and Schroit, A. J. (1988). *Biochemistry*, **27**, 848.
9. Sims, P. J., Wiedmer, T., Esmon, C. T., Weiss, H. J., and Shattil, S. J. (1989). *J. Biol. Chem.*, **264**, 17049.

10. Owen, W. G., Esmon, C. T., and Jackson, C. M. (1974). *J. Biol. Chem.*, **249,** 594.
11. Fujikawa, K., Legaz, M. E., and Davie, E. W. (1972). *Biochemistry*, **11,** 4892.
12. Wroblewski, R. and La Due, J. S. (1955). *Proc. Soc. Exp. Biol. Med.*, **90,** 210.
13. Bevers, E. M., Comfurius, P., Nieuwenhuis, H. K., Levy-Toledano, S., Enouf, J., Belluci, S., *et al.* (1986). *Br. J. Haematol.*, **63,** 335.
14. Lindhout, T., Govers-Riemslag, J. W. P., van de Waart, P., Hemker, H. C., and Rosing, J. (1982). *Biochemistry*, **21,** 5495.
15. Crompton, M. R., Moss, S. E., and Crumpton, M. J. (1988). *Cell*, **55,** 1.
16. Klee, C. B. (1988). *Biochemistry*, **27,** 6645.
17. Creutz, C. E. (1992). *Science*, **258,** 924.
18. Geisow, M. J., Fritsche, V., Hexham, J. M., Dash, B., and Johnson, T. (1986). *Nature*, **320,** 636.
19. Huber, R., Römisch, J., and Paques, E.-P. (1990). *EMBO J.*, **9,** 3867.
20. Huber, R., Schneider, M., Mayr, I., Römisch, J., and Paques, E.-P. (1990). *FEBS Lett.*, **275,** 15.
21. Reutelingsperger, C. P. M., Kop, J. M. M., Hornstra, G., and Hemker, H. C. (1988). *Eur. J. Biochem.*, **173,** 171.
22. Andree, H. A. M., Reutelingsperger, C. P. M., Hauptman, R., Hemker, H. C., Hermens, W. Th., and Willems, G. M. (1990). *J. Biol. Chem.*, **265,** 4923.
23. Tait, J. F., Gibson, D., and Fujikawa, K. (1989). *J. Biol. Chem.*, **264,** 7944.
24. Andree, H. A. M., Stuart, M. C. A., Hermens, W. Th., Reutelingsperger, C. P. M., Hemker, H. C., Frederik, P. M., *et al.* (1992). *J. Biol. Chem.*, **267,** 17907.
25. Thiagarajan, P. and Tait, J. F. (1990). *J. Biol. Chem.*, **265,** 17420.
26. Comfurius, P., Bevers, E. M., and Zwaal, R. F. A. (1985). *Biochim. Biophys. Acta*, **815,** 143.
27. Thiagarajan, P. and Tait, J. F. (1991). *J. Biol. Chem.*, **266,** 24302.
28. Shapiro, H. M. (1988). *Practical flow cytometry*, 2nd edn. Alan R. Liss, Inc., New York.

The study of platelet function in other species

ALASTAIR W. POOLE

1. Introduction

Research into platelet function has largely concentrated upon human platelets for readily apparent reasons. There are however special reasons for the study of platelet function in other species. In particular *ex vivo* pharmacological and toxicological studies are undertaken in experimental animals, in addition to work involving animal models of human platelet-derived disease or work of primary veterinary interest.

This chapter will deal mainly with techniques used to obtain platelet preparations from the various domesticated and laboratory species. In addition information is given about species variation in surface receptor populations. This will enable the researcher to better choose the appropriate animal model for their area of research. Useful further reading for information about laboratory animal handling, including bleeding techniques, includes the recent report of a joint working group on refinement in laboratory animal techniques (1), and a newly published handbook of laboratory animal management (2).

2. Blood sampling techniques

There are several pertinent points to bear in mind when sampling blood from animals for platelet research.

(a) Bleeding is a potentially stressful procedure for the animal if not performed correctly. This is undesirable for two reasons. It is clear that minimizing the pain and distress which animals suffer is important. Moreover stress may also induce unpredictable changes in platelet function due to release of mediators such as adrenaline.

(b) Animals are generally less amenable to being bled than we are, and some form of restraint is usually required. Restraint may take the form of physical or chemical methods, the latter commonly involving general anaesthesia of the animal. The majority of substances used for anaesthesia however have some effect upon platelet function and should therefore be restricted to cases in which they are unavoidable. It is important that the animal is restrained gently by an experienced handler who, whenever possible, should be known to the animal. It is also important that blood withdrawal be performed skilfully and positively rather than hesitantly. It is recommended that the procedure be practised on cadavers so that the relevant anatomy becomes familiar to the operator in order to avoid repeated unsuccessful attempts resulting in undue stress to the animal.

(c) Most platelet functional studies require relatively large volumes of blood (> 1 ml). The total blood volume (TBV) of most animal species averages about 70 ml/kg (see *Table 1* for details of animal TBVs) and it is recommended that no more than 10% of the TBV be taken in any one sampling procedure and that no more than 15% TBV should be taken during a four-week period. For these reasons, enough blood is obtained from the small mammals (rats, mice, and guinea-pigs) only by inducing euthanasia through exsanguination. Most other experimental animals however have TBVs large enough to accommodate being bled on a regular basis.

2.1 Blood sampling from small mammals

Protocol 1 describes the procedure for blood sampling from small mammals (mice, rats, and guinea-pigs) by exsanguination under terminal general anaesthesia. Schedule 1 of the United Kingdom Animals (Scientific Procedures) Act 1986 lists standard methods of humane killing of laboratory animals, for which neither a project nor a personal licence is required. It is however required that the operator be competent to carry out the killing without causing undue distress to the animals involved. The methods include overdose of volatile anaesthetic agent, concussion by striking the back of the head, and exposure to a rising concentration of carbon dioxide, all followed by exsanguination. For the purposes of assessment of platelet function, the procedure should minimize unwanted effects from the anaesthetic upon these cells and therefore the latter two methods become the procedures of choice for sampling from mice, rats, and guinea-pigs.

Protocol 1. Euthanasia of small mammals by exposure to CO_2 followed by exsanguination by cardiac puncture[a]

Equipment and reagents

- Carbon dioxide restraining chamber[b] (International Market Supply Ltd)
- 21 gauge 1.5 inch needle
- Carbon dioxide cylinder (BOC Ltd)
- Collection pot, e.g. 25 ml Universal (Bibby Sterilin)
- Anticoagulant (see Chapter 1 and below)

Method

1. Place the animal in the chamber and turn on the flow of carbon dioxide (2–3 litres/min is sufficient). Ensure that the carbon dioxide concentration is atmospheric when the animal is placed in the chamber and allow it to rise slowly. The animal gradually becomes hypoxic and loses consciousness.

2. Exsanguinate the unconscious animal by placing it on its right side in the chamber and puncturing the left ventricle using a 21 gauge 1.5 inch needle passed through the sixth intercostal space, one-third of the way up the chest from the sternum.

3. Collect the blood into the collection pot with appropriate anticoagulant.

4. Wash out and invert the chamber after use so as to tip out residual carbon dioxide. This is important, since if animals are subsequently placed in the chamber when the CO_2 concentration is too high, they will rapidly exhibit respiratory distress and discomfort before unconsciousness ensues.

[a] This method is suitable for the euthanasia of rodents over ten-days-old and under 1.5 kg.
[b] Use a suitable chamber so that the animal may be easily observed throughout the procedure, and which can be easily and thoroughly cleaned so as to remove all faeces and urine which may contain pheromones by which the animals communicate fear. Also for this reason, it is important that animals are removed to a room away from their group before being killed, so as not to stress the other animals.

2.2 Blood sampling from larger mammals

Under the United Kingdom Animals (Scientific Procedures) Act 1986, the sampling of blood from live animals requires both a personal and project licence. *Protocol 2* describes the general procedure for regular blood sampling from larger species, with specific comments for each species made in the following paragraphs. Light physical restraint is all that is required for this procedure. Many animals can be trained to accept the handling necessary to take blood samples, and although this training process is initially time-consuming, it is worthwhile as an investment for the future. In some circumstances frequent repeated blood samples may be required over a period of 24–48 hours, and in this case cannulation of the vein is preferred to repeated venepuncture. This procedure will not be described, but is adequately dealt with elsewhere (2,3).

Protocol 2. General technique for blood sampling of larger laboratory species

Equipment and reagents
- Syringe (10, 20, or 50 ml, e.g. Becton Dickinson Ltd)
- Needle (see Section 2.2.1)
- Anticoagulant (see Chapter 1 and below)
- Ethanol (70%)

Method
1. Clip up the sampling site,[a] clean with warm water, and dry before swabbing with 70% ethanol.
2. Fill the syringe with the appropriate quantity of anticoagulant (see below) and firmly attach a needle of an appropriate size to the syringe.
3. Raise the vein by applying light pressure to the thoracic inlet with the thumb of one hand whilst holding the syringe and needle in the other. Insert the needle in the direction of the animal's head, bevel uppermost, into the vein at an angle of approximately 30° to the skin. Once in the lumen, a drop of blood will appear at the hub of the needle, at which point advance the needle at a shallower angle, almost parallel to the skin.
4. *Slowly* draw back on the syringe to extract the blood.[b]
5. After taking the sample, withdraw the needle from the vein and apply gentle pressure to the site for 30–60 sec to prevent haemorrhage. Do not apply pressure until the needle is fully removed, otherwise it is possible to lacerate the vessel.

[a] With the exception of the rabbit and pig (details for these species below), the jugular vein is the preferred site for bleeding. A site half-way from thoracic inlet to the angle of the jaw is suitable and minimizes the risk of puncturing vital structures.
[b] Platelets respond to shear stress and the greater the pressure applied to draw the syringe, the greater the turbulence of the blood flow, and the more likely it is that platelets will be activated by the procedure. For this reason also, bleeding using evacuated tubes, although convenient, is not recommended for platelet studies.

2.2.1 Choice of needle

The required needle size varies with species. In order to minimize the pressure required to draw the syringe, the needle length should be the minimum required to access the vein (usually 1–1.5 inches, except in pigs) and the gauge should be as large as possible. There is however an upper limit on needle gauge so as to avoid excessive damage to the lining of a frequently bled vessel. As a guide-line, the recommended maximum diameter of needles used to regularly bleed rabbits should be 23 gauge, for dogs, cats, and sheep it should be 21 gauge, whilst for pigs, cattle, and horses it should be 19 gauge. For larger blood samples from the larger species (pig, ox, and horse) however, where the maximum allowable single bleed (10% of TBV) may be several litres, needles of greater diameter (12 or 14 gauge) will be necessary so as to acquire the blood within a reasonable period of time. In this case local anaesthetic (e.g. lignocaine, Astra) should be infiltrated intradermally at the site 10 min prior to venepuncture or alternatively a local anaesthetic cream (e.g. EMLA, Astra) may be applied 30–60 min prior to venepuncture so as to prevent discomfort. For convenience, bleeding into standard blood packs (Tuta Laboratories) is recommended since the needle is directly sealed on to the collection tubing, allowing collection of large volumes by gravity. If volumes larger than the pack size (500 ml) are required, the set may be modified by cutting the bag from the tubing and collecting the blood into a larger container with anticoagulant already present.

2.3 Special species considerations

2.3.1 Rabbit

For the rabbit, blood may be collected from the marginal ear vein using a 23 gauge over-the-needle cannula or butterfly needle and blood allowed to drip into a collection pot with anticoagulant. Bleeding from the central ear artery is possible but is not recommended as it can lead to the development of a large haematoma with consequent ear damage and potential necrosis of the ear.

2.3.2 Pig

The pig is probably the most difficult of the domesticated species to bleed since it has no large peripheral vein. The cranial vena cava is therefore the preferred site for bleeding and is accessed using a long needle (19 gauge, 3 inch) inserted in the thoracic inlet and passed caudally at a slight dorso-medial angle to enter the vein.

2.3.3 Horse

Horses are commonly 'needle-shy' and may move violently upon insertion of the needle. For this reason it may be preferable to insert the needle (19 gauge, 1–1.5 inch) in the vein prior to attaching the syringe. This precaution is rarely necessary however if the horse is trained to accept the needle.

2.3.4 Dog, cat, and bovine

Blood may be drawn from dogs and cats using the cephalic vein. Cattle may also be bled from the ventral coccygeal vein.

3. Preparation of platelet suspensions

The anticoagulant of choice for blood collection in most of the laboratory species is sodium citrate (0.11 M or 3.8% (w/v) solution; 1 : 9 citrate vol. :

Table 1. Characteristics of animal blood and platelet preparation[a]

Species	Blood volume (ml)	Platelet count (whole blood) (x 10^3 /mm^3)	Mean platelet volume (fl)	PRP preparation centrifugation
Human	5000–7000	200–400	6.7	200 *g*, 15 min
Mouse	1.3–2.7	160–410	3.3	250 *g*, 10 min
Rat	18–30	500–1300	4.7	250 *g*, 10 min
Guinea-pig	58–85	250–850	4.5	250 *g*, 10 min
Rabbit	60–350	250–270	3.3	250 *g*, 10 min
Dog (Beagle)	900–1400	200–900	7.5	180 *g*, 15 min
Cat	140–200	300–700	12.0	180 *g*, 15 min
Sheep	3000–4500	300–600	4.4	400 *g*, 20 min
Pig (Large White)	13 000–15 500	350–700	6.9	200 *g*, 15 min
Bovine	30 000–50 000	100–800	5.0	400 *g*, 20 min
Horse	20 000–50 000	120–360	5.1	160 *g*, 15 min

[a] Note that a safe volume for a single bleed is 10% of the total blood volume, that the total blood volume is approximately 70 ml/kg body weight, and that the final bleed out volume for the small laboratory species is approximately 50% of the total blood volume.

blood vol.). Exceptions to this rule apply in the case of the dog and rat. Canine platelets are notoriously variable in their responsiveness and for this reason a higher concentration of sodium citrate has been recommended (0.18 M or 6.2% (w/v) solution; 1 : 9 citrate vol. : blood vol.) which is reported to reduce this variability (4). Rat platelet responses are, on the other hand, reduced often to nil in the presence of citrate, and it is therefore recommended that they should be anticoagulated either with heparin (15 U/ml blood) or that the citrate concentration be reduced (0.09 M or 3.0% (w/v) solution; 1 : 9 citrate vol. : blood vol.).

Preparation of platelet-rich plasma from blood is a one-step centrifugation procedure as for human platelet preparation. The sedimentation rate of blood cells from different species varies and optimal centrifugation parameters are given in *Table 1*.

4. Platelet surface receptor populations: pertinent species comparisons

Amongst the range of platelet agonists and responses, there are some generalizations which apply to platelets from all species.

(a) All animal platelets respond to thrombin and collagen by undergoing shape change, aggregation, and release of granule contents.

(b) In some species (rodents and carnivores) the arachidonic acid pathway is well developed, whereas in the larger domesticated species this pathway is rudimentary.

Table 2. Effect of common mediators upon animal platelet function

Species	PAF	AA	5-HT	ADP	ATP	Adrenaline
Human	Ir	Ir	R	Ir	Antag	Var
Mouse	X	Ir	–	Ir	–	P
Rat	X	Ir	P	Ir	Ir	P
Guinea-pig	Ir	Ir	X	Ir	Ir	X
Rabbit	Ir	Ir	R	R	Antag	P
Dog	–	Var	Ir/R	Ir	Antag	Var (Ir, P)
Cat	–	Ir	Ir	Ir	–	Ir, P
Sheep	–	–	P	Ir	–	X
Pig	Ir	X	–	R	–	X
Bovine	Ir	SC	P	Ir	–	X
Horse	Ir	R	R	Ir	–	X

Ir, irreversible aggregation; R, reversible aggregation; SC, shape change only; P, potentiatory action only; Antag, antagonist of ADP response; Var, variable response; X, no effect. Note that all animal platelets respond to thrombin and collagen by undergoing shape change, irreversible aggregation and release of dense granule contents.

(c) ADP is a universal agonist, whereas 5-HT, the other dense granule constituent, has a potentiatory role except in carnivores where it acts as a potent agonist in its own right.

(d) PAF may play an important role in the larger domesticated species and rabbits and guinea-pigs, but has no role in rats and mice.

(e) Platelet function in all species is inhibited by prostacyclin.

A brief description follows of major differences between species regarding platelet ultrastructure, receptor population, and signalling pathways, in particular in comparison to human platelets. This is not intended to be a review of the literature but merely to emphasize the differences in platelet structure and function in different species so as to enable the researcher to select an experimental species with appropriate knowledge of its special idiosyncrasies. *Table 2* summarizes the functional differences detailed below.

4.1 Rat

(a) Although ADP induces irreversible aggregation of rat platelets, ATP is also an agonist and the response to ADP is unaffected by AMP (4).

(b) 5-HT induces no direct response in rat platelets, although it does potentiate responses to other agonists.

(c) The thromboxane pathway is well developed since rat platelets form relatively large quantities of TxB_2 upon stimulation and respond to arachidonic acid by irreversibly aggregating. There is however breed variation in the response to AA, with the sensitivity in rank order NBR > Hoffman > Sprague-Dawley = Lewis.

(d) Rat platelets, like mouse platelets, are unresponsive to platelet activating factor.

(e) Adrenaline is only capable of potentiating responses to other agonists rather than inducing activation in its own right. Rat platelets possess both α_2 and β_2 adrenoceptors (5,6).

(f) Unlike most other species except the rabbit, free extracellular fibrinogen is not required for aggregation of rat platelets induced by ADP (7).

(g) Kinlough-Rathbone *et al.* (8) and Cook *et al.* (9) also found that despite potent activation of rat platelets by thrombin, the free thrombin receptor peptide (TRP; SFLLRNPNDKYEPF) derived from the human thrombin receptor sequence induced no activation of rat platelets.

(h) Measurement of cytosolic calcium in rat platelets using fura-2 is hampered by a plasma factor which inhibits loading of the dye in its acetoxymethyl ester form (10). Loading of the dye takes place satisfactorily however in washed platelets or platelets resuspended in heat treated plasma.

4.2 Guinea-pig

(a) ADP and ATP both induce irreversible platelet aggregation which is commonly biphasic in nature.

(b) Guinea-pig platelets are exquisitely sensitive to PAF, responding maximally to concentrations as low as 100 pM (11).

4.3 Rabbit

(a) The secretable fraction of adenine nucleotides in rabbit platelets is high (> 4 μmol/10^{11} platelets) and in common with human platelets, the ADP response in rabbit platelets is inhibited by both ATP and AMP.

(b) Rabbit platelets have the largest secretable pool of 5-HT of any of the domesticated species, and unusually their dense granules also contain secretable histamine.

(c) Rabbit platelets synthesize relatively large quantities of TxB_2 upon stimulation, and AA induces irreversible platelet aggregation.

(d) As for the rat however, although thrombin is a potent activator of rabbit platelets, the human thrombin receptor peptide induces no response (8).

(e) Rabbit platelets lack Fc receptors for IgG, unlike human platelets, and do not respond to immune complexes (12).

4.4 Dog

(a) The response of canine platelets to AA shows much inter-individual variability.

(b) Canine platelets are unusual in being the only laboratory species to undergo aggregation and secretion to acetylcholine, mediated by a muscarinic receptor (4).

(c) Although the major role for adrenaline in platelet function is as a potentiator, there are some reports of it inducing aggregation responses in its own right (13). This response is also unusual in that it is preceded by a lag phase of 8–12 min.

(d) Canine platelets are reported to be approximately tenfold more sensitive to thrombin than human platelets (14).

4.5 Cat

(a) In feline platelets ADP induces irreversible platelet aggregation which is commonly biphasic in nature.

(b) Cats are the only domesticated species in which the aggregation response to 5-HT is consistently irreversible and is coupled to secretion of granule contents and formation of TxB_2.

(c) Arachidonic acid metabolism is important for normal platelet aggregation in feline platelets, and because it is an essential fatty acid in this species, the platelet response may be modified by dietary change.

(d) As for the dog, adrenaline induces an aggregation response in feline platelets. This response, like that in canine platelets, is unusual in that it is preceded by a lag phase of 8–12 min (15).

4.6 Pig

(a) The secretable fraction of adenine nucleotides of pig platelets is high (> 4 μmol/10^{11} platelets) and in common with human platelets, the ADP response in pig platelets is inhibited by AMP.

(b) In common with the rabbit, pig platelets are unusual in that their dense granules contain secretable histamine.

4.7 Bovine

(a) The 5-HT content of ox platelet dense granules is high and therefore these granules have a core which is intensely electron dense.

(b) Structurally the most striking difference between bovine platelets and those from other species is the lack of a surface-connected cannalicular system, which may explain their lack of spreading on glass surfaces.

(c) The secretable fraction of adenine nucleotides of bovine platelets is low (< 1 μmol/10^{11} platelets) (16).

(d) Arachidonic acid induces only a small shape change response in bovine platelets, without subsequent platelet aggregation.

4.8 Horse

(a) The secretable fraction of adenine nucleotides of horse platelets is low (< 1 µmol/10^{11} platelets) (16).

(b) Arachidonic acid and TxA$_2$ analogues induce only a small reversible aggregation response, and the dose–response curve to AA is often bell-shaped.

(c) Equine platelets are exquisitely sensitive to PAF, responding to picomolar concentrations of the agonist.

References

1. BVA/FRAME/RSPCA/UFAW Joint working group on refinement. (1993). *Lab. Animals*, **27**, 1.
2. Wolfensohn, S. and Lloyd, M. (1994). *Handbook of laboratory animal management and welfare*. Oxford University Press, Oxford.
3. Hall, L. W. and Clarke, K. W. (1991). *Veterinary anaesthesia*. Baillière Tindall, London.
4. Meyers, K. M. (1985). *Adv. Vet. Sci. Comp. Med.*, **30**, 131.
5. Kerry, R. and Scrutton, M. C. (1983). *Br. J. Pharmacol.*, **79**, 681.
6. Kerry, R., Scrutton, M. C., and Wallis, R. B. (1984). *Br. J. Pharmacol.*, **81**, 91.
7. Harfenist, E. J., Packham, M. A., and Mustard, J. F. (1988). *Blood*, **71**, 132.
8. Kinlough-Rathbone, R. L., Rand, M. L., and Packham, M. A. (1993). *Blood*, **82**, 103.
9. Cook, N. S., Zerwes, H. G., Tapparelli, C., Powling, M., Singh, J., Metternich, R., *et al.* (1993). *Thromb. Haemost.*, **70**, 531.
10. Cavallini, L., Francesconi, M. A., Ruzzene, M., Valente, M., and Deana, R. (1991). *Thromb. Res.*, **63**, 47.
11. Cargill, D. I., Cohen, D. S., Van Valen, R. G., Kimek, J. J., and Levine, R. P. (1983). *Thromb. Haemost.*, **49**, 294.
12. Sinha, R. K., Santos, A. V., Smith, J. W., Horsewood, P., Andrew, M., and Kelton, J. G. (1992). *Platelets*, **3**, 35.
13. Clemmons, R. M. and Meyers, K. M. (1984). *Am. J. Vet. Res.*, **45**, 137.
14. Soslau, G., Arabe, L., Parker, J., and Pelleg, A. (1993). *Thromb. Res.*, **72**, 127.
15. Hwang, D. H. (1985). In *The platelets: physiology and pharmacology* (ed. G. L. Longenecker), pp. 289–308. Academic Press, London.
16. Meyers, K. M., Holmsen, H., and Seachord, C. L. (1982). *Am. J. Physiol.*, **243**, R454.

A1

Addresses of suppliers

Amersham International plc
Amersham International plc, Amersham Place, Little Chalfont, Buckinghamshire HP7 9NA, UK.
Amersham Corporation, PO Box 92708, Chicago, IL 60675, USA.
Amersham Canada Ltd., 1166 South Service Road West, Oakville, Ontario L6L 5T7, Canada.
Astra Pharmaceuticals Ltd, Home Park Estate, King's Langley, Hertfordshire WD4 8DH, UK.
Baxter Diagnostics Corporation, CanLab Division 11620-181 Street, Edmonton, Alberta T5S 1M6, Canada.
BDH Laboratory Supplies
BDH Laboratory Supplies, Magna Park, Lutterworth, Leicestershire LE17 4XN, UK.
BDH Chemicals Canada Limited, VWR Scientific, 77 Enterprise Drive, London, Ontario N6N 1S5, Canada.
Beckman Instruments
Beckman Instruments UK Ltd Oakley Court, Kingsmead Business Park, London Road, High Wycombe HP11 1JU, UK.
Beckman Instruments Inc. 2470 Faraday Street, Carlsbad, CA 92008, USA.
Becton Dickinson
Becton Dickinson UK Ltd, 21 Between Towns Road, Cowley, Oxford OX4 3LY, UK.
Becton Dickinson, Rutherford, New Jersey 07070, USA.
Becton Dickinson Immunocytochemistry Systems, PO Box 7375, Mountain View, CA 94039, USA.
Bellco Biotechnology, PO Box b 340, Vineland, NJ 08360, USA.
Bender Medsystems, PO Box 73, A-1121 Vienna, Austria.
Bibby-Sterilin, Tilling Drive, Stone, Staffordshire ST15 0SA, UK.
Biolog Life Science Institute, Flughafendamm 9a, 28199 Bremen, Germany.
Biomol Research Lab
Affiniti Research Products Ltd, GPT Business Park, Technology Drive, Nottingham NG9 2ND, UK.
Biomol Research Lab Inc, 5166 Campus Drive, Plymouth Meeting, PA 19462, USA

Biomol, Waidmannstr. 35, 22769 Hamburg, Germany.

Bio-Rad Laboratories Ltd

Bio-Rad Laboratories Ltd, Maylands Avenue, Hemel Hempstead, Hertfordshire HP2 2TD, UK.

Bio-Rad Laboratories Ltd , Life Sciences Group, Chicago, IL 60673, USA.

Biozym Nederland BV, PO Box 31087, 6370 AB Landgraaf, The Netherlands.

BOC Ltd, Priestley Road, Worsley, Manchester M28 2UT, UK.

Boehringer Mannheim

Boehringer Mannheim UK Ltd, Bell Lane, Lewes, East Sussex BN7 1LG, UK.

Boehringer Mannheim Biochem., PO Box 50414, Indianapolis, IN 46250, USA.

Boehringer Mannheim GmbH, Sandhofer Strasse 116, D-68298 Mannheim, Germany.

Boehringer Mannheim, 201 Boulevard Armand Frappier, Laval, Quebec H7V 4A2, Canada.

Brinkman Instruments Inc, Cantiague Road, Westbury, NY 11590, USA.

Cairn Research Ltd, Cairn House, Newnham, Sittingbourne, Kent, UK.

Calbiochem-Novabiochem, 701 B Street, San Diego, CA 92101, USA.

Chromogenix AB, Taljegardsgatan 3, S-431 53 Molndal, Sweden.

Chrono-log

Chrono-log, 2 West Park Road, Havertown, Pennsylvania 19083-4691, USA.

Biopol Canada Inc,1016 Sutton Drive, Unit C8, Burlington, Ontario L7L 6B8, Canada.

Costar, U.K. Limited, Victoria House, 28–38, Desborough Street, High Wycombe, Bucks HP11 2NF, UK.

Coulter Electronics Ltd

Coulter Electronics Ltd, Northwell Drive, Luton, Bedfordshire LU3 3RH, UK.

Coulter Electronics of Canada Ltd, 905 Century Drive, Burlington, Ontario L7L 5J8, Canada.

Dade International, Bonnstrasse 9, CH-3186 Dudingen, Switzerland.

Dako Ltd

Dako Ltd, 16 Manor Courtyard, Hughenden Avenue, High Wycombe, Buckinghamshire HP13 5RE, UK.

Dako Ltd, Produktionsvej 42, DK-2600 Glostrup, Denmark.

Desaga GmbH, PO Box 101969, D-6900, Heidelberg 1, Germany.

Dupont,

Dupont (UK) Ltd, NEN Products Division, Wedgewood Way, Stevenage, Hertfordshire SG1 4QN, UK.

Dupont Biotechnology Systems, NEN Research Products, 549 Albany Street, Boston, MA 02118, USA.

New England Nuclear, Mississauga Road, Mississauga, Ontario L5M 2H3, Canada.

Dynal (UK) Ltd, Station House, 26 Grove Street, New Ferry, Wirral, Merseyside L62 5AZ, UK.

Dynatech Laboratories Inc, Daux Road, Billingshurst, West Sussex RH14 9SJ, UK.

Electron Microscopy Science, PO Box 251, Fort Washington, PA 19034, USA.

Eppendorf North, PO Box 5433, Madison, WI 53705, USA.

Fisher Scientific Co

Fisher Scientific Co, Dept. 191137-01, Pittsburgh, PA 15230, USA.

Fisher Scientific Co, 112 ch. Colonnade Road, Nepean, Ontario K2E 7L6, Canada.

G. Bopp & Co, 115 Brunswick Park Road, New Southgate, London N11 1LJ, UK.

Gibco BRL, see **Life Technologies Ltd.**

Helena Laboratories

Helena Laboratories, 1530 Lindbergh Drive, PO Box 752, Beaumont, Texas 77704-0752, USA.

Helena Laboratories, Unit 2 6725 Millcreek Drive, Mississauga, Ontario L5N 5V3, Canada.

Hi-Tech Scientific, Brunel Road, Salisbury, Wiltshire SP2 7PU, UK.

Hoefer Scientific Instruments UK

Hoefer Scientific Instruments UK, Unit 12, Croft Road Workshops, Hempstall Lane, Newcastle-under-Lyme, Staffordshire ST5 0TW, UK.

Hoefer Scientific, 654 Minnesota Street, San Francisco, CA 94107, USA.

Hormon Chemie, Nycomed Arzneimihel GmbH, Freisinger Landstrasse 74, Postfach 450361, D-8000, Munchen, Germany.

Horwell Ltd, 73 Maygrove Road, London NW6 2BP, UK.

Hybaid Ltd, 111-113 Waldegrave Road, Teddington, Middlesex TW11 8LL, UK.

Hyclone Laboratories Inc, 1725 South Hyclone Road, Logoan, Utah 84321-6212, USA.

ICN Biomedicals

ICN Biomedicals Ltd, Thame Park Business Centre, Wenham Road, Thame, Oxon OX9 3XA, UK.

ICN Biomedicals, PO Box 60018, Los Angeles, CA 90060, USA.

Ingram and Bell Surgical Supply, Toronto, Canada.

International Market Supply Ltd, Dane Mill, Broadhurst Lane, Congleton, Cheshire CW12 1LA, UK.

Jackson ImmunoResearch, West Grove, PA, USA.

Janssen Pharmaceutica, Turnhoutseweg 30, B-2340 Beerse, Belgium.

J. B. EM Services, Box 693, Pointe-Claire, Dorval, Quebec H9R 4S8, Canada.

Life Technologies Ltd, PO Box 35, Trident House, Renfrew Road, Paisley PA3 4EF, Scotland, UK.

London Resin Co, 10 Church Road, Reading RG7 4LT.

Luckham Ltd, Victoria Gardens, Burgess Hill, Sussex RH15 9QN, UK.

Merck, Darmstadt, Germany.

Millipore (UK) Ltd, The Boulevard, Blackmore Lane, Watford, Hertfordshire WD1 8YW, UK.

Miltenyi Biotec GmbH, Friedrich-Ebert-Straße 68, D-5060 Bergisch Gladbach 1, Germany.

Molecular Dynamics Ltd, 4 Chaucer Business Park, Kemsing, Sevenoaks, Kent TN15 6PL, UK.

Molecular Probes Inc, PO Box 22010, Eugene, OR 97402-0414, USA.

Nalgene Co, 75 Panorama Creek Drive, Box 20365, Rochester, NY 14602, USA.

National Diagnostics, Unit 4, Fleet Business Park, Itlings Lane, Hessle, Hull HU13 9LX, UK.

New England Nuclear, see **Dupont**.

Nikon UK Ltd, 380 Richmond Road, Kingston-Upon-Thames, Surrey KT2 5PR, UK.

Nuchek Prep Inc, PO Box 295, Elysian, Minnesota, 56028, USA.

Nunc, see **Life Technologies Ltd.**

Oncogene Science Inc, 106 Charles Lingbergh Boulevard, Uniondale, NY 11553, USA.

Organon-Teknika Corp, PO Box 751087, Charlotte, NC 28275, USA.

Ortho Diagnostic Systems, Raritan, NJ, USA.

Payton Scientific, (Ion-Trace Inc), 115 Heatherside Drive, Scarborough, Ontario M1W 1T6, Canada.

Peninsula Laboratories, Belmont, 611 Taylor Way, Belmont, CA 94002, USA.

Pharmacia Biotech, 23 Grosvenor Road, St. Albans, Hertfordshire AL1 3AW, UK.

Pharmacia LKB Biotechnology, Box 776, S-19127, Sollentuna, Sweden.

Photon Technology International Inc, Suite 3, The Sanctuary, Oakhill Grove, Surbiton, KT6 6DU, UK.

Pierce Chemical, PO Box 117, Rockford, IL 61105, USA.

Polysciences Inc, 400 Valley Road, Warrington, PA 18976, USA.

Porton Products Ltd, Porton Down, Salisbury, Wiltshire SP4 0JG, UK.

Rank Bros Ltd, 56 High Street, Bottisham, Cambridge CB5 9DA, UK.

Reichert-Jung, c/o Leica Instruments, GmbH Nussloch, Germany.

RMC, 4400 South Santa Rita Avenue, Tucson, Arizona 85714, USA.

Sandoz Products Ltd, Sandoz House, 23 Great Castle Street, London W1, UK.

Schleicher & Schuell

    Schleicher & Schuell, Keene, NH 03431, USA.

    Schleicher & Schuell, CH-8714 Feldbach, Switzerland.

Scotlab, Kirkshaws Road, Coatbridge, Strathclyde ML5 8AD, Scotland, UK.

Shionogi Research Laboratories, Fukushima-ku, Osaka, Japan.

Sigma Chemical Co Ltd
  Sigma Chemical Co. Ltd, Fancy Road, Poole, Dorset BH17 7NH, UK.
  Sigma Chemical Co., PO Box 14508, St. Louis, MO 63178, USA.

SPI Supplies, Box 656 West Chester, PA 19381-0656, USA.

Stirling Winthrop, 81 Columbia Purn Pike, Rensselaer, NY 12144, USA.

Terochem Laboratories, 2740-A Slough Street, Unit 3, Mississauga, Ontario L4T 1G3, Canada.

Thorn-EMI, Bury Street, Ruislip, Middlesex HA4 7TA, UK.

Transduction Laboratories, 2134 Nicholasville Road, Suite 18, Lexington, KY 40503, USA.

Tuta Laboratories Ltd, 74 Smithbrook Kilns, Cranleigh, Surrey GU6 8JJ, UK.

UBI, 199 Saranac Avenue, Lake Placid, NY 12946, USA.

Ultrasonic Engineering Ltd, Sonic House, Singapore Road, Ealing, London W13 0UW, UK.

Upjohn Scientific Co, Fine Chemical Marketing, 7000 Portage Road, Kalamazoo, MI 49001, USA.

Upstate Biotechnology Inc, 199 Saranac Avenue, Lake Placid, NY 12946, USA.

UVP Ltd, Science Park, Milton Road, Cambridge CB4 4FH, UK.

Vector Laboratories Inc, 1429 Rollins Road, Burlingame, CA 94010, USA.

VWR Scientific Inc, PO Box 777, Philadelphia, PA 19175, USA.

Dr. Weber Gmbh, Am Enlischen Garten 6, D-85737 Ismaning, Germany.

Whatman International Ltd, St. Leonards Road, 20/20 Maidstone, Kent ME16 0LS, UK.

Wellcome Foundation, Langley Court, Beckenham, Kent BR3 3BS, UK.

Index

Index